HYPERBARIC NURSING

HYPERBARIC NURSING

VALERIE LARSON-LOHR
HELEN C. NORVELL

EDITORS

BEST PUBLISHING COMPANY

Cover photos: The cover features hyperbaric chamber systems manufactured by Perry Baromedical Corporation, Riviera, Florida, USA. Their complete product line includes monoplace, duoplace and multiplace systems. For more information, contact Perry Baromedical at 800-741-4376 or by e-mail at baromed@aol.com or by visiting their web site at: www.perrybaromedical.com.

Cover Design: Vanessa Palacio
Text Layout and Design: Jill McAdoo
Editorial: James Joiner

International Standard Book Number:1-930536-00-3

Library of Congress catalog card number:2001093221

Published by:
Best Publishing Company
Post Office Box 30100
Flagstaff, AZ 86002-0100, USA

CONTENTS

PREFACE

Since beginning work in hyperbaric medicine, we have heard baromedical nurses say, "we need a book for nurses about hyperbaric medicine." Without a nursing textbook, information was acquired by communication between peers and sharing of nursing articles. Finally, after brainstorming, many phone calls, e-mails, planning, assigning, nudging, long nights, editing and re-editing, we have a textbook on hyperbaric nursing.

Through the combined efforts of the Baromedical Nurses Association membership and many other dedicated individuals, this first edition contains the essential and practical information about our specialty for all nurses. We would like to express gratitude to the contributing authors for taking time from their busy schedules to make this publication possible.

Valerie Larson-Lohr
Helen C. Norvell

CONTRIBUTORS

BARRY BAKER
TOM BAKER
ANN CHARLOTTE-GRONQVIST
DEBORAH LEE CRITZ
SUE DeSANTIS
CAROLINE E. FIFE
STEPHEN V. FABUS
JULIO GARCIA
REZA GORJI
RICHARD B. GUSTAVSON
LAURA JOSEFSEN
PATRICK N. KIMBRELL
CAROLYN LAND
VALERIE LARSON-LOHR
CHIN-THANG LEE
WENDY McGINN-MERRITT
WAYNE McHOWELL
KAREN MINKIEWITZ WHITE
MARCO NICASIO
HELEN C. NORVELL
KAREN PARKER
SVEN VAN POUKE
E. CUAUHTEMOC SANCHEZ
MONICA SKARBAN
HARRY G. VINCENT
WILBUR (TOM) WORKMAN
CLAUDE WRENFORD-BROWN
ANN L. ZIEMBA

CHAPTER I

BAROMEDICAL NURSES ASSOCIATION HISTORY

K. MINKIEWITZ WHITE AND T. BAKER

The Baromedical Nurses Association provides nurses with a professional organization in order to define, develop, maintain, and promote the status and standards of practice in Baromedical nursing according to our Mission Statement. But what did nurses do before the organization was founded? The Undersea Medical Society (UMS) was available at that time (before they added Hyperbaric to their name) and nurses could be associate members. Nurses were involved in developing hyperbaric programs, training nurses and others in the care of patients receiving hyperbaric oxygen therapy and starting to write in nursing and other scientific journals about the baromedical nursing experience. This did not seem to meet the need, however, to talk nursing with colleagues. We had a desire to come together as nurses, to discuss the problems and patients that we were dealing with on a daily basis, usually by ourselves or with just a few other co-workers. So, after much ground work by Diana Greenberg assisted by Valerie Messina, a meeting was held in Long Beach California as part of the 1985 Joint Conference, Undersea Medical Society Annual Scientific Meeting/Tenth Annual Conference on Clinical Application of Hyperbaric Oxygen. At the meeting 35 nurses voted to establish the Baromedical Nurses Association. The enthusiasm and energy at the initial meeting was fantastic! We were a nursing organization, for nurses by nurses. The mission statement was approved. The functions were identified as:

- To define and implement standards of practice
- To promote ongoing educational endeavors for nurses practicing in the specialty of Baromedical nursing and to educate other nurses regarding the specialty
- To support research validating the concepts inherent in Baromedical nursing and the publication and dissemination of these findings
- To promote professional activities that enhance the effectiveness of Baromedical nursing in the overall healthcare system

We elected Diana De Jesus-Greenberg as our first president and established standing committees—most with chairpersons and some even with committee members. The date and site of the first annual meeting was determined. We decided to try to meet with the UHMS scientific meeting to promote attendance and room space. We also voted to obtain the services of a legal firm to ensure we were setting up our new organization correctly. Plans began immediately for a credentialing system and all present went home with a sense of pride and wonderment that a new organization had been born.

The next few years were busy ones as the organization sought to grow in a fluid universe. Diana served for two years as president and laid a foundation. Each future president, and especially the people working with her (and him), helped the organization grow. We formally incorporated and sought out other small specialty organizations to see what they did, and we continued to grow. By 1988, we had 176 members including several international members, 23 affiliate members, and 5 corporate members. The BNA Update, our official newsletter, was published quarterly by the Editorial committee and received an official masthead in 1998. Members worked hard on certification, membership, and benefits. There is now a BNA Certification Board that verifies and oversees three levels of certification in hyperbaric nursing. The BNA members established by-laws and rules, which are reviewed and updated annually by the By-Laws committee. The Safety committee has BNA representation at NFPA meetings and the Program committee organizes a BNA meeting each year, sometimes in combination with the UHMS Associates. The Nominations committee calls for recommendations for election of new officers, sends out ballots, and tallies the results. The Education committee has established a video library for nurses in hyperbaric medicine to obtain continuing education. Continuing Education is through the State of California and maintained by the CEU committee. The newest committee is Research. It has established a research grant to promote research in the field of hyperbaric nursing. Finally, the Diane Norkool Award was established in 1997 to recognize a nurse's research and leadership contribution in the field of hyperbaric nursing.

The face of the Baromedical Nurses Association has aged but is essentially unchanged in its mission to serve nurses practicing in the field of clinical hyperbaric medicine. Even some of the names continue to be the same after16 years. The biggest difference is that now most of us have someone we can call when we have a question. We know other nurses all over the country. We have a directory full of other nurses who provide care for the same kinds of patients that we do, and who experience the same issues. We have a voice and it is the Baromedical Nurses Association.

PAST PRESIDENTS OF BAROMEDICAL NURSES ASSOCIATION

YEAR	PRESIDENT
1985	Diana De Jesus-Greenberg
1986	Diana De Jesus-Greenberg
1987	Linda Mones
1988	Karen Minkiewitz
1989	Beth Whittaker
1990	Toni Kempner
1991	Lynn Scoggins
1992	Susan Clary
1993	Cathy Todd-Kersey
1994	Michael Hartsell
1995	Carolyn Land
1996	Laura Josefsen
1998	Helen Norvell
2000	Valerie Larson-Lohr
2002	Harry Vincent

CHAPTER I

DOCUMENTATION

H.G. VINCENT

DOCUMENTATION

Documentation refers to the preparation and maintenance of records that describe a patient's care. Detailed documentation can demonstrate the quality of patient care, outcome of that care, and the treatment or therapy still required. Nurses need to have a good understanding of what is required for "good" documentation, and survive scrutiny by many reviewers which include but are not limited to:

- Other healthcare team members,
- Accrediting, certifying, and licensing organizations,
- Performance improvement monitors,
- Peer reviewers,
- Medicare and insurance reviewers,
- Attorneys and judges, and
- Researchers and educators working to improve patient care and provide continuing education.
  (3, 5, 6, 13)

OVERVIEW

Historically, nurses recorded their observations of patients, creating documents only under the direction of physicians. The primary focus of these documents was to demonstrate that the physician's orders had been followed, the facility's policies and procedures had been observed, and all requisite care had been provided. Charting began as a checklist of cursory observations, such as whether the patient "ate well" or "slept well." Florence Nightingale is customarily regarded as the founder of nursing documentation. In "Notes on Nursing," the importance of gathering patient information in a clear, concise, and organized manner was stressed and identified. Nurses gradually began to be trained in her concept of lucid, formal nursing documentation. Gradually, nurses' perceptions and observations about patient care gained credence and respect.

By the 1970s, nurses began creating their own vocabulary for documentation based on nursing diagnoses. Although reimbursement for nursing diagnoses has failed to gain acceptance, the current reimbursement trend is to compensate nurses, especially nurse practitioners and home health agency nurses, for skilled care that meets eligibility requirements. Nursing documentation increasingly plays a role in ensuring reimbursement by verifying and justifying a nurse's actions. (1, 3, 5, 6, 7, 13)

UNDERSTANDING THE MEDICAL RECORD

Purpose

The medical record is an accounting of a patient's course of treatment, care, and/or therapy through an episode or course of injury or disease. Although some may see the process of documentation and charting as a dry summary of the accounts that take place, this should not be the case. It should be an accounting or incremental record of the patient's daily care, actual and potential problems, the interventions that took place, and the results of those interventions. Each medical record should be an individual story with a beginning, middle, and end, each including many sub-stories. It could be considered a "story" of the patient during his or her admission, whether inpatient or outpatient.

Elements of Sound Documentation

Typically a patient's medical record contains many forms that are organized by category, and often place an undue focus on format over content. Categories of a medical record may include, but are not limited to:

Face Sheet: is usually the first form and includes identification of the patient by name, date of birth, social security number, marital status, and insurance information. The closest living relative or guardian, drug allergies, admitting diagnosis, assigned diagnosis-related group (inpatient), and primary (admitting) physician are usually included. These may be updated during the course of stay or treatment to reflect additional diagnoses, procedures (surgeries), and additional physicians.

History and Physical: contains the initial medical examination and evaluation, and may answer questions of why the patient is here and what has taken place up to this point. The Joint Commission on Accreditation of Healthcare Organizations (JCAHO) has mandated that this should be completed and placed into the medical record within 24 hours of admission.

Initial Nursing Assessment: often will include the patient's health history, physical and psychosocial assessments (nutritional status, age, and educational level), baseline functional status (mobility, disabilities, and prosthesis), and pertinent social environment information (family and significant others).

Physician Order Sheet: is the record of physician orders, which may be directly or indirectly written by the physician. Standing and verbal orders still require the physician to sign off on them as his own and there are usually time limits as to when this should occur.

Problem List, Nursing Diagnosis List, and/or Summary List: problem lists or nursing diagnoses lists are used in healthcare facilities that follow problem-oriented charting. This is where nurses note individual problems until resolution or discharge. A summary list is a

JCAHO requirement for outpatients (and can be utilized for inpatients) where four areas are required to be current on one form or location. The four areas are diagnoses, medications, allergies, and significant invasive procedures. Additional information may be noted such as: other services consulted or involved (physical therapy, occupational therapy, dietary, etc.), all involved or consulted physicians, and significant non-invasive procedures (lab, x-ray, etc.). The key to the summary list is to review and update the information at every visit, so that it remains current.

Plan of Care: may be a nursing care plan (or a statement) which is sometimes in the patient's chart, or separately maintained at the nurse's station until the patient's discharge. Another form of care planning may be "team planning," which utilizes a treatment team or reviewers (physicians, nurses, therapists, dieticians, etc.). This team approach designates a certain frequency or time period in which specified patients (by diagnosis) are reviewed and a plan of care and goals are set that best meet the patient's needs. On subsequent reviews, the improvement (or lack thereof) is noted as compared to the plan and goals. Subsequent changes in care, up to and including patient discharge, are set at these reviews and noted on a specific form or location. The team planning approach may be most familiar in rehabilitation facilities.

Graphic Sheet: usually tracks the patient's vital signs and possibly daily weight. Additional forms may note (track) information such as blood glucose levels, urinalysis results, neurological assessment data, and patient intake and output. These forms identify and give a continuous record of certain assessment tasks that would have to be recorded elsewhere if not here.

Medication Administration Record (MAR): contains a complete record of all medications, dosages, and administration routes and sites for a specific patient and usually for a given date and time period. Many MARs are for a twenty-four-hour period beginning at midnight or whenever the facility sets as the standard time to start over (the beginning of the day shift). The current MAR may actually be separate from the patient's medical record for the actual time period that it is in effect due to the use of medication carts or specific medication administration personnel. At the end of the specified time period (that day) the original with all appropriate signatures and notations is added to the patient's permanent record.

Nurses' Progress Notes (Nurses' Notes): the detailed record of patient care information performed by the nursing staff. The record should also contain specific nursing intervention and the patient's responses. This may take on many different formats and will be discussed later.

Physician Progress Notes: similar to the nurses' notes, this record contains the physician's observations and notes on the patient's progress. It may also include treatment data, responses to treatment, whether specific goals of care have been obtained, and changes in these goals or specific treatments.

Diagnostic Findings: may be combined or subdivided into laboratory, radiology, and other areas of diagnostic reports.

Healthcare Team Records: if not specifically noted within a separate section, this is where other healthcare professionals would record their information, therapy, interventions, assessments, and results. Such professionals would include physical therapists, respiratory therapists, and social workers. If there is not a specific section for each, all may utilize one form sometimes referred to as a multidisciplinary progress note.

Consultation Sheets: forms include evaluations made by physicians, clinical specialists, and other professionals consulted for diagnostic and treatment/therapy recommendations. These may be handwritten or dictated in a standard format of the facility.

Discharge Plan and/or Summary: a brief accounting of the patient's stay or treatment course at your facility and the plans for care following discharge. Pertinent data may include dietary and medication regimens and follow-up appointments or referrals.

Requirements and Policies Affecting Documentation

When we look at the requirements of documentation, who has the established right and authority to set such requirements? First, Federal and State agencies have been empowered to make laws and regulations governing the care, storage, and confidentiality of medical records. These agencies have set legal limits on how long and under what conditions medical records must be kept. In addition, regulations and guidelines have been set on who has access to and how information can (when appropriate) be obtained from these records.

Once the laws and regulations are known, Federal and State intermediaries establish requirements for a facility to receive fees for services rendered under those programs. Following along closely are the private insurance companies, which make up the remainder of healthcare reimbursement. Many, if not most, intermediaries and insurance companies, health maintenance organizations (HMOs), preferred provider organizations (PPOs), and managed care groups enlist and follow guidelines and standards set for levels of care and the documentation of such care. Organizations, which have recognized standards for documenting patient information, include the American Nurses Association (ANA) and the JCAHO. The National Committee for Quality Assurance (NCQA) is an approved organization for accrediting managed care plans and certification of quality assurance specialists. Federal and State agencies have approved organizations such as the JCAHO to accredit facilities and agencies. Such accreditation may also ensure eligibility to receive reimbursement from Federal (Medicare) and/or State (Medicaid) programs.

Within a facility or agency, self-governing policies and standards are mandated and required in order to maintain accreditation. These internal policies are intended to establish systems which develop, monitor, and evaluate the quality of patient care. Policies are also established to oversee and facilitate the documentation of that patient care and to determine who is responsible to see that it is done. Facility quality management programs have evolved from risk management and quality assurance, to measuring the outcomes of the care rendered. Many accreditation organizations now require outcome measurements and tracking. Facilities are recognizing the cost-effectiveness of doing such tracking so as to offer the patient the best course of therapy/treatment in the shortest amount of time and at the lowest cost.

In the past ten years we have also seen the requirement by both the federal government and state nursing boards to have peer review systems which evaluate the quality and appropriateness of care by individuals.

Current Trends of Documentation

Sound documentation utilizes a logical approach to problem solving that includes assessment, the planning of patient care, nursing interventions, and the patient's response and progress. Legible, accurate, and clearly written charts that demonstrate professionalism and diligence will withstand litigation, ensure reimbursement, and satisfy reviewer requirements. Three "C's" of charting are: Clarity, Conciseness, and Consistency. It is imperative that spelling, abbreviations, and use of symbols be in approved and standardized formats. Avoid altering notations, and ensure legibility and neatness. Signatures should include the date and time of posting. Nursing documentation should include the nursing process, and must comply with standards established by accrediting and licensing organizations, state and federal agencies, intermediaries, and your healthcare facility.

Most pure narrative charting has been replaced with more efficient systems such as Subjective-Objective-Assessment Plan (SOAP), Problem-Intervention-Evaluation (PIE), and focus charting. Activities of daily living (ADL) flow sheets are often used along with these types of charting to improve efficiency. A more comprehensive comparison of charting systems, including the trend toward computerized charting, will be reviewed later in the chapter. Part of the motivation for newer documentation tools has been changes in reimbursement guidelines, such as diagnosis-related groups (DRGs) and ambulatory payer classifications (APCs) for Medicare. (1, 5, 6, 7, 13, 16)

LEGAL AND ETHICAL IMPLICATIONS OF DOCUMENTATION

Legal Relevance

Accurate and complete documentation helps members of the healthcare team confirm their impressions of the patient's condition and progress, and gives indications for adjustments to the therapeutic regimen. The medical record could be thought of as clinical communication, which if completed accurately and concisely, will stand the test of time, legal scrutiny, and an intermediary review.

Nursing documentation is dictated by state legislatures, state boards of nursing and/or nurse examiners, and professional organizations such as JCAHO and ANA. Intermediaries establish minimum requirements of documentation for reimbursement of procedures, therapy, and care provided by facilities and healthcare providers. The goal of nursing documentation has changed little since its inception, but the methods and techniques have changed and continue to change quite dramatically. Although narrative charting is still acceptable, time constraints and the need for efficiency have condensed and abbreviated the process into flow sheets, graphic records, checklists, and charting by exception (where only exceptions are noted), to name a few.

Timely communication is the key to today's documentation processes. Timeliness involves the care of the patient and communicating changes and/or reactions to that care in an appropriate manner to the appropriate party (physician), the response to that communication, and actions dictated to that response. Many legal cases involve failure to notify the physician, documentation of that notification, and the timeliness of that communication. These failures often involve extreme situations, which may result in death or permanent disability.

Individual credibility can be severely undermined when errors and omissions are present in documentation. The old adage of "if it wasn't charted, it didn't happen" applies especially when in the middle of a court proceeding. Late entries must be dated the date entered. Corrections should be made *only* by drawing a line through the initial note, signing and dating it, and making the appropriate entry. *Never erase, obliterate, or otherwise alter a record.*

Malpractice

Depending on the documented accuracy and the quality of the care delivered, the medical record may or may not support a plaintiff's complaint of malpractice. Malpractice focuses on four elements: *duty, breach of duty, causation, and damages.* A nurse has a *duty* to provide care once a nurse-patient relationship is established. The relationship may be established in person or at a distance (by telephone). *Breach of duty* indicates a failure to fulfill nursing obligations and may be difficult to prove due to the overlap of responsibilities of doctors, nurses, and other healthcare providers. A key question that is asked when breach of duty is investigated: "How would a reasonable, prudent nurse with comparable training and experience have acted in the same or similar circumstances?" The proof normally depends on whether or not the nurse failed to provide the appropriate care.

Once a plaintiff establishes breach of duty, he must then prove *causation* and injury. For a nurse to be liable, he/she must have proximately caused the injury by an act, omission, or oversight. Proximity may be difficult to prove due to the number of caregivers involved in a patient's care.

Once breach of duty and causation is established, the plaintiff must then prove *damages* occurred as a result. To provide for this, one must establish the difference between a bad outcome and malpractice. If the medical record indicates that all policies and procedures were properly followed, and the hospital policy established a reasonable standard, the patient has no cause for claim. This may be simply a bad outcome. It is usually the burden of the plaintiff to establish the standard of care was not met. Many complaints can be prevented by good communication between the healthcare providers and their patients to establish realistic expectations and awareness of the risks involved. It is not sufficient that a patient is disgruntled or dissatisfied. Damages or injury must be established, which are usually physical and not just emotional or mental. Physical damages may lead to a monetary award by the courts.

Risk Management

To reduce injuries and accidents, minimize financial loss, and meet the guidelines of the JCAHO and other regulatory agencies, healthcare facilities have instituted risk management programs. The primary objectives of risk management programs are:

- To ensure optimal patient care,
- To reduce the frequency of preventable injuries and accidents leading to liability claims by maintaining or improving quality of care,
- To decrease the chance of a claim being filed by promptly identifying and following up on adverse events (incidents or variances), and
- To help control costs related to claims by identifying trouble spots early and intervening with the patient and his family.

Many facilities now coordinate risk management with quality improvement to ensure they fulfill their legal duty to provide reasonable care.

A coordinated system usually consists of a dual focus on different aspects of healthcare delivery. Risk management focuses more on the patients' and families' perceptions of the care provided, while quality improvement focuses on the role and functions of the healthcare provider. A reputation for safe, reliable, effective service is a healthcare facility's primary defense against liability. Systematic, coordinated risk management and quality improvement programs demonstrate legal responsibility.

Bioethical Dilemmas

Nurses routinel[illegible] ociated decisions. These may r[illegible] patient confidentiality to deci[illegible] thical dilemmas have grown p[illegible] ology in healthcare. At the sa[illegible] llent resources for addressing t[illegible] and societies as well as written [illegible] that hospitals address ethical i[illegible] ave incorporated patient rights [illegible] ng home patients. The ANA [illegible] fic codes of conduct for nurses.

Ethical Codes for Nurses

The ***ANA code of ethics*** [illegible] following actions:

- Provide services with re[illegible] uniqueness of the patie[illegible] social or economic statu[illegible] of health problems.
- Safeguard the patient's ri[illegible] protecting information of a confiden[illegible]
- Act to safeguard the patie[illegible] and the public when healthcare and safety are affected by the incompetent, unethical, or illegal practice of any person.
- Assume responsibility and accountability for individual nursing judgements and actions.
- Maintain competence in nursing.
- Exercise informed judgment and use of individual competence and qualifications as criteria in seeking consultation, accepting responsibilities, and delegating nursing activities to others.
- Cooperate in activities that contribute to the ongoing development of the profession's body of knowledge.
- Participate in the profession's efforts to implement and improve standards of nursing.
- Take part in the profession's efforts to establish and maintain conditions of employment conducive to high-quality nursing care.

- Share in the profession's efforts to protect the public from misinformation and misrepresentation and to maintain the integrity of nursing.
- Collaborate with members of the healthcare professions and other citizens in promoting community and national efforts to meet the health needs of the public.

The ***code for LPNs and LVNs*** seeks to provide a motivation for establishing, maintaining, and elevating professional standards. It includes the following imperatives:

- Know the scope of maximum utilization for the LPN and LVN, as specified by the nurse practice act, and function within this scope.
- Safeguard the confidential information acquired from any source about the patient.
- Provide healthcare to all patients regardless of race, creed, cultural background, disease, or lifestyle.
- Refuse to give endorsement to the sale and promotion of commercial products or services.
- Uphold the highest standards in personal appearance, language, dress, and demeanor.
- Stay informed about issues affecting the practice of nursing and delivery of healthcare, and, where appropriate, participate in government and policy decisions.
- Accept the responsibility for safe nursing by keeping oneself mentally and physically fit and educationally prepared to practice.
- Accept responsibility for membership in the National Federation of Licensed Practical Nurses, and participate in its efforts to maintain the established standards of nursing practice and employment policies that lead to quality patient care.

According to the ***International Council of Nurses code of ethics***, the fundamental responsibility of the nurse is fourfold: to promote health, prevent illness, restore health, and alleviate suffering. It is further stated that inherent in nursing is respect for life, dignity, and human rights and that nursing is unrestricted by considerations of nationality, race, creed, color, age, sex, politics, or social status. The key points of the code are:

Nurses and People

- The nurse's primary responsibility is to those who require nursing care.
- The nurse, in providing care, respects the beliefs, values, and customs of the individual.
- The nurse holds in confidence personal information and uses judgment in sharing this information.

Nurses and Practice

- The nurse carries personal responsibility for nursing practice and for maintaining competence through continual learning.
- The nurse maintains the highest standards of nursing care possible within the reality of a specific situation.
- The nurse uses judgment in relation to individual competence when accepting and delegating responsibilities.
- The nurse, when acting in a professional capacity, should at all times maintain standards of personal conduct that would reflect credit upon the profession.

Nurses and Society

- The nurse shares with other citizens the responsibility for initiating and supporting action to meet the health and social needs of the public.

Nurses and Coworkers

- The nurse sustains a cooperative relationship with coworkers in nursing and other fields.
- The nurse takes appropriate action to safeguard the individual when a coworker or any other person endangers his care.

Nurses and the Profession

- The nurse plays a major role in determining and implementing desirable standards of nursing practice and nursing education.
- The nurse is active in developing a core of professional knowledge.
- The nurse, acting through the professional organization, participates in establishing and maintaining equitable social and economic working conditions in nursing.

Other bioethical issues involving documentation include the following:

- Informed consent (including witnessing informed consent and informed refusal),
- Advance directives (also known as living wills),
- Power of attorney,
- Do-not-resuscitate orders,
- Withdrawal of Treatment (associated with patient noncompliance), and
- Confidentiality of the medical record.

INFORMED CONSENT

Informed consent is required before most treatments and procedures, and indicates that the patient understands the proposed therapy and its risks and agrees to undergo it by signing a consent form. The physician (or other practitioner) who will perform the procedure is legally responsible for obtaining the patient's informed consent. The duty may be delegated to a nurse, but the responsibility remains with the physician or practitioner. Facility policies will dictate the actual process for obtaining and witnessing informed consents.

For informed consent to be legally binding, the patient must be mentally competent and the physician or practitioner must:

- Explain the patient's diagnosis as well as the nature, purpose, and likelihood of success of the treatment or procedure,
- Describe the risks and benefits associated with the treatment or procedure,
- Explain the possible consequences of not undergoing the treatment or procedure,
- Describe alternative treatments and procedures,
- Inform the patient that he/she has the right to refuse the treatment or procedure without having other care or support withdrawn (this includes withdrawing his consent after giving it),
- Identify who will perform the procedure,
- Identify who is responsible for the patient's care, and
- Obtain consent without coercing the patient.

Informed consent has two elements: the information and the consent. To be *informed,* the patient must be provided with a description of the treatment or procedure, the name and qualifications of the person who will perform it, and an explanation of risks and alternatives. All this must be in language that is appropriate to the age, education, and cultural level of the patient to ensure understanding. The JCAHO mandates elements of the informed consent, while some states only require the physician to explain the procedure and ask the patient if there are any questions. In life-threatening emergencies, informed consent may not be required as the law implies consent due to everyone's right to live and the physician's responsibility to intervene and save life without consent.

When witnessing a patient signing an informed consent document, you are not witnessing that he/she received or understood the information. You are simply witnessing that the person signing the consent is in fact the person he/she says he/she is.

- Always verify the patient's identity (armband) prior to witnessing.
- You need not be present when the physician informs the patient because you are only witnessing that the patient is signing the document, not the information given.
- A signed informed consent must be in the patient's medical record prior to the procedure being performed.

- If a patient questions or expresses concern about a procedure, notify your supervisor and/or the physician.
- The patient may change his/her mind about a procedure. If this happens:
  - Notify the physician, and
  - Document the date and time of the refusal, the date and time you notified the physician, and the physician's response.

Patient Participation

Occasionally, patients do or fail to do things which may contribute to injury or cause failure of therapy or care to reach intended goals. Document these behaviors and the outcomes. Patients do have the right to refuse medical and nursing care. Nurses are responsible for documentation of any behavior which contradicts medical instruction and the fact that the patient is informed of the possible consequences of his/her actions.

- A patient has the right to ***refusal of treatment.*** With a few exceptions, a competent patient has a right to refuse mechanical ventilation, tube feedings, antibiotics, fluids, and other treatments that will clearly result in death if withheld. In healthcare, the patient must also have capacity (legally considered an adult for consent purposes under state law) for legal competency to be present. Documentation is essential in this situation, not only to note that the patient was given the information, but that the patient refused the treatment. Some facilities have developed informed refusal forms. Exceptions to the right to informed refusal include pregnant women where the life of the unborn child is at risk, and parents who may withhold treatment or care from their children.
- ***Against medical advice (AMA) discharges*** may occur when a patient decides to leave the hospital. When this is imminent, notify your supervisor, the patient's physician, and possibly a member of the patient's family who may be able to persuade the patient to stay. The physician may attempt to inform the patient of the risks posed by refusing treatment. If the patient leaves, the nurse is responsible to complete the paperwork required by the facility and note: the time and patient's condition, any reasons stated by the patient for leaving, and how the patient left.
- ***Elopements*** can occur when a patient leaves the facility without any prior notification or any witness to the departure. Search the unit immediately and notify security, your supervisor, the physician, and the patient's family. If the patient is at risk for harming himself or others, notify the police. The nurse is responsible to document the time of discovery, attempts to locate the patient, and the times and people notified.

- ***Patient noncompliance*** is the unwillingness of a patient to practice prescribed health-related behavior(s). Nurses are responsible to document noncompliance of behavior, or any patient behavior that goes against instructions. The behavior must then be reported to the appropriate person and documented. Note any attempts to encourage the patient's compliance, even if unsuccessful.
- ***Discharge instructions to patients*** with noncompliance and/or patients released AMA should include:
  - Review the discharge instructions and discuss the date on which the patient should have a follow-up evaluation. Address the need for continued medical care.
  - Document the date that the patient is expected for follow-up, the location, and the date and time this was discussed with him/her.
  - Document any related teaching that was performed and any written instructions provided.
  - Copies of mailed instructions and reminders are also to remain in the medical record.

Power of Attorney

Power of attorney is a legal document where a competent person designates another to act or conduct legally binding transactions on his behalf. If the power of attorney covers health matters, it allows the designated person to express an opinion and make decisions about the kind of healthcare the patient would want. Power of attorney ends if the patient becomes incompetent or revokes the document, unless a *durable power of attorney* has been executed. This act designates another person to act on his behalf if he should become incapable of managing his own affairs. Any written power of attorney or advance directives should be placed in a conspicuous place within the medical record and must be honored.

Do-Not-Resuscitate (DNR) Orders

Physicians write DNR orders when medically indicated and should be reviewed as policy indicates or whenever significant change occurs in the patient's clinical status. DNR orders may be temporarily suspended during surgery. Partial resuscitation orders are legally precarious since the standard of care is to attempt full resuscitation. Family members or friends do not have legal authority to write an advance directive or advise a physician regarding DNR unless they have legal power of attorney or durable power of attorney.

Withdrawal of Treatment

Healthcare facilities are usually reluctant to withdraw futile treatment unless the patient (or legal designee) agrees. Many facilities and academic medical centers are struggling to balance the ethical, practical, and legal pitfalls of *withdrawal of treatment* without suffering additional cost through lawsuits. In any event, documentation of the patient's condition and prognosis is the chief nursing responsibility.

Confidentiality

Nurses have a legal and professional responsibility to protect the *confidentiality* of the patient's medical record. The nurse's role is primary in maintaining this confidentiality and must be constantly on guard for inadvertent conversation in areas where they can be overheard (elevators, halls, cafeterias, etc.). Copies of medical records should go through Medical Records and follow facility policies and procedures. Increasing use of computers creates a new avenue for unauthorized release of patient information.

The patient has a right to the information within the medical record, although the facility owns the record. Most states allow for patient access to their medical records. Special state statutes may cover the release of psychiatric records, records of minors, records with adoptive parent information, and records addressing drug and alcohol treatment or communicable diseases. Federal facilities and many states must give patients access to their records under "Freedom of Information Acts" while these same acts control access by third parties. Other statutes come in when dealing with criminal law, domestic abuse, and third-party payer or Medicare claims.

COMMON CHARTING FLAWS

Ideally, every chart should be complete and accurate. Unfortunately, this is not always the case.

Blank Spaces in Chart or Flow Sheet

A *blank space* may imply that complete care or assessment did not occur. Facility policies often specify how to address items that do not apply. Usually, writing "N/A" or drawing a line through the empty spaces will leave no doubt that this was addressed and not applicable. This also prevents information being inserted that could change the meaning of the original document.

Care Given by Someone Else

Care provided by another individual other than the one entering the notation should include the name and titles of who provided the care. If unlicensed personnel are allowed to chart, you may have to countersign the entry. Care should be taken to countersign only care observed. You can document that you reviewed the notes and consulted with the technician or assistant on certain aspects of care. Any follow-up care provided by the nurse should be fully documented.

Late Entries

Late entries are appropriate in several situations:

- If the chart was unavailable when you needed it,
- If you need to add important information after completing your notes, and
- If you forget to write notes on a particular chart.

Late entries should be identified to indicate they are out of sequence. Record the date and time of the entry, and within the entry record the date and time it should have been made.

Corrections

Never erase, cover, completely scratch out, or otherwise obscure an erroneous entry. This may imply a cover-up. Erasures, use of correction fluid, or heavy black ink to obliterate an error are usually unacceptable. Always treat the medical record as a legal document. (1, 2, 3, 4, 5, 6, 7, 8, 12, 16)

QUALITY MANAGEMENT AND REIMBURSEMENT

Documentation and Quality Management

The impact of nursing documentation on patient care quality and reimbursement for that care extends through and beyond the patient's stay. It is normally the nursing documentation that makes up the majority of the medical record, and proves or disproves if acceptable care was delivered and qualifies for reimbursement. Parties that are interested in the quality of care delivered, reimbursement standards, and legal practices include but are not limited to JCAHO, Medicare and Medicaid auditors, peer review organizations (PROs), and quality management or quality improvement committees. The JCAHO, PROs, case managers, quality management committees, and NCQA are just a few of the groups that will periodically evaluate quality of care, service, and competence.

JCAHO Quality Standards

A facility may be eligible to receive Medicare and Medicaid reimbursement and not be a member of and accredited by the JCAHO. It is the JCAHO that is the most widely known accreditation process involved in healthcare facilities. To be accredited by JCAHO, a healthcare facility must have an organized, systematic, and ongoing method for documenting quality. Documenting to reflect JCAHO standards ideally should show that your facility:

- Monitors and evaluates healthcare activities and caregivers,
- Defines the scope of care provided,
- Recognizes the most important aspects of care provided,

- Identifies indicators (a sign or symptom or set of signs or symptoms) and appropriate clinical criteria for monitoring the important aspects of care,
- Establishes thresholds (or limits) for the indicators to trigger evaluation of care,
- Collects and organizes data for each indicator to analyze and monitor the important aspects of care,
- Evaluates healthcare when thresholds are reached to identify problems or opportunities to improve care,
- Acts to correct identified problems or to improve care, and
- Assesses the effectiveness of corrective actions and documents improvements of care, and communicates the results of the monitoring and evaluation to relevant individuals, departments or services, quality improvement administrators, and, in general, the entire healthcare staff.

To meet these standards, JCAHO recommends a 10-step process of monitoring and evaluation. These steps are:

Step 1: Assigning responsibility - The ultimate responsibility for quality lies with the hospital's governing body which may include the board of directors and administrator. The board normally charges the administrator to appoint an individual to oversee monitoring and evaluation activities throughout the facility. This individual oversees the facility's programs for quality management through all departments and chains of command.

Step 2: Delineating scope of care and service - Each group within the facility must clearly define its function and scope of service. To do so, they consider the types and numbers of patients treated, the patient's diagnoses, the treatments performed, the staff members providing the service, and the locations and times of care.

Step 3: Identifying key aspects of care - Team members must identify the most important functions in order to pinpoint where quality management activities will begin. These functions are routinely evaluated as high risk, high volume, and problem-prone activities. The functions are organized to allow for systematic evaluation of all functions, and usually within or over specific time periods.

Step 4: Identifying indicators - Each function to be evaluated or monitored in a specific time period is broken down into specific indicators which measure structures, processes, and outcomes of care. These indicators are based on the latest information from research, journals, and professional organizations in relation to local, state, and national standards of care.

Step 5: Establishing a means to trigger evaluations - Before data collections begin, team members must set a threshold (percentage of this standard that is met) for each function. A threshold is a boundary alerting team members that intensive review is required. Depending on the threshold, the staff may need to review resources, staff education, or even a doctor's response time. Not all thresholds are, or should be, set at 100%. Occasionally, failing to meet a threshold may be justifiable, such as 95%, 90%, etc. However, a pattern of noncompliance points to a problem requiring correction.

Step 6: Collecting and organizing data - Once the aspects of care to be monitored, specific indicators for each aspect of care, and the threshold for each indicator have all been identified, collection of data for a specific time period may begin. The specific time period may vary, but commonly seen are three to six month periods. If three months or one quarter is used, then four different aspects of care can be evaluated in a year. The previous year can then be summarized into an annual report.

Step 7: Initiating evaluation - The team members review the data, looking for trends or patterns to determine whether a problem exists or if further investigation is warranted. If no problem exists or if acceptable care is found, no further action is warranted. If unacceptable care is found, a specific threshold is not met, or a problem is identified, the team proceeds with appropriate action.

Step 8: Taking action to improve care and service - When corrective action is required, the team recommends and initiates the corrective action themselves. If the required action is beyond their authority, the team makes recommendations to the person or department that does have the authority to act. A corrective action plan should identify:

- Who or what needs to change,
- Who is responsible for implementing the action,
- The specific action required in view of the problem's cause and severity, and
- When the change should occur.

Step 9: Assessing the effectiveness of actions - After suggesting or taking action, the team members continue to monitor and evaluate the problem area. This may cause a specific aspect of care to be continued into the next time period to measure the effects of action taken, or the aspect of care may be continued until the threshold is met.

Step 10: Communicating results - Whatever the findings, the quality management team members must report their findings to the quality management program director and to relevant staff members, departments, and services. Reporting periods will depend on what the facility has agreed is appropriate.

Quality management teams or committees generate documentation to confirm the care provided meets acceptable standards, to identify areas that need improvement, and to draw attention to problems. In today's increasingly competitive markets, comparing outcome data has gained a greater focus. Additionally, quality management teams review nursing performance as it relates to standards of care. The nursing standards as identified by JCAHO outline the documentation required to assess clinical competence of nursing staff members, nursing personnel from outside agencies, and specialty unit nursing staff.

Other Focus and Efforts

In addition to the JCAHO's 10-step model, several other models and foci exist. Some that may be utilized are:

PDCA cycle
- *Plan*: Study a process by collecting data and evaluating results.
- *Do*: Carry out the plan on a small-scale pilot.
- *Check*: Check results of the change. (Some now use "S" for "study.")
- *Act*: Implement the change or abandon the plan and go through the cycle again.

FOCUS
- **F**ind a process to improve.
- **O**rganize a team that knows the process.
- **C**larify current knowledge.
- **U**nderstand variation.
- **S**elect a potential process improvement.

FADE
- **F**ocus: Narrow a list of problems to one.
- **A**nalyze: Collect data and determine influential factors.
- **D**evelop: Formulate a plan to solve the problem.
- **E**xecute: Gain an organizational commitment, put plan into action, and monitor effect.

IMPROVE
- **I**dentify and define the problem.
- **M**easure the impact on customers.
- **P**rioritize possible causes.
- **R**esearch and analyze root causes.
- **O**utline alternative solutions.
- **V**alidate that solutions will work.
- **E**xecute solutions and standardize.

PROs focus - PROs were developed to assist the utilization process, and consist of groups of doctors and nurses to monitor and evaluate the quality and appropriateness of care given. When reviewing medical records, PROs use special screening criteria to evaluate the intensity of services and severity of illness. These factors may directly relate to Medicare and Medicaid reimbursement. PROs look at varying criteria, which look at the care given, and rely heavily on documentation in the medical record. The primary focus is quality patient care carried out within cost-containment guidelines. PROs scrutinize documented care as a means for determining reimbursements.

Case Management focus - Case management is a three-part process that consists of identifying individuals with specific healthcare needs, formulating and implementing a plan which efficiently utilizes healthcare resources, and measuring patient outcomes along a continuum of care. A case management system provides healthcare facilities with another way to improve quality while containing costs. Case managers direct and coordinate patient care to the most cost-effective healthcare services while meeting quality standards.

Fiscal Implications

What the nurse documents in the medical record and how it is documented has direct impact not only on the quality of patient care, but also on the facility's revenue. Specific and complete nursing records are the keys to ensuring financial reimbursement. Not only must care and treatment be validated, but also items must be billed. Today's healthcare system includes multiple, complex structures with multiple, complex requirements for reimbursement.

Caregivers and healthcare facilities must deal with quality management teams, case managers, and required reimbursement structures (for Medicare and Medicaid). In addition, reimbursement intermediaries for Medicare, Medicaid, HMOs, PPOs, and independent practice associations (IPAs). Reviewers from these groups examine the medical record for discrepancies in the treatment ordered and the treatment provided. When a discrepancy cannot be explained to satisfaction or reconciled reasonably, payment is denied.

How Documentation Affects Costs

Facilities have invested time and effort to calculate costs of delivering care and how to control them. Historically, the cost of nursing care was included in the patient's daily room rate. Recently, facilities have applied standard cost-accounting techniques to nursing care. Some facilities have taken this a step further to actually billing for nursing care. This requires a determination of the cost of nursing time and detailed documentation, which results in a detailed financial record.

How Documentation Affects Revenues

Documentation must confirm that the nursing staff is meeting certain standards:

- Adhering to the nursing process,
- Timely recording of changes in the patient's condition and care needs,
- Using medical equipment judiciously and appropriately to meet the patient's needs, and
- Adequately teaching the patient about his condition and treatment plan.

The nursing process involves problem-solving and decision-making that nurses do to provide patient care. The process is systematic and composed of five steps: assessment, nursing diagnosis, planning, implementation, and evaluation. These steps are sequential and cyclical. When the fifth step is reached, you return to the first step for reassessment. This process continues until patient discharge. JCAHO requirements are evident throughout the nursing process.

Changes in the patient's condition places documentation are at the forefront of quality, reimbursement, and legal issues. Improvement in the patient's condition may signal a successful outcome and the need for discharge, while deterioration demands concise, factual recording of events. On admission, a baseline assessment is recorded, and later changes are noted against the presenting signs and symptoms, health history, physical examination, and ancillary test results. Admission, transfer, and discharge notes must accurately reflect changes in the patient's condition. Condition changes justify changes in care and subsequent reimbursement. The appropriateness of admission, transfer, and discharge are all evaluated on the patient's condition, while JCAHO standards guide the recording of changes of the patient's condition and care.

Documentation provides evidence that certain equipment is essential to patient care, verifies that the equipment has been used appropriately, and justifies reimbursement. Reviewers require this documentation before approving reimbursement.

Patient education has become an important requirement of JCAHO accreditation. Documented teaching can also protect a healthcare facility and its nurses from legal problems. Patient education should include medication use, medical equipment, pain assessment, nutrition, etc. Patient teaching must be interdisciplinary and related to the plan of care. Discharge instructions and planning are also a part of this interdisciplinary approach and are initiated from admission.

Finally, inconsistencies may hinder reimbursement. Medicare and other intermediaries will always request explanations for conflicting data in the medical record. Accurate details may be very difficult to obtain retrospectively. The result of inconsistent data could be denial of payment. (1, 3, 5, 6, 7, 8, 9, 14, 16)

DOCUMENTATION SYSTEMS

Although each healthcare facility determines its own documentation and evaluation requirements, it must comply with legal, accreditation, and professional standards. Likewise, a nursing department can select the documentation system it wants as long as the system demonstrates adherence to standards and care requirements. Regardless of the system used, specific policies and procedures for documentation must be in place and known. Understanding these policies and procedures will not only help to document accurately, but will also serve the facility well when evaluating or modifying your documentation system or selecting a new one.

Healthcare facilities are striving for greater efficiency and quality of care. When evaluating your current documentation system, you must structure your system to reflect not only the patient's response to care, but also the quality of that care which must meet the profession's accepted standards. Facility committees and structures utilize well-defined, objective, and readily measurable indicators that allow them to assess the structure, process, and outcome of patient care within the medical records. Intermediaries review nursing documentation to verify the use of procedures and supplies when auditing charts.

Evaluating Your Documentation System

When reviewing the usefulness of your current documentation system, consider the following questions. If the answer is "NO" to any of them, you may consider a closer review of your current system.

- Does your current system reflect the patient's progress and the interventions based on recorded evaluations?
- Is there evidence within the record of the patient's response to nursing care (such as analgesic administration), and care modification as a result of that response?
- Does the record note continuity of care or exhibit unexplained gaps with late or absent entries?
- Are patient daily activities documented?
- Is the nursing process of nursing diagnoses, written assessments, interventions, and evaluation of response to those interventions clearly portrayed within the medical record?
- Does the current documentation system facilitate and document interdisciplinary communication among health team members?
- Is discharge planning clearly demonstrated to show evidence of interdisciplinary coordination, team involvement, patient and/or family teaching, and discharge instructions?
- Is patient and/or family education age, education level, and cultural background appropriate, and provided by individuals with documented training of such?
- Does the record reflect the administration of care within the current standards of care and the policies and procedures of the facility?
- Are all entries complete and legible according to facility policies and procedures, and if not, is the documentation of the omission and why it occurred complete?

- Does the documentation make sense and allow for the patient's care and hospital course to be tracked?
- Can the record be read for the previous 24 hours of documentation and demonstrate his problem, the interventions provided, and the outcomes obtained?

If after asking these questions you determine that you need a new system, form a group or committee to do the following:

- Review all available systems;
- Consult other facilities for systems that work better;
- Assess the likely cost, time, and commitment and effects on staff; and
- Evaluate possible alternative systems for how well professional standards and regulation requirements are met.

TRADITIONAL NARRATIVE CHARTING

Traditional narrative charting systems document ongoing assessment data, nursing interventions, and patient responses in chronological order. Few facilities rely on narrative charting alone, and most combine it with other systems.

Format and Components

Narrative charting is a straightforward, chronological accounting of the patient's status, nursing interventions performed, and the patient's response to those interventions. Flow sheets may supplement the narrative notes. Progress notes require knowledge of how to organize the data and what to document.

Current JCAHO standards direct healthcare facilities to establish policies and procedures about the frequency of patient reassessment. ***Specific and descriptive notes should be recorded whenever the following are observed:***

- Changes in the patient's condition (progression, regression, or new problems),
- A response by a patient to treatment or medication,
- Lack of improvement in the patient's condition, and
- A patient or family member's response to teaching, such as return demonstrations.

Documentation includes exactly what is heard, observed, inspected, done, or taught. As much specific descriptive information as possible should be included. Always document how the patient responds to care given and progression toward desired outcomes. ***In order to write meaningful notes:***

- Read the narrative notes written by other healthcare professionals before writing your own.
- Read notes recorded by nurses on other shifts and make additional comments on those findings to demonstrate continuity of care.
- Within facility policies, use flow sheets to document repetitious procedures or measurements, and summarize the information in the narrative notes.
- Record specific information and the exact times of the events when observing changes in your patient's condition, a lack of progress in his/her condition, or a response to treatment, medication, or patient teaching.
- When possible, document an event immediately after it occurs, and if you cannot, make notes to help you remember.

Before writing anything, always organize your thoughts so paragraphs will be coherent. Referring to the plan of care, unresolved problems, prescribed intervention, and expected outcomes can help one organize thoughts. ***If still having difficulty with organizing thoughts, follow this sequence of questions:***

- How did the problem first become evident?
- What has the patient stated about the problem that is significant?
- What has been observed that is related to the problem?
- What is the plan for dealing with the problem?
- What steps have been taken to intervene?
- How has the patient responded to current interventions?

Advantages

The traditional narrative charting is the most flexible of all charting and can suit any clinical setting. This type of charting strongly conveys nursing interventions and the patient's responses. Training time is usually brief, and allows for easy review by other team members. The narrative format easily lends itself to presenting information collected over an extended time period, and is easily combined with other documentation devices such as flow sheets to decrease charting time.

Disadvantages

Narrative charting can be weak when recording patient outcomes, tracking problems, and identifying trends. The weakness lies in the volume of documentation that may need to be covered in order to find answers to these. Because the narrative format has no inherent guide to document what is important, the tendency is to document everything in long, rambling, repetitive, subjective, and time-consuming notations.

PROBLEM-ORIENTED MEDICAL RECORD SYSTEM

The problem-oriented medical record (POMR) system was originally developed by physicians and was later adapted by nurses. The POMR system focuses on specific patient problems, and describes each on a multidisciplinary progress note, not progress notes containing only nursing information.

Format and Components

The POMR has five components: database, problem list, initial plan, progress notes, and discharge summary. Interventions and evaluations are recorded in the progress notes and discharge summary.

The ***database*** is usually completed by a nurse and is a collection of subjective and objective information about the patient; it forms the foundation for the plan of care. This initial assessment contains the reason of admission, medical history, allergies, medication regimen, physical and psychosocial findings, self-care ability, educational needs, and other discharge planning concerns.

After analyzing the database, the nurse, physician, and other relevant health team members identify and list the patient's current problems in chronological order according to date identified, or ***problem list.*** Usually physicians and nurses will maintain separate lists. Each problem should be numbered and this number referred to in all future notations of the POMR. The problem list must be kept current with new numbers corresponding to new problems. When a problem is resolved, a line is drawn through it or it is highlighted with a felt-tip pen or highlighter to show it as inactive. This information becomes the foundation for a problem list. The JCAHO also calls for a "summary list" to be kept current with the diagnoses, medication regimen, allergies, and significant invasive procedures on all outpatients. The two could be combined.

An ***initial plan*** should be constructed for each problem after the problem list is complete. This plan should include expected outcomes, plans for future data collection (if needed), patient care, and teaching plans. Mutual goal setting is essential for your interventions to be effective.

The most prominent feature of the POMR system is ***progress notes.*** You may see several formats, such as the SOAP, SOAPIE, or SOAPIER.

SOAP format: document information in the following manner:

- **S**ubjective data: information told to you by the patient or family,
- **O**bjective data: factual, measurable data gathered during the assessment, such as signs and symptoms, vital signs, and laboratory values,

- **A**ssessment data: conclusions based on subjective and objective data, and formulated as patient problems and nursing diagnoses, and
- **P**lan: the strategy for relieving the patient's problem(s).

SOAPIE format: utilizes the SOAP format and adds:

- **I**ntervention: measures taken to achieve an expected outcome, and
- **E**valuation: an analysis of intervention effectiveness.

SOAPIER format: utilizes the SOAPIE format and adds:

- **R**evision: any changes from the original plan of care.

The ***discharge summary*** completes the POMR format and covers each problem on the list and notes whether resolution was reached. Any unresolved problems should be discussed and a plan specified for dealing with them after discharge. Any communications with other facilities or agencies should be included here.

Advantages

POMR documentation organizes information about each problem into specific categories which all healthcare team members understand, thus promoting interdisciplinary communication and data retrieval. The problem list serves as an index to the medical record. POMR documentation also illustrates the continuity of care and unification of the care plan and progress notes into a full record of care planned and delivered.

The POMR also promotes documentation of the nursing process, facilitates consistent documentation, and eliminates documentation of nonessential data and the need for task documentation. This format can also serve as a checklist to draw attention to problems needing intervention. The POMR format is most effective in acute care or long-term care settings.

Disadvantages

Analyzing trends with the POMR format is particularly difficult with its emphasis on chronology of problems rather than their priority. The SOAPIE format commonly produces repetitious charting of assessment findings and interventions, because both assessments and interventions commonly apply to more than one problem. This resulting overlap makes the POMR system time-consuming to perform and read, and due to the emphasis on problems, routine care may remain undocumented unless flow sheets are utilized.

Difficulties may arise if teammates fail to update the problem list regularly, or if they are confused about which problems should be listed. It requires considerable time and cost to train new personnel to use SOAP, SOAPIE, or SOAPIER formats or significant considerations. The POMR format is not well-suited for areas with rapid turnover, short procedure units, or emergency departments.

PROBLEM-INTERVENTION-EVALUATION SYSTEM

The problem-intervention-evaluation (PIE) documentation system was developed to simplify the charting process. PIE charting organizes information according to problems as defined by a group of nurses in 1985 at Craven Hospital in New Bern, NC. This approach considers three categories: problem (P), intervention (I), and evaluation (E). This format requires the staff to keep daily patient assessment flow sheets and progress notes. By integrating the plan of care into the nurses' progress notes, PIE format eliminates the need for a separate plan of care. This results in a concise, efficient record of patient care that has a nursing focus.

Format and Components

The PIE documentation system is initiated with an assessment of the patient documented on a daily patient assessment flow sheet. The flow sheet list defines assessment terms under major categories, along with routine care and monitoring. Space is typically included to record pertinent treatments within the flow sheet. Assessment terms which apply to your patient are initialed, while abnormal findings are noted with an asterisk. Detailed information is recorded in the progress notes.

Problem

After documenting the initial assessment, identify pertinent nursing diagnoses with the data gathered. There should be an accepted list of diagnoses approved by your facility and this usually corresponds with the North American Nursing Diagnosis Association (NANDA) approved list. A problem statement can be used when no diagnosis from the approved list fits. Each diagnosis is documented in the progress notes and identified with a "P" and an identifying number (P#1).

This labeling system allows you to refer back to a specific problem by label only. Some facilities use a separate problem-list form to keep a running account of nursing diagnoses for a particular patient.

Intervention

Nursing actions taken for each diagnosis are documented in this section. Actions are documented on the progress notes, labeled as "I" followed by the problem number.

Evaluation

Related effects are charted after interventions are noted in the progress notes. A label of "E" followed by the problem number identifies the entry. One nurse must evaluate each problem every eight hours. After every three shifts, the notes from the previous 24 hours are reviewed to identify the patient's current problems and responses to interventions. Continuing problems are documented daily, along with relevant interventions and evaluations. Resolved problems are crossed out from the daily documentation.

Advantages

The PIE format can ensure that your documentation includes nursing diagnoses, related interventions, and evaluations. JCAHO standards can be readily met due to the PIE requirements of organizing thoughts and writing, and incorporating the plan of care into the progress notes. Continuity of care is promoted by tracking the patient from admission to discharge. The PIE method also improves the quality of progress notes by highlighting care interventions and requiring a written evaluation of the patient's response to those interventions.

Disadvantages

PIE format may require in-depth training for staff members. It is also very time-consuming to reevaluate each problem during each shift, which leads to repetitive entries. Some problems don't require this frequency of evaluation. The planning step of the nursing process which addresses outcomes is omitted, and that is an essential component of evaluating the patient's responses. PIE charting does not incorporate multidisciplinary charting.

Focus Charting

Nurses at Eitel Hospital in Minneapolis, MN developed focus charting. They found the SOAP format awkward, while focus charting encourages you to organize your thoughts into patient-centered topics or foci of concern and then to document precisely and concisely. This format encourages the use of assessment data to evaluate patient care concerns. It helps with identifying necessary revisions to the plan of care as you document each entry. Focus charting works well in acute care settings, and where the same care and procedures are repeated frequently.

Format and Components

Focus documentation requires the use of a progress sheet with categories for date, time, focus, and progress notes.

Foci

Typically, each focus is noted as a nursing diagnosis, whether it is a particular condition, signs and symptoms, a particular behavior, special need, acute change of condition, or a significant event.

Progress Notes

In the progress notes column (of the progress sheet), information is organized into three categories and labeled: data (D), action (A), and response (R). In the data category, include subjective and objective information that relates to the focus. The action category should include immediate and future nursing actions based on the patient assessment. Any changes to the plan of care would also be noted in the action category.

The response category is used to describe the patient's response to any aspect of nursing or medical care. All three categories, if used appropriately, ensure complete documentation based on the nursing process. Routine tasks and assessment data are recorded on flow sheets and checklists.

Advantages

Focus charting is flexible and can be adapted to fit any clinical setting while centering on the nursing process. The data-action-response style provides cues that direct documentation in a process-oriented manner. By separating the focus statement from the narrative in the progress notes, it is easy to locate information on a particular problem, which saves time and promotes communication among healthcare team members.

This format also highlights the nursing process in documentation of daily care, encourages regular documentation of patient responses to medical and nursing care, and ensures that JCAHO standards for documenting patient responses and outcomes are met. This format can be used for many topics in addition to those on the problem list or plan of care. Focus charting also helps organize thoughts and encourages precise documentation.

Disadvantages

Focus charting may require in-depth training, and requires the use of many flow sheets and checklists which can lead to inconsistent documentation and difficulty in tracking problems. If the patient's response to interventions is not specifically noted, the focus format can become a large narrative note.

Charting-By-Exception System

Nurses at St. Luke's Hospital in Milwaukee designed the charting-by-exception (CBE) documentation system to overcome long-standing charting problems, such as lengthy and repetitive notes, poorly organized information, difficult-to-retrieve data, and a high risk of errors of omission. To avoid these problems, CBE radically departs from traditional systems by requiring documentation of only significant or abnormal findings in a narrative portion of the record. The CBE system also uses military time to help prevent misinterpretations and errors.

Format and Components

You must know and adhere to established guidelines for nursing assessments and interventions to use CBE documentation effectively. The CBE nursing assessment has printed guidelines for each body system and relies on written standards of practice that identify the nurse's basic responsibilities to patients. Because the standards are clear and concise, all charting related to routine nursing care is eliminated. You document only deviations from the standards, which omits repetitive charting of routine procedures. Intervention guidelines for the CBE system derive from these sources:

- Nursing diagnosis-based standardized plans of care - identifies patient problems, desired outcomes, and interventions,
- Patient care guidelines - standardized interventions established for specific patient populations that outline the nursing interventions, treatments, and time frame for repeated assessments,
- Doctor's orders - prescribed medical interventions,
- Incidental orders - normally one-time, miscellaneous nursing or medical orders or interdependent interventions related to a protocol or a piece of equipment, and
- Standards of nursing practice - defined, acceptable level of routine nursing care for all patients.

Nursing Diagnosis-based Standardized Plans of Care

Preprinted plans of care are utilized whenever a nursing diagnosis is identified. A separate form is used for each pertinent diagnosis. Spaces are present so each form can be individualized, and when completed, each form is placed in the nursing progress notes section.

Nursing Care Flow Sheet

Nursing care flow sheets are utilized to document patient assessments and interventions. Each flow sheet is designed for a 24-hour period of care for the patient. Following the nursing assessment, findings are compared to normal parameters defined in printed guidelines on the form. If the findings are within normal limits, place a check mark with your initials in the appropriate category box. If findings are not within normal limits, put an asterisk in the category box and explain your findings in the comments section.

A finding that is not defined in the guidelines may be normal for a particular patient. If the patient's condition hasn't changed from the last assessment, a horizontal arrow is drawn from the previous category box to the current one. Following the nursing assessment, the previous nurse's note and symbol is reviewed to determine if the patient's condition changed. Significant or abnormal findings are indicated with an asterisk and an explanation in the comment section. If the findings were unchanged, an arrow is used.

When an entire column of assessments and interventions is documented, initial the column. All comments are initialed and the page is signed. Some facilities use nursing care flow sheets that combine all necessary sections (graphic record, daily nursing care activities checklist, and a patient care assessment section).

Graphic Record

The flow sheet or section of a flow sheet is used to document trends in the patient's vital signs, weight, intake and output, and stool, urination, appetite, and activity levels. Check marks are used to indicate expected findings and asterisks to indicate abnormal findings. Comments on abnormalities are recorded in the nurse's progress notes. Established nursing care interventions are checked off in the box labeled "Routine standards."

Patient-Teaching Record

Use this form or section to identify the knowledge, psychomotor skills, and social or behavioral measures that your patient or his caregiver must learn by a predetermined date. The record includes teaching resources, dates of patient achievements, and other pertinent observations. A patient with multiple learning needs may require more than one form.

Patient Discharge Note

This is similar to other discharge forms, and utilizes a flow sheet for documenting ongoing discharge planning.

Progress Notes

Another portion of the CBE format is the progress notes, which are used to document revisions to the plan of care and interventions that don't lend themselves to the nursing care flow sheet. Because CBE format permits most assessments and interventions to be documented on the nursing care flow sheet, the progress notes typically contain little.

Advantages

The CBE format has many advantages. Including only information that deviates from expected findings decreases the amount of documentation needed, eliminates redundancies, and clearly identifies abnormal data. This results in less time needed to document normal and abnormal findings. Guidelines, including normal findings, are pre-printed on the form. Abnormal findings are highlighted for quick reference to significant changes and trends in the patient's condition. Documentation of routine care is eliminated through the use of nursing standards.

All flow sheets are kept at the patient's bedside for ready reference, which encourages immediate documentation. This eliminates the need for temporary notes. Other caregivers have access to the data, and because of standardized assessments, evaluations and documentations are consistent. Finally, documentation previously recorded isn't repeated.

Disadvantages

The primary drawback to the CBE format is the large time commitment required to develop clear guidelines and standards of care. To be legally sound, the guidelines and standards must be in place and understood by all nursing staff before the format can be implemented. Consistent use of the appropriate documenting procedures is key to the format. If a facility uses multiple forms that combine CBE components, the documenting process can be confusing and the records incomplete.

CBE format does not accommodate integrated or multidisciplinary charting. Unexpected events or isolated occurrences may not be fully documented and require a narrative. The CBE format was developed for registered nurses, and must be evaluated and modified if licensed practical or vocational nurses use the system due to their separate scope of practice. Due to the limited use of CBE format, this type of charting may draw additional questioning when brought to court for legal proceedings.

FACT SYSTEM

The FACT system is named for its individual elements and incorporates many CBE principals. This format was designed to avoid the documentation of irrelevant data, repetitive notes, and inconsistencies among departments, and to reduce the amount of time spent charting.

Format and Components

The Fact system has four key elements:

- **F**low sheets are individualized to specific services.
- **A**ssessment features are standardized with baseline parameters.
- **C**oncise, integrated progress notes and flow sheets are utilized to document the patient's condition and responses to therapy and care.
- **T**imely entries are recorded when the care is given.

The FACT system requires documentation of exceptions to the norm or significant information about the patient. This eliminates the need to chart normal findings while still incorporating each step of the nursing process. FACT documentation begins with a complete initial baseline assessment of each patient utilizing standardized parameters. The system uses an assessment-action flow sheet, a frequent assessment flow sheet, and progress notes. The flow sheet's content may be individualized to some extent and covers a 24 to 72 hour period, which requires all entries to note date and time.

Assessment-Action Flow Sheet

This form is used to document ongoing assessments and interventions. Normal assessment parameters for each body system are printed on the form along with planned interventions. The assessment action flow sheet may be individualized according to the patient's needs.

Frequent Assessment Flow Sheet

This form is used to chart vital signs and frequent assessments.

Progress Notes

The progress notes include an integrated progress record where you will use narrative notes to document the patient's progress and any significant incidents. As in focus charting, narrative notes are written using the data-action-response method. Progress notes are updated in relationship to patient outcomes every 48 hours.

Advantages

The computer-ready FACT charting system has the advantages of eliminating repetition and encouraging consistent language and structure. The system is outcome-oriented and communicates patient progress to all healthcare team members. It also permits immediate recording of current data and is readily accessible at the patient's bedside. The system eliminates the need for many different forms and reduces the time spent writing narrative notes.

Disadvantages

FACT charting does require a major time commitment to developing standards and implementing the system across all departments of the healthcare facility. Narrative notes may be too brief, and the nurse's perspective on the patient's status may be overlooked. It may also be difficult to identify all the portions of the nursing process in this system.

CORE SYSTEM

The core system focuses on the nursing process, which is the *core* or most important part of documentation

Format and Components

This system consists of a database, plans of care, flow sheets, progress notes, and discharge summaries. The core system requires an assessment and records a patient's functional and cognitive status within eight hours of admission.

Database and Plans of Care

The initial assessment focuses on the patient's body systems and activities of daily living, and includes a summary of the patient's problems along with appropriate nursing diagnoses. The completed database and plan of care are then entered on the patient's medical record card, also known as the "Kardex."

Sheets

Flow sheets are used to document the patient's activities and responses to nursing interventions, diagnostic procedures, and patient teaching.

Progress Notes

The progress notes are used to record the following information (DAE) for each problem:

- Data,
- Action, and
- Evaluation or response.

Discharge Summary

The discharge summary of core documentation incorporates information related to nursing diagnoses and patient teaching. It also includes recommended follow-up care.

Advantages

Core documentation incorporates the entire nursing process into a single documentation system by grouping diagnoses and functional status assessments together. It is complemented by the DAE component, and promotes concise documentation with minimal repetition while encouraging daily recording of psychosocial information. The core system is useful in acute care and long-term care facilities.

Disadvantages

The core system of documentation may require in-depth training for staff members who are familiar with other documenting systems. The development of forms may be costly and time-consuming. The DAE format does not always present information chronologically, which may make it difficult to perceive the patient's progress quickly. One other difficulty is ensuring that the progress notes relate to the plan of care. It may take additional time to monitor this last item to ensure quality care and documentation.

Outcome Documentation System

The outcome documentation system is a process-oriented system focused on the patient's behaviors and responses to nursing care and patient teaching. The system presents the patient's condition in relation to predetermined outcomes on the plan of care, focusing on desired outcomes rather than problems.

Format and Components

This documentation system utilizes progress notes, flow sheets, and plans of care for documentation. Typically, this system combines with another documentation system and features three components: a database, a plan of care, and expected outcome statements.

Database

An initial information database is obtained which includes subjective and objective data identifying the patient's problems and learning needs. The collected information serves as a foundation for ongoing evaluations of the patient's status. The teaching sheet should include the patient's and family's problems, special learning needs, and any barriers to learning which have been identified.

Plan of Care

Utilizing the information in the initial database, a patient plan of care is developed that establishes priorities, identifies expected outcomes and nursing interventions, and documents the plan. This plan gives the healthcare team a central information source about the patient's needs and goals. All the following types of plans of care include expected outcomes:

- Traditional individual patient handwritten plans of care,
- Standardized plans of care with preprinted categories such as nursing diagnoses, outcome statements, and recommended interventions with blank spaces for individualization of the plan,
- Patient care guidelines which include specific sequential instructions for treating patients with specific problems, and
- Clinical pathways (healthcare maps) that outline expected outcomes on a timeline and provide key interventions for patients with specific diagnoses.

Expected Outcome Statements

Also known as goals or objectives, expected outcome statements are drawn from the patient's nursing diagnoses. Expected outcomes serve as the basis for identifying nursing actions to help the patient achieve goals by describing the desired results of nursing care. Nursing care and patient teaching effectiveness are also evaluated through these statements. Specific expected outcomes must be stated because nursing diagnoses may each have many expected outcomes. Once this is done, specific criteria must be established to determine whether outcomes have been achieved.

Outcome Criteria

To objectively evaluate outcomes, these four components must be included:

- Specific behaviors which show the patient has progressed toward or reached the established goal,
- Standards for measuring the patient's behaviors,
- Conditions under which the behavior should occur, and
- A target date or time the behaviors should occur.

When writing outcome criteria, these guidelines should be followed:

- The statement must be specific.
- Focus should be on the patient's behavior and not a nursing action.
- The patient should be encouraged to participate in developing outcomes.
- Outcomes must be adapted to the patient.

Learning Outcomes

The patient-teaching plan identifies what a patient (and possibly a family) needs to learn, how you will teach him/her, and ways to evaluate what has been learned. Some teaching plans are included as part of the patient's plan of care. However, many healthcare facilities require the teaching plan to be separate because of the JCAHO's and other regulatory agencies' emphasis on interdisciplinary patient teaching and documentation of learning responses. Learning outcomes should describe observable and measurable behavior and must focus on the patient. A patient's learning behaviors fall into three categories: cognitive (knowledge), affective (attitudes), and psychomotor (movement and coordination).

Evaluation

Expected outcomes are evaluated by gathering assessment data, comparing the finding with the outcome criteria, determining the extent to which the goals were achieved, writing evaluation statements, and revising the plan of care. If a patient meets his or her goals and the problem is resolved, the plan of care or teaching plan is discontinued. If the goals are not met, continue the plan but set new target dates.

Factors which may work against successful goal completion include unrealistic outcome statements, unrealistic target dates, outcomes that are unacceptable to the patient, and ineffective strategies.

Advantages

With outcome documentation, all phases of the nursing process are used and recorded, making this system ideal for determining continuous quality improvement. The system additionally fosters mutual goal-setting and clear documentation of performed patient teaching and achieved learning.

Disadvantages

If the nursing process is not used consistently, adequately carrying out outcome documentation will be difficult.

COMPUTERIZED CHARTING

Charting with computers can significantly reduce the amount of time you spend on documentation. Computers can facilitate accurate and quick documentation, help complete nurse management reports, provide patient classification data, and make staffing projections. In addition, computers can identify patient teaching needs and supply data for nursing research and education. Patient vital signs can be tracked electronically on some bedside terminals.

Computer systems for healthcare documentation are still developing. Currently, there may be a stand-alone unit or a subsystem of a facility-wide network. Personal computers or terminals may be located at workstations, allowing staff quick access to vital information (lab, order entry, reports, etc.). Terminals are now being placed at the patient bedside, which makes obtaining and entering data much easier.

Systems and Functions

Computers and software are diversified, and a keyboard, light pen, touch-sensitive screen, mouse, or even a voice may access information. Some computerized documentation systems provide a menu of words or phrases you can choose from to produce individualized documentation or complete narrative notes. A problem may be elaborated on or flow sheet documentation clarified in the comment section of a computerized form by entering standardized phrases or typing comments. Some current systems are the Nursing Information System, the Nursing Minimum Data Set, the Nursing Outcomes Classification, and voice-activated systems.

Nursing Information Systems

Nursing Information Systems (NIS) software allows nurses to record actions electronically, making nursing documentation easier. The NIS reflects all the components of the nursing process and meets the standards of the ANA and JCAHO. Each NIS can be customized to conform to a facility's documentation forms and formats.

Most NISs manage information passively by collecting, transmitting, organizing, formatting, printing, and displaying information that can help make decisions without suggesting decisions. Some newer systems can suggest nursing diagnoses based on predefined assessment data entered. More sophisticated systems provide standardized patient status and nursing intervention phrases that can be used to construct progress notes. Standardized phrases can be changed if necessary to allow room for individualized notes.

The most recent development in NIS is individual interaction, prompting the nurse with questions and suggestions about the information entered. This sequential decision-making format should lead to more effective nursing care and documentation. After a brief narrative, the questioning and diagnostic suggestions provided make documentation thorough and quick, while still allowing for individualization of the record.

Nursing Minimum Data Set

The Nursing Minimum Data Set (NMDS) system attempts to standardize nursing information. NMDS contains three categories of data: nursing care, patient demographics, and service elements.

The NMDS allows the collection of *nursing diagnosis and intervention data to identify the nursing needs* of various patient populations. Patient outcomes can be tracked along with the nursing care in various settings (including home care). This system helps establish accurate estimates of nursing costs and data, which may help influence healthcare policy and decision making. It allows comparison of nursing trends locally, regionally, and nationally to compare data from various clinical settings, patient populations, and geographic areas.

The NMDS can also help you provide *better nursing care.* Examining the outcomes of patient populations will help set realistic outcomes for an individual patient as well as formulate accurate nursing diagnoses and plan interventions.

The standardized format of NMDS encourages *more consistent documentation.* All data are coded, making documentation and information retrieval faster and easier. Currently, NANDA assigns numerical codes to all nursing diagnoses and is compatible with the NMDS.

Nursing Outcomes Classification

The Nursing Outcomes Classification (NOC) system is the first computerized, comprehensive, and standardized method of measuring nursing-sensitive patient outcomes. The NOC can make a major impact on nursing administration and patient care delivery. The system allows comparison of patient outcomes to larger outcomes of larger groups according to such parameters as age, diagnosis, or healthcare setting.

NOC implementation is important for supporting ongoing nursing research. The system allows inclusion of patient data-related outcomes that have been lacking from computerized medical information databases.

Voice-Activated Systems

Voice-activated nursing documentation systems are beginning to appear in some facilities. This system is most useful in hospital departments with a high volume of structured reports (operating room). This is possible due to the system's specialized knowledge base of nursing words, phrases, and report forms, combined with automated speech recognition (ASR) technology. The ASR system allows for complete nursing notes by voice with little or no keyboard use. You simply speak into the handset and text appears on the computer screen.

The software program includes a database on the nursing process, nursing theory, nursing standards of practice, report forms, and a logical format. Trigger phrases cue the system to display passages of report text while still allowing word-for-word dictation and editing. The speed of reporting is increased and the nurse is freed from some of the paperwork to allow for more time at the bedside.

Advantages

Computerized documentation systems make recording, storing, and retrieving information fast and easy. These systems allow for efficient and constant updating of data and help link diverse sources of patient information. They also store valuable data on patient populations that can help improve the quality of nursing care. Using standard terminology, computerized documentation promotes better communication among healthcare disciplines and promotes more accurate comparisons. It also improves legibility. Finally, computerized documentation provides for the quick and efficient transfer of requests and patient information from one source to another.

Disadvantages

If not properly monitored and administered, patient information can be scrambled, and improper security could allow patient privacy to be threatened. Inaccurate or incomplete information may be yielded due to standardized, limited vocabulary or phrases. Computers breaking down, and too many nurses trying to use too few terminals, can both make the system unavailable. Finally, a computerized documentation system may be cost prohibitive for many facilities. (1, 3, 5, 6, 7, 8, 9, 11, 16)

DOCUMENTATION OF THE NURSING PROCESS

Regardless of which documentation system used, documentation must reflect the nursing process. The updated charting guidelines of the JCAHO reaffirm this emphasis. The nursing process follows a scientific method based on theories of nursing and other disciplines. The problem-solving process systematically organizes nursing activities to ensure the highest quality of care. This process allows you to determine which problems you can help alleviate and which potential problems you can help prevent. The nursing process also helps identify what kind of and how much assistance a patient requires, who can best provide that assistance, which desired outcomes the patient can achieve, and whether they are achieved.

To get a complete picture of the patient's situation, systematically follow the five steps of the nursing process: assessment, nursing diagnosis, planning, intervention, and evaluation. All of these must be documented effectively.

Fundamentals of Nursing Documentation

To ensure clear communication and complete, accurate documentation of nursing care, keep in mind the fundamentals of documentation. Follow these guidelines:

Write Neatly and Legibly

Documentation of nursing care serves the purpose of communicating with other members of the healthcare team. Sloppy or illegible handwriting confuses team members and wastes their time trying to decipher it. More seriously, the patient may be injured if other team members cannot understand crucial information.

If there is not enough room to chart something legibly, leave that section blank, place a bracket around it, and write "See progress notes." The information can then be recorded fully and legibly in the progress notes.

Write in Ink

The medical record is a permanent document and therefore must be completed in ink or printed from a computer. Most facilities require the use of black or blue ink since other colors may not photocopy well. Also, the use of felt-tipped pens is discouraged because facilities which utilize multi-part forms (carbon or carbon-less) require enough pressure when written to carry the impression through to all forms.

Use Correct Spelling and Grammar

Documentation filled with misspelled words and incorrect grammar create the same negative impression as illegible handwriting. To avoid spelling and grammatical errors:

- Keep a dictionary in charting areas, and
- Post a list of commonly misspelled words, especially terms and medications regularly used on the unit.

This is where computerized charting would have a great advantage. Many systems incorporate both spell and grammar correction packages.

Use Standard Abbreviations

An approved abbreviation list is required by JCAHO and many state regulations to prevent confusion. The use of unapproved abbreviations can result in ambiguity, which may endanger a patient's health.

Write Clear, Concise Sentences

Long words should not be used when a short word will do. The subject of the sentence should be clearly identified. The use of "I" can help differentiate your actions from those of the patient, physician, or other healthcare team members.

Say What You Mean

The best approach is to say clearly and succinctly what you see, hear, and do. Don't sound tentative. Qualified observations with such words as "appears" and "apparently" may cause other healthcare team members to conclude that one was not sure of what was being described.

Chart Promptly

Charting should be completed as soon as possible after observations or care provided to promote the clearest recollection of circumstances. Charting left to the end of the shift may cause important details to be forgotten. Bedside flow sheets facilitate charting all through the shift. Bedside computers also allow you to chart and document promptly.

Some nurses are uncomfortable about leaving written flow sheets or notes at the bedside, and understandably so. Flow sheets usually don't contain confidential information as progress notes do. The records should be kept in a safe and secure place to protect confidentiality. Local charting stations near patients' rooms (fold-down desks) can facilitate timely and legible charting. These may also be constructed to allow for a secure place to keep the chart.

When bedside flow sheets or computers are not available, make notes on worksheets or pads that are kept in a pocket. Noting key phrases, occurrences, and times may allow accurate transcription later. These notes are a reminder and not part of the medical record.

Note the Time

Times must be specific in the chart. The exact time of sudden changes in the patient's condition, significant events, and nursing actions are noted. A block of time should not be noted (i.e., 0700 to 1500) because it sounds vague and implies inattention to the patient.

Chart in Chronological Order

Assessments and observations are most useful as a part of a pattern of assessments and observations. An isolated assessment may give very little information, while in chronological order a pattern is revealed of either improvement or deterioration. Taking the time to note observations and assessments when made will allow for chronological order. Nurses often wait until the end of the shift, then record groups of assessments that omit important variations.

Document Accurately and Completely

The facts should be recorded, not opinions or assumptions. Although routine tasks don't need to be charted, you do need to chart all relevant information relating to patient care and reflecting the nursing process.

Document Objectively

Exactly what is seen, heard, and done should be recorded. Patient statements should be recorded in the patient's exact words. Subjective statements should be avoided; instead, include the facts that led to this conclusion. Document only the data you witness or data from a reliable source. When information is included from another source, cite the source.

Sign Each Entry

Each entry you make in the progress notes should be signed with your first name or initial, full last name, and professional licensure. When a last entry is unsigned, the nurse who made the entry should be contacted immediately. If the nurse can not be found, simply write the next entry and sign the progress notes. The time differences and change in handwriting should dispel confusion as to the author.

ASSESSMENT

A nurse's assessment of a patient begins when the patient is first encountered and continues throughout the hospitalization as more information is obtained on the changes of condition. As the initial step of the nursing process, assessment includes collecting relevant information from various sources and analyzing it to form a complete picture of the patient.

The assessment is recorded accurately and this will help guide you through the rest of the nursing process. The nursing diagnosis can then be formulated, along with the patient problem list and nursing plans of care. A well-documented assessment serves as a vital communication tool for other healthcare team members, and forms the baseline from which a patient's progress is evaluated. This is required to meet JCAHO and other regulatory agencies' expectations. It also provides a means of indicating that quality care has been rendered which PROs and quality assurance reviewers often use as proof. In case of litigation, the assessment can be used as evidence in court.

Initial Assessment

The initial assessment is performed when first meeting the patient. Before starting, consider two questions:

- Which information will be the most relevant for this patient?
- How much time is there to gather the information?

The answers to these questions will help you collect meaningful information and make comprehensive, goal-directed nursing interventions possible.

Collecting Relevant Information

The initial assessment may begin with signs and symptoms, chief complaint, or medical diagnosis. It also may focus on the type of care already received, such as from the emergency department (ED) or another unit. Start by identifying basic information:

- Why has the patient sought healthcare?
- What are the immediate problems?
- Are these problems life-threatening?
- Does a potential for injury exist?
- What other influences may affect treatment outcomes (advanced age, fear, cultural differences, lack of understanding, etc.)?
- Is the patient allergic to anything (medications, latex, etc.)?

Complying with the Time Frame

The policy of your facility will establish the time limit for completing the initial assessment. The JCAHO requires facilities to establish a time frame for assessment of each type of patient served. This may range from minutes to hours. Normally, the more acute the care delivered, the shorter the time frame. Thus, the ED would have a shorter period than would an elective medical surgical unit.

Categorizing Assessment Data

When collecting and analyzing assessment information, distinguish between subjective and objective information. Subjective information is the patient's perception of their problem, while objective information is something observed and/or verified (vital signs). Both types will be gathered from both primary and secondary sources.

Subjective Data

Subjective data during the initial assessment includes the patient's chief complaint or concern, current health status, health history, family history, psychosocial history, activities of daily living (ADLs), and a review of body systems. This may be your most important source of information, but remember that the patient is embodying his/her perception of the problem(s).

When documenting subjective data, record it as such. Whenever possible, note the patient's own words in quotation marks as "Patient states." Pain is an important assessment area and it is important to note not only the patient's description of the pain and how it is relieved (if relieved), but also define it on a numeric scale which is identified by facility policies. Unfamiliar words or slang used by the patient needs to be clarified and documented in both the phrase and the patient's definition.

Objective Data

Objective data normally involves no interpretation. Healthcare team members should avoid using subjective descriptions such as "large," "small," or "moderate" when documenting findings. When possible, use measurements, and specify color, size, and location. Also, avoid interpretation of the data or reflecting a personal opinion.

Sources of Data

Information collected directly from the patient (primary source data) is usually the most accurate reflection of the situation. Additional data may be obtained from secondary sources, which include family members, friends, and other healthcare team members. Written records such as past admissions, transfer summaries, and personal documents (living will) also provide important information.

Secondary source information often gives alternative viewpoints to those of the patient. Because of the patient's condition or age, it may be necessary to establish a complete baseline. Family members and friends give important indications of family dynamics, educational needs, and available support systems.

Performing the Initial Assessment

An initial assessment consists of general observations, the health history, and the physical examination.

General Observations

Observing the patient can yield a wealth of information. These observations begin at the initial meeting and continue throughout the admission. By looking critically at the patient, valuable information can be collected about the emotional state, immediate comfort level, and general physical condition. Observations should be objective and refrain from drawing conclusions. Initial conclusions are often wrong because they are based on too little evidence. Proper documentation should record facts.

Health History

The health history is a guide to subsequent physical assessment and organizes pertinent physiological, psychological, cultural, and psychosocial information. The history consists of subjective data about the patient's current health status and provides clues that point to actual or potential health problems. It also reveals the patient's ability to comply with healthcare interventions and patient expectations for treatment outcomes. Finally, the health history yields details about the patient's lifestyle, family relationships, and cultural influences that may affect his healthcare needs.

The health history is used to identify patient problems that nursing interventions can help resolve. Once the problems are identified, nursing diagnoses can be formulated and subsequently the plan of care based on those problems.

Preparing to Take the Health History. The health history is obtained through an interview that needs to be in a comfortable environment for the patient. The interview should include family members and close friends when appropriate. The patient's willingness to participate is a crucial factor and should be evaluated. If the patient is sedated or confused, hostile or angry, or experiencing pain or dyspnea, ask only the essential questions. A more in-depth interview can be performed later when conditions are improved. Secondary sources can often provide much needed information during this time.

The patient's discomfort and anxiety should be alleviated as much as possible during this time, and an attempt should be made to create a quiet, private environment for the interview. Interruptions should be avoided, and interest in and respect for the confidentiality of the information being shared should be shown. Inform the patient of the expected time involved with the interview at the forefront. Explain the purpose of doing the history, so the asking of personal questions will be understood. Lastly, be calm, relaxed, and unhurried in order to convey patience and the importance of the health history interview.

Conducting the Interview. Empathy, compassion, self-awareness, and objectivity are necessary to promote a trusting relationship with the patient. To obtain a comprehensive health history, a variety of interviewing techniques are needed. Some of these techniques are:

- Using general leads,
- Restating (summarizing) information,
- Using reflection,
- Stating the implied meaning,
- Focusing the discussion, and
- Asking open-ended questions.

Techniques to Avoid. Avoid alienating the patient and/or the family during the interview and thus hindering communication. Refrain from the following techniques:

- Judgmental or threatening questions,
- Probing and persistent questions,
- Inappropriate language,
- Advice, and
- False reassurances.

Timesaving Measures. Increased patient acuity and staff shortages sometimes make conducting a thorough interview difficult, but certain strategies can help make the most of the time without compromising quality. In some cases, ask the patient to complete a questionnaire about his past and present health status instead of conducting a patient interview. The document can then be quickly and easily reviewed to obtain the health history. This method may be more successful in short procedure units and before admission for elective procedures. Although this method saves time, it does not allow the development of a positive relationship with the patient.

Physical Examination

The physical examination is performed by using assessment techniques of inspection, palpation, percussion, and auscultation. During this phase of the assessment, obtain objective data that may confirm or rule out suspicions raised during the health history interview. These findings will enable planning of care and teaching the patient about their condition.

The scope of physical examination depends on the patient's condition, the clinical setting, and policies and procedures established by the healthcare facility. A routine examination that notes abnormal findings would then call for a more in-depth assessment. The major components of a physical examination include height, weight, vital signs, and a review of major body systems. A routine review for an adult patient on a medical-surgical unit includes the following body systems:

- Respiratory system,
- Cardiovascular system,
- Neurologic system,
- Eyes, ears, nose, and throat,
- GI system,
- Musculoskeletal system,
- Genitourinary system,
- Reproductive system, and
- Integumentary system.

Meeting JCAHO Requirements

JCAHO requires that accredited facilities meet certain standards for healthcare professionals performing patient assessments. One key requirement of JCAHO is that assessment information from family and friends be obtained when appropriate. For individuals interviewed that are not family members, the nature of the relationship and length of time knowing the patient must be properly noted.

Assessment Requirements

JCAHO standards require that each patient's initial assessment include three key categories: physical, psychological, and social status. The standards further state that the scope and intensity of any further assessments are based on the patient's diagnosis, the care setting, the patient's desire for care, and his response to previous care. The patient's nutritional and functional statuses are assessed if appropriate. The patient's educational and discharge planning needs should also be assessed in the admission process.

Documenting the Initial Assessment

Documentation styles and formats vary, depending on the policy and procedures of the facility and the patient population served. Facilities will also have policies and procedures for documentation of education needs, discharge planning, and incomplete initial assessment data. Familiarity with facility documentation standards of the initial assessment is required.

Documentation Styles

Initial assessment findings are usually documented in one of three basic styles: narrative notes, standardized open-ended style, and standardized closed-ended style. Many assessment forms utilize a combination of all three styles.

Narrative Notes. (See Traditional Narrative Charting) Although narrative notes allow the listing of findings in order of importance, there are problems. These notes are time-consuming and tend to mimic the medical model by focusing on a review of body systems. Because narratives require the remembering and recording of all significant information in a detailed, logical sequence, this is often unrealistic in today's hectic world. Legibility also comes into play and may lead to misinterpretation.

Narrative notes are probably most used by independent practitioners. Within healthcare facilities, narrative initial assessments are a waste of time and may jeopardize quality of care.

Standardized Open-Ended Style. This is a typical "fill-in-the-blanks" assessment form with preprinted headings and questions. Time is saved with information being categorized under specific headings which allows information to be easily recorded and retrieved. Also, the use of partial phrases and approved abbreviations speeds things along.

Unfortunately, open-ended forms don't always provide enough space or instructions to obtain thorough descriptions. Nonspecific responses may lead to misinterpretation.

Standardized Closed-Ended Style. This type of assessment form provides preprinted headings, checklists, and questions with specific responses that simply allow the appropriate one to be checked off. This type also saves time and eliminates legibility problems. The form can also be easily incorporated into most computer systems. The type of information which the facility requires uses established and nonspecific terminology with clearly defined terms such as "within normal limits" or "no alteration."

The disadvantage to closed-ended forms is the lack of space to note relevant information that doesn't fit preprinted choices. These forms also tend to be lengthy, especially when a facility's policy calls for in-depth physical assessment data.

Documentation Formats

Historically, the nursing assessment followed the medical format. As previously noted, a narrative form of the nursing assessment has disadvantages. Some facilities have adopted formats that more readily reflect the nursing process. This format is based on either human response patterns or functional healthcare patterns. Other formats are modeled on specific conceptual frameworks based on published nursing theory.

Human Response Patterns. NANDA has developed a classification system for nursing diagnoses based on human response patterns. These patterns relate directly to actual or potential health problems, as identified or indicated by assessment data. This allows for the establishment of appropriate diagnoses while the assessment form is recorded. The main drawback is that these forms tend to be lengthy.

Functional Healthcare Patterns. Functional healthcare patterns, developed by Marjory Gordon, classify nursing data according to the patient's ability to function independently. Many nurses consider this system easier to understand and remember than the human response system.

Conceptual Frameworks. Some healthcare facilities have modeled assessment forms on nursing philosophies that the nursing departments follow. Assessment forms based on specific nursing philosophies reflect the theories of individuals such as Dorothea Orem, Imogene King, and Sister Callista Roy.

Documenting Learning Needs

Most initial assessment forms have an identified section assessing or documenting the age, education, and cultural level and/or needs of the patient. When these needs are later reassessed, they can be documented within the progress notes or specific education flow sheets designed as such. These may be open-ended, closed-ended, or specifically designed flow sheets.

Documenting Discharge Planning Needs

Effective discharge planning begins when you identify and document the patient's needs during the initial assessment or on admission. Discharge needs should be noted on the initial assessment form, on a specifically designed discharge planning form, or any number of other forms. The significant factors are to begin documentation from admission and follow the appropriate process.

Documenting Incomplete Initial Data

Whenever this occurs, and for whatever reason, base the initial assessment on observations and physical examination of the patient. Be sure to note "Unable to obtain complete data at this time." If you do not, this could indicate a failure to obtain a complete assessment. Missing information should be obtained as soon as possible. Be sure to note how and when the missing information was obtained. The facility standards for documentation must be adhered to, whether the initial assessment form is added to or the information is documented in the progress notes.

When the information is added to complete the initial assessment, be sure to revise the nursing plan of care accordingly.

Ongoing Assessment

Patient assessment is a continuous process. Reassessment evaluates the effectiveness of nursing interventions and determines the patient's progress toward desired outcomes. Effective documentation of these further assessments facilitates communication with other healthcare team members and allows the planning of the most appropriate patient care.

The frequency of reassessment depends on the patient's condition, but JCAHO requires each patient be reassessed at appropriate intervals as defined by the facility's policies and procedures. Care should be planned accordingly.

Planned Reassessment

A planned reassessment provides routine data needed to evaluate a patient on a regular basis. This reevaluation must include not only physical, but also psychosocial, educational, environmental, and discharge needs. This could occur in the previously noted "team planning" format (see Understanding the Medical Record). Records of these meetings are maintained in the medical record to ensure communication with other healthcare team members.

Unplanned Reassessment

This occurs whenever the patient's condition or circumstances change unexpectedly. In many instances, a complete assessment would occur along with scheduling further diagnostic evaluations according to the new revised plan of care.

Documenting Ongoing Assessment

Ongoing assessments are documented on flow sheets and/or narrative progress notes. Ideally, flow sheets would contain all the routine assessment data and nursing interventions, which allows for shorter narrative notes and less documentation time. Flow sheets come in all shapes and sizes and can allow for ease of charting and show patient progression.

Because flow sheets are legally accepted as a component of the medical record, they must be completed correctly and according to facility policies and procedures.

When additional documentation is required, note such in the appropriate location, such as in the progress notes. If additional information is not necessary, draw a line through the unnecessary portions of the flow sheet. Never leave blanks.

Nursing Diagnosis and Plan of Care

Once the nursing diagnoses are formulated, a written plan of care plays a key role in returning (or attempting to return) the patient to a state of wellness. Careful selection of the diagnoses is essential for the plan of care to be solid. A plan can then be written that not only fits the nursing diagnoses, but also fits the patient. The diagnoses and plan must take into account the needs, age, developmental level, culture, strengths, and weaknesses of a patient, and a patient's willingness and ability to take part in his or her care.

The plan of care should help patients reach their highest functional level with minimal risk and without new problems. If complete recovery is unlikely or impossible, the plan of care should help the patient cope physically and emotionally with his/her impaired or declining health. All of this must be well documented.

Formulating the Nursing Diagnoses

A nursing diagnosis focuses on the patient's responses to illness, while a medical diagnosis focuses on the pathophysiology or illness.

Types of Nursing Diagnoses

According to the facility policies and procedures, standardized diagnoses should be used or formulated by the nursing staff.

Using Standardized Diagnoses

Several organizations have developed standardized lists of diagnoses for consistency. NANDA has developed the most complete and widely accepted lists of nursing diagnoses. NANDA classifies nursing diagnoses according to the human response patterns: exchanging, communicating, relating, valuing, choosing, moving, knowing, and feeling. The association meets every two years to consider new diagnoses.

Diagnoses can also be categorized according to nursing models such as the one developed by Marjory Gordon, where nursing diagnoses correspond to functional health patterns. The self-care model of Orem may also be used. Or, the facility or unit may establish its own list of nursing diagnoses, categorizing them according to medical diagnoses and invasive (surgical) procedures.

No accrediting organization requires the use of standardized diagnoses; however, by using such, facilities establish a common language, making communication easier and diagnoses more precise.

Formulating Your Own Nursing Diagnoses

This takes more time than utilizing standardized ones. Some nurses prefer formulating their own diagnoses because they find the standardized lists incomplete or the language overly formal or abstract. This approach can help characterize a problem that standardized diagnoses don't really address.

Deciding on a Diagnosis

Before developing or utilizing nursing diagnoses, evaluate relevant assessment data. The data are normally taken from the standardized assessment form that groups related information into categories. Reviewing the data in these groupings lets you determine which patient needs require nursing intervention. Some assessment forms list relevant nursing diagnoses alongside the assessment findings. Traditional narrative charting does not facilitate this well.

Components of the Diagnosis

After reviewing the assessment data, formulate the nursing diagnoses. Each diagnosis usually has three components: the human response or problem, related factors, and signs and symptoms.

1. Human Response or Problem

The human response is the first step of identifying a diagnosis, and identifies actual or potential problems that can be affected by nursing. If the NANDA complete list (Taxonomy, see Appendix) doesn't provide a label that fits a particular problem, or the facility doesn't use standardized diagnoses, create a label for the patient's condition.

2. Related Factors

The second step of the nursing diagnosis identifies related factors, which may precede, contribute to, or simply be associated with the human response. However they relate, these make the diagnosis more closely fit the particular patient and help choose the most effective interventions. When a related factor cannot be determined, write "related to unknown etiology" and modify the diagnosis as more information is obtained. The standard abbreviation "R/T" for "related to" may be used.

3. Signs and Symptoms

Finally, to complete the nursing diagnosis, the signs and symptoms that led to the diagnosis must be noted. NANDA refers to these as the "defining characteristics" which will be drawn from the assessment data. Signs and symptoms can be included in this. Choose only the key characteristics which relate to formulating the nursing diagnoses. This will contribute to brevity.

The signs and symptoms can be joined to the first step of the nursing diagnosis with the words "as evidenced by," abbreviated "AEB."

Setting Priorities

Once the nursing diagnoses have been determined, they will need to be ranked, based on which problems require immediate attention. Whenever possible, include the patient in this process. The generally accepted basis for setting priorities is Maslow's hierarchy of needs. The first nursing diagnosis will typically stem from the primary medical diagnosis or the patient's chief complaint. This first diagnosis normally points out a threat to the patient's well-being and sometimes his/her life.

Related nursing diagnoses follow in order to define problems of less immediate threats. Then the nursing diagnoses, which pertain to the patient's psychosocial, emotional, or spiritual needs, are listed. Although a nursing diagnosis may have a lower priority, don't wait to intervene with this problem. Helping with a lesser priority problem such as anxiety may have direct effect on resolving the primary problem (such as congestive heart failure).

Developing Expected Outcomes

After nursing diagnoses have been established and ranked, relevant expected outcomes can be developed, which is an increasingly important planning step. Expected outcomes are goals that the patient should reach based on the nursing diagnoses and nursing interventions. There may be more than one outcome for each nursing diagnosis.

An outcome can specify improvement in the patient's ability to function or amelioration of a problem. Each outcome should call for the maximum realistic improvement.

Writing Specific Outcome Statements

An ideal outcome statement should include four components: the specific behavior that will demonstrate the patient has reached his goal, criteria for measuring the behavior, the conditions under which the behavior should occur, and the time by which the behavior should occur. When writing outcome statements, the following guidelines should be used:

Make your Statements Specific

Action verbs such as *walks, demonstrates, consumes,* and *expresses* should be used to make specific statements. Vague statements should be avoided because they give colleagues little to go on. Clearly state which behaviors the patient is expected to exhibit and when.

Focus on the Patient

The outcome statement should reflect the patient's behavior and not the nursing intervention.

Let the Patient Help You

Patients are more motivated when they take part in developing outcome statements. More realistic goals can be set when there is input from the patient and family members.

Take Medical Orders into Account

Don't write outcome statements that ignore or contradict medical orders. Make sure the medical orders are not more restrictive than the outcome statement.

Adapt the Outcomes to the Circumstances

Outcomes must take into account the patient's coping ability, age, educational level, cultural influences, support systems, living conditions, and socioeconomic status. The anticipated length of stay must also be considered when deciding on time limits for achieving goals.

Change Your Statements as Necessary

Written outcome statements may occasionally need to be revised. When a patient is having difficulty reaching a goal, the date may need to be adjusted or the goal changed to one which the patient can more easily reach.

Use Shortcuts

Including only the essential can save time in formatting outcome statements. Simply write, "Patient will demonstrate. . .by (*date*)."

Selecting Interventions

Interventions are nursing actions that the patient and staff agree will help him/her reach expected outcomes. Interventions are based on the second part of the nursing diagnosis – the related factors. These could be interventions which reduce or eliminate the related factors as stated by the patient. At least one intervention must be written for each outcome.

Interventions can be determined in several ways. Initially consider ones that the patient or staff has successfully tried before. Interventions can also be selected from standardized plans of care, interventions successfully used by colleagues, or nursing journals that discuss interventions for standardized nursing diagnoses.

Writing Intervention Statements

The intervention statements must communicate your ideas clearly to other staff members. Follow these guidelines when writing interventions:

Clearly State the Necessary Action

As much specific detail as possible should be included in interventions to promote continuity of care. Document how and when to perform the intervention as well as any special instructions.

Tailor the Intervention to the Patient

Interventions should be written with the patient's age, condition, developmental level, environment, and value system in mind.

Keep the Patient's Safety in Mind

The patient's physical and mental limitations should be taken into account so as to not worsen existing problems or create new ones. Make sure the patient is physically capable of doing a new task or exercise without injury prior to teaching the patient how to perform it.

Follow the Rules of Your Health Facility

The facility's rules, policies, and procedures cannot be ignored or contradicted by interventions.

Take Other Healthcare Activities into Account

Other necessary activities, such as diagnostic tests, may interfere with planned interventions. In this case, the intervention would have to be adjusted.

Include Available Resources

Make full use of the facility's resources and outside resources to make interventions effective. Education material and programs from both the facility and outside agencies can be of good use in writing interventions and being effective to the patient.

Writing the Plan of Care

The plan of care is the blueprint for concise, meaningful charting. A well-written plan of care will be reflected in the nurse's progress notes and will almost allow them to write themselves. A good plan of care consists of the following:

- Patient problems identified during the admission interview and hospitalization,
- Realistic, measurable expected outcomes and target dates, and
- Nursing interventions that will help the patient or patient's family achieve the set outcomes.

Either a traditional or standardized plan of care can be used to document nursing diagnoses, expected outcomes, and interventions. Protocols may be used along with the plans or alone to demonstrate the planned care. Patient-teaching and discharge plans are included in the plan of care.

Types of Nursing Plans of Care

There are two basic types of plans of care: traditional and standardized. With either, the plan of care should cover all nursing care from admission to discharge and be a permanent part of the patient's medical record. The plan should be written and placed into action as soon as possible after the initial assessment. This will allow for revision and updates throughout the patient's hospitalization.

Traditional Plan of Care

The traditional plan of care, also called the *individually developed plan of care,* is written from scratch for each patient. This is written following an analysis of the assessment data. Although this type is rarely used due to the time required to perform, it is worthwhile to understand how it is developed.

The basic form utilizes columns. The three main columns are for nursing diagnoses, expected outcomes, and interventions. Other columns are for the date the plan of care was initiated, the target date for expected outcomes, and the dates for reviews, revisions, and resolution. There is also space for signatures or initials.

The outcomes and notations will vary as the expected length of admission varies. Shorter stays would see outcomes that could be reached by discharge. Long-term care facilities would have outcomes that reflect the maximum functional level the patient could reach.

Standardized Plan of Care

Standardized plans of care provide a series of standard interventions for patients with similar diagnoses, and were developed to save time and improve quality of care. The standardization easily lends itself to computerized charting. Most standard plans also supply root outcome statements. Medical diagnoses and some nursing diagnoses classify some plans.

Current versions allow for customization where earlier versions didn't make much allowance for differences in patient needs. The current versions require an explanation of how the plan was individualized. To use such a plan, the following information is usually required:

- Related factors and signs and symptoms for a nursing diagnosis,
- Time limits for the outcomes,
- Frequency of interventions, and
- Specific instructions for interventions.

A patient with more than one diagnosis could create quite a cumbersome amount of standardized care plans. This is where computers could be of great value. Computers can allow plans to be combined and edited, where only the applicable portions of each plan are used to make one manageable plan. Some computers utilize checklists for interventions that allow the building of a custom plan. Standardized plans usually include only essential information but allow space for customization.

Practice Guidelines

The practice guidelines system is a newer documentation tool which gives sequential instructions for treating patients with particular problems. This system was developed to help nurses manage equipment and provide specific treatments. Practice guidelines are also used to manage patients with specific nursing diagnoses.

Practice guidelines offer several advantages because they spell out the steps to follow for a patient with a particular diagnosis, can help provide thorough care, and ensure that the patient receives consistent care from all caregivers. Many practice guidelines are detailed to specify what to teach the patient and what to document. They even include a reference section that lets you quickly reference how current the guideline is.

Some practice guidelines identify the role of other healthcare professionals, which helps all team members coordinate efforts. This feature can also serve as a teaching tool to inexperienced staff members. Whether used alone or in conjunction with other plans, practice guidelines can also save documentation time.

Using Practice Guidelines

The practice guidelines that best fit your patient are the ones to use. You may have several different practice guidelines, depending on the number of problems identified. When there is not a specific guideline for a particular problem, this is the opportunity to develop one. Once a practice guideline is selected, it must be tailor-fit to the patient's needs, and any modifications made to the plan of care are documented.

Documenting Practice Guidelines

When a practice guideline is documented on a plan of care, use the intervention section and indicate that the guideline will be followed. The practice guideline to be used can also be listed on a flow sheet. Always document any modifications made to the guideline. When complete, the use of the practice guideline can be noted in the progress notes or on the flow sheet. The guidelines themselves usually remain at the nurses' station as a reference.

Clinical Pathways

Clinical pathways, also known as critical pathways or care maps, are one of the newest documentation tools. The tool draws input from all disciplines involved with the care of a similar group of patients, and defines the care to be provided and the anticipated length-of-stay.

Patient-Teaching Plan

Patient-teaching plans are now needed in the plan of care. This can be included in the main plan of care or written separately. Many facilities require a separate plan due to the emphasis placed on patient teaching by accrediting and regulatory organizations. With shorter lengths-of-stay, patients are requiring more extensive teaching plans to support follow-up and home care regimens.

In addition to identifying what the patient needs to learn and how this information is to be taught, a teaching plan sets criteria for evaluating how well it was learned. This plan also allows educators from different areas to coordinate efforts. The teaching plan serves as legal proof that the patient has received the appropriate instruction and meets the requirements of regulatory organizations such as JCAHO.

The teaching plan needs to be carefully organized to ensure that it is all it should be. This will help identify what the needs of the patient are, how the instruction will be provided, and how the results will be measured. For the content of the plan to be realistic and attainable, other healthcare team members and family members will need to be worked with. Provisions for follow-up teaching at home must be included. Lastly, the teaching plan needs to have flexibility, taking into account variables that will act as obstructions to learning as well as the healthcare team member's own time limits.

Components of the Plan

Although the scope of each teaching plan differs, each should contain the same elements:

1. Patient-Learning Needs
2. Expected Learning Outcomes
3. Teaching Content
4. Teaching Methods
5. Teaching Tools
6. Barriers to Learning and Readiness to Learn

1. Patient-Learning Needs

Identifying learning needs helps decide which outcomes should be established for the patient. This should include not only what the health team wants the patient to learn, but also what the patient wants to learn.

2. Expected Learning Outcomes

Expected learning outcomes should focus on the patient and be readily measurable. The patient's learning behaviors and outcomes developed fall into three categories:

- Cognitive - relating to understanding,
- Psychomotor - covering manual skills, and
- Affective - dealing with attitudes.

In order to formulate precise, measurable outcomes, evaluation techniques which will best reveal the patient's progress must be identified. Questions and answers may be best for cognitive learning, while return demonstration may be best for psychomotor learning.

3. Teaching Content

In order to teach the patient what he will need in order to achieve expected outcomes, the content of the teaching must be identified. Family members and other healthcare team members must be included in these decisions. In many situations, the family members themselves may be included in part of the teaching. This is especially true when the family member will be the caregiver at home and will need to continue the progress made during hospitalization.

Once the content has been set, it must be organized from simplest content to more complex. This will facilitate patients and/or family members with little education or those who don't learn well by listening.

4. Teaching Methods

The appropriate teaching method(s) will need to be decided on for the patient. Many learning tasks can be taught on a one-on-one basis, which not only allows the patient to be better known, but also builds a relationship and tailors the teaching to the patient's needs.

Other methods may be utilized either in place of or in conjunction with one-on-one teaching. Demonstrations, practice, and return demonstrations may be incorporated into the teaching plan. Role-playing may help involve the patient, while self-monitoring may involve the patient in assessing his/her own situation. When several patients need similar instruction, group teaching or therapy may be appropriate.

5. Teaching Tools

Teaching tools ranging from printed pamphlets to television or video programs can facilitate learning. Focus on what will work best for a particular patient when choosing a tool. This will vary from a patient who responds best to video, versus one who prefers hands-on. In some instances a computerized program may be best, while others may just want to read and study about the procedure or treatment.

The patient's abilities and limitations must be kept in mind when choosing teaching tools. Staff-development instructors and/or access to an education or even a patient education department will make this decision process easier. If the facility does not have the tools or resources, look into the community for various suppliers, and associations and foundations that may have access to local and/or national resources.

6. Barriers to Learning and Readiness to Learn

Assessing any barriers to learning and the patient's readiness to learn is another important aspect of the teaching plan. The impediment may be physical or psychological. If the patient is not receptive to teaching efforts, it will be difficult to meet his needs. Document any learning barriers as well as the patient's willingness to learn.

Documenting the Patient-Teaching Plan

There are several forms available for documenting the patient teaching plan. Many include phases of the nursing process as it relates to patient education. A number of facilities are being encouraged to create systematic interdisciplinary approaches to patient teaching.

Patient-teaching plans are normally found in two basic types. One type provides the format and calls for the plan to be written. The other type is known as the standardized plan and utilizes checked-off items or closed-ended notations to note and date items. Items can then be added or deleted from the standardized plan.

Depending on the plan's format, space may be included for problems that hinder learning, comments and evaluations, and dates and signatures. This information may also be included in the progress notes. The plan that is used becomes a permanent part of the medical record.

Discharge Planning

Discharge planning is the final plan of the process and has increased in importance because of the trend toward shorter hospital stays. Optimally, discharge planning is started prior to admission (for pre-planned admissions), or, at the minimum, from the day of admission.

Responsibility for Discharge Planning

In some facilities the responsibility for discharge planning resides with the social services department. Some facilities may have a nurse discharge planner to facilitate home care planning, but staff nurses play a major role in preparing patients and caregivers for the responsibility of ongoing care.

All healthcare team members need to coordinate efforts with the discharge planners or social services department. This may best be completed at a multidisciplinary discharge conference or at a "team planning" meeting. At these meetings, team members evaluate the patient's discharge needs, discuss appropriate plans, and evaluate patient progress.

Components of the Plan

A discharge plan should note the anticipated length-of-stay and identify education needs including:

- Diet,
- Medications,
- Treatments,
- Physical activity limitations,
- Signs and symptoms to report to the physician,
- Follow-up medical care,
- Equipment, and
- Appropriate community resources.

The plan should include an instruction sheet for the patient to reinforce what he/she learns and what he/she needs to remember about follow-up care. Future care should be identified to include the setting, the intended caregiver and support systems, actual or potential barriers to care, and any referrals.

Documenting the Discharge Plan

How you document the discharge plan will depend on the policies and procedures of your facility. This may vary from assessing discharge needs on admission and then documenting the discharge plan on a separate form, to documenting the discharge plan as a component of the discharge summary. Some forms use discharge planning from several different team members.

Case Management

Case management goes a step beyond planned care to managed care, and is a method of delivering healthcare that controls cost while ensuring quality care. This system came about in the 1980s after the federal government introduced the prospective payment system, also known as Diagnostic Related Groups (DRGs). Basically, the facility receives a flat rate per admission, and if the patient has a lengthy stay or develops complications, the facility loses money.

DRGs forced healthcare facilities to deliver cost-effective care without decreasing the quality of care. The case management system proposes to assist by managing each patient's care to meet both clinical and financial goals.

The Case Manager's Role

The case manager's role is expanded beyond giving nursing care. This involves the management of closely controlled systems and multidisciplinary care. The case manager is also responsible for outcomes, length-of-stay, and use of resources throughout the patient's illness.

How the System Works

In many instances, when a patient is assigned a particular DRG, they are also assigned a case manager. Optimally, this occurs shortly after admission, but in some instances it doesn't occur until discharge. In the latter situation, the case manager is making an educated guess as to what DRG the patient will be in. Each DRG case management plan has standard outcome criteria and includes both medical and nursing interventions as well as interventions from other disciplines.

The case manager may be augmented with a multidisciplinary team to evaluate the patient's progress and suggest any necessary revisions, keeping in mind the need for continuity of care and efficient use of resources. Case management documentation would include variations in the time line, processes, outcomes, and the reasons for the variations. One major task for the case manager is to keep duplication of services and medical orders to a minimum.

Another major task is to start and continue discharge planning throughout the admission so that discharge needs are anticipated. Coordinating home health, other agencies and facilities, and equipment are keys to meeting anticipated discharge dates and the patient's needs while ensuring quality care.

Types of Case Management Systems

Several systems and various adaptations exist while facilities continue to create new case management systems. Most systems are patterned after the New England Medical Center (NEMC) system, which was one of the first facilities to use case management in an acute care setting. Most facilities adapt the NEMC model to meet their own needs and philosophy of care.

Tools for Case Management

Most case management tools are patterned after those of the NEMC system. These are the *case management plan* and the *clinical pathways,* which allow one to direct, evaluate, and revise patient progress and outcomes.

Case Management Plan. The case management plan is the basic tool of case management systems and spells out the standardized care that a patient with a specific DRG should receive. The plan includes:

- Nursing-related problems,
- Patient outcomes,
- Intermediate patient outcomes,
- Nursing interventions,
- Medical interventions, and
- Target times.

Each care unit that the patient may be admitted to during an illness is covered in a subsection of the plan.

Clinical Pathway. Because case management plans are lengthy, they are not usually used on a daily basis. The clinical pathway or abbreviated form of the case management plan is used instead. This clinical pathway or healthcare map covers only the key elements which must occur for the patient to be discharged within the target date. These events include consultations, diagnostic tests, physical activities the patient must perform, treatments, diet, medications, discharge planning, and patient teaching.

Once a pathway has been established, any variance is noted and grouped by cause. Variances may result from the system, the caregivers, or a patient problem that has developed. The clinical pathways should be reviewed at shift report each day with other nurses. Any changes in the expected length of stay should be noted, and point out critical events scheduled for the next shift to the nurses coming on duty. Any variances that occurred during the shift should also be discussed.

Drawbacks of Case Management

The case management system normally works with patients that have one primary diagnosis, no secondary diagnoses, and few if any complications. Patients with multiple diagnoses or patients with multiple variances will likely have expected course of treatment changes and the length of stay will likely change. Documentation for these types of patient admissions becomes lengthy and complicated.

NURSING INTERVENTIONS

Documenting nursing interventions has long been standard practice, but methods have changed dramatically over the years due to frustration with tedious traditional methods and the urgency of economics with hospital operations. Instead of lengthy narrative notes, flow sheets or "refer to practice guidelines" has greatly streamlined the process. This section will review how to perform and document interventions, including patient teaching and discharge summary.

Performing Interventions

Nursing interventions put the plan of care into action, which is a crucial step in the nursing process. Implementation begins once the plan of care is established and recorded. Interventions fall into two general categories of *interdependent* and *independent.* A brief assessment must be made before performing either.

Need for Reassessment

Just before performing a particular intervention, reassess the patient quickly to ensure the plan of care is still appropriate.

Types of Interventions

Interdependent interventions include ones performed in collaboration with other healthcare professionals to help achieve a patient outcome. Interdependent interventions also include activities you perform at a physician's request to help implement the medical regimen.

Independent interventions are measures taken at your own discretion, independent of other healthcare team members. Such interventions would include instituting common comfort measures and teaching routine self-care techniques.

Documenting Interventions

Interventions must be documented along with the time performed, the patient's response, and additional interventions taken based on the response (including the reasons for the additional interventions). This makes your documentation outcome-oriented.

The documentation may take place on graphic records, patient care flow sheets, progress notes, or other specialized documentation forms such as MARs. Facility policies and procedures will dictate the specific method of documentation. Document interventions when administering routine care, observing changes in the patient's condition, providing emergency care, and administering medications.

Routine Care

JCAHO has encouraged healthcare facilities to utilize flow sheets for documentation of routine care measures for years. In response, flow sheets have been developed for just about everything. Due to their brevity, flow sheets make documenting and reviewing material quick and easy. Patient trends can be evaluated at a glance. Caution should be maintained, because flow sheets can lead to fragmented documentation and obscure the patient's clinical picture.

Changes in Condition

Any changes in a patient's condition require documentation in the progress notes. The narrative format of the progress notes allows for more detailed documentation of the event. The note can then direct the reader to the effects the event has had on the plan of care. The MAR may also lead to valuable information.

Patient Teaching

The teaching implemented for each patient must be recorded clearly and completely along with the results. Clear documentation of patient teaching can not only protect the healthcare team from charges of insufficient care, but also help administrators gauge the overall value of the particular patient-education program being employed.

Direct Benefits

Proper documentation can save time for other team members by not duplicating education tasks already performed. Documentation can also help motivate the patient by sharing success and progress with him/her.

Documentation Tools

In many facilities, patient education is documented on preprinted forms that are part of the medical record. These forms not only speed documentation but also facilitate complete documentation. Whenever preprinted forms or narrative notes are used, keep these tips in mind:

- Check the facility's policies and procedures regarding when, where, and how to document teaching.
- Each shift, ask these questions: "What part of the teaching plan did I complete?" and "What other teaching have I given this patient or his or her family members?" Then note your answers.
- Make sure the documentation indicates that the patient's ongoing educational needs are being met.
- Before discharge, document the patient's remaining learning needs.

Patient Discharge

An assessment of continuing care needs as well as referrals for such care must be documented when preparing a patient for discharge. This is a JCAHO requirement. Many facilities have developed forms that combine both discharge summaries and patient instructions to facilitate this process. Of course, not all facilities use these forms. Some still use narrative discharge forms summaries. If narrative forms are used, be sure to include the following information:

- Patient's status on admission and discharge,
- Significant highlights of the hospitalization,
- Outcomes of your interventions,
- Resolved and unresolved patient problems, continuing care needs for unresolved problems, and specific referrals for continuing care, and
- Instructions given to the patient or family member about medications, treatments, activity, diet, referrals, and follow-up appointments, as well as any other special instructions.

Evaluation

The current emphasis on evaluating interventions has changed documentation. Today, progress notes must include an assessment of the patient's progress toward expected outcomes established in the plan of care. This is called *outcomes and evaluation documentation*, which focuses on the patient's response to nursing care and thus enables the nurse to provide high-quality, cost-effective care. This form of charting is replacing narrative charting and lengthy, handwritten plans of care.

Outcomes and evaluation documentation force nurses to focus on patient responses to determine if interventions and the plan of care are working. Evaluation of care gives the nurse a chance to:

- Determine if the original assessment findings still apply,
- Uncover complications,
- Analyze patterns or trends in the patient's care and his/her responses to it,

- Assess the patient's response to all aspects of care, including medications, changes in diet or activity, procedures, unusual incidents or problems, and teaching,
- Determine how closely care conforms with established standards,
- Measure how well the patient has been cared for,
- Assess the performance of other members of the healthcare team, and
- Identify opportunities to improve the quality of care.

When to Perform Evaluation

Although outcome evaluation is an ongoing process, how often you are required to make evaluations is influenced by several factors. These factors depend on the acuity setting and the acuity of your patient. Acute care facilities may require plans to be reviewed every 24 hours while long-term care facilities may require the plan to be evaluated only every 30 days. Facility policies and procedures will direct this.

Evaluating Expected Outcomes

Evaluations include gathering reassessment data, comparing findings with the outcome criteria, determining the extent of outcome achievement, writing evaluation statements, and revising the plan of care. Revisions start with the determination of whether the patient has achieved the expected outcomes. If the outcomes have been fully met, decide if the problem is resolved and whether the plan can be discontinued. If the problem persists, the plan continues with new target dates until the desired status is achieved.

When outcomes are partially met or unmet, you must identify interfering factors, such as misinterpreted information, and revise the plan accordingly. This may involve the following:

- Clarify or amend the database to reflect newly discovered information,
- Reexamine and correct nursing diagnoses,
- Establish and correct criteria that reflect new information and new or amended nursing strategies,
- Add the revised nursing plan of care to the original document, and
- Record the rationale for the revisions in the nurse's progress notes.

Documenting Evaluation

Evaluation statements should indicate whether expected outcomes were achieved and should list evidence supporting the conclusion. The statements are based on outcome criteria from the plan of care, and use action verbs such as "demonstrate" or "ambulate." Include the patient's response to specific treatments, and describe the conditions under which the response occurred or failed to occur. Patient teaching and palliative or preventive care are documented as well.

After the outcomes are evaluated, be sure to record them in the medical record with clear statements that demonstrate the patient's progress toward meeting the expected outcomes. (1, 3, 5, 6, 7, 8, 9, 10, 16)

APPENDIX

NANDA Taxonomy I, Revised

The North American Nursing Diagnosis Association (NANDA) endorsed its first nursing diagnosis taxonomic structure, NANDA Taxonomy I, in 1986. This taxonomy was revised in 1989, 1994, and, most recently, 1988. The taxonomy that appears here represents the currently accepted classification system for nursing diagnoses.

This classification system, which appears below, consists of nine human response patterns and their definitions: Exchanging: Mutual giving and receiving; Communicating: Sending messages; Relating: Establishing bonds; Valuing: Assigning worth; Choosing: Selection of alternatives; Moving: Activity; Perceiving: Reception of information; Knowing: Meaning associated with information; and Feeling: Subjective awareness of information.

Pattern 1: Exchanging

1.1.2.1	Altered nutrition: More than body requirements
1.1.2.2	Altered nutrition: Less than body requirements
1.1.2.3	Altered nutrition: Risk for more than body requirements
1.2.1.1	Risk for infection
1.2.2.1	Risk for altered body temperature
1.2.2.2	Hypothermia
1.2.2.3	Hyperthermia
1.2.2.4	Ineffective thermoregulation
1.2.3.1	Dysreflexia
1.2.3.2	Risk for autonomic dysreflexia
1.3.1.1	Constipation
1.3.1.1.1	Perceived constipation
1.3.1.1.2	Colonic constipation
1.3.1.2	Diarrhea
1.3.1.3	Bowel incontinence
1.3.1.4	Risk for constipation
1.3.2	Altered urinary elimination
1.3.2.1.1	Stress incontinence
1.3.2.1.2	Reflex urinary incontinence
1.3.2.1.3	Urge incontinence
1.3.2.1.4	Functional urinary incontinence
1.3.2.1.5	Total incontinence
1.3.2.1.6	Risk of urinary urge incontinence
1.3.2.2	Urinary retention
1.4.1.1.1	Altered (specify type) tissue perfusion (renal, cerebral, cardiopulmonary, gastrointestinal, peripheral)
1.4.1.2	Risk for fluid volume imbalance
1.4.1.2.1	Fluid volume excess
1.4.1.2.1.1	Risk for fluid volume deficit
1.4.2.1	Decreased cardiac output
1.5.1.1	Impaired gas exchange
1.5.1.2	Ineffective airway clearance
1.5.1.3	Ineffective breathing pattern
1.5.1.3.1	Inability to sustain spontaneous ventilation
1.5.1.3.2	Dysfunctional ventilatory weaning response
1.6.1	Risk for injury
1.6.1.1	Risk for suffocation
1.6.1.2	Risk for poisoning
1.6.1.3	Risk for trauma
1.6.1.4	Risk for aspiration
1.6.1.5	Risk for disuse syndrome
1.6.1.6	Latex allergy
1.6.1.7	Risk for latex allergy
1.6.2	Altered protection
1.6.2.1	Impaired tissue integrity

1.6.2.1.1	Altered oral mucous membrane
1.6.2.1.2.1	Impaired skin integrity
1.6.2.1.2.2	Risk for impaired skin integrity
1.6.2.1.3	Altered dentition
1.7.1	Decreased adaptive capacity: Intracranial
1.8	Energy field disturbance

Pattern 2: Communicating

2.1.1.1	Impaired verbal communication

Pattern 3: Relating

3.1.1	Impaired social interaction
3.1.2	Social isolation
3.1.3	Risk for loneliness
3.2.1	Altered role performance
3.2.1.1.1	Altered parenting
3.2.1.1.2	Risk for altered parenting
3.2.1.1.2.1	Risk for altered parent/ infant/ child attachment
3.2.1.2.1	Sexual dysfunction
3.2.2	Altered family processes
3.2.2.1	Caregiver role strain
3.2.2.2	Risk for caregiver role strain
3.2.2.3.1	Altered family process: Alcoholism
3.2.3.1	Parental role conflict
3.3	Altered sexuality patterns

Pattern 4: Valuing

4.1.1	Spiritual distress (distress of the human spirit)
4.1.2	Risk for spiritual distress
4.2	Potential for enhanced spiritual well being

Pattern 5: Choosing

5.1.1.1	Ineffective individual coping
5.1.1.1.1	Impaired adjustment
5.1.1.1.2	Defensive coping
5.1.1.1.3	Ineffective denial
5.1.2.1.1	Ineffective family coping: Compromised
5.1.2.2	Family coping: Potential for growth
5.1.3.1	Potential for enhanced community coping
5.1.3.2	Ineffective community coping
5.2.1	Ineffective management of therapeutic regimen (individual)
5.2.2	Noncompliance (specify)
5.2.3	Ineffective management of therapeutic regimen: Community
5.2.4	Effective management of therapeutic regimen: Individual
5.3.1.1	Decisional conflict (specify)
5.4	Health-seeking behaviors (specify)

Pattern 6: Moving

6.1.1.1	Impaired physical mobility
6.1.1.1	Risk for peripheralneurovascular dysfunction
6.1.1.1.2	Risk for perioperative positioning injury
6.1.1.1.3	Impaired walking
6.1.1.1.4	Impaired wheelchair mobility
6.1.1.1.5	Impaired wheelchair transfer ability
6.1.1.1.6	Impaired bed mobility
6.1.1.2	Activity intolerance
6.1.1.2.1	Fatigue
6.1.1.3	Risk for activity intolerance
6.2.1	Sleep pattern disturbance
6.2.1.1	Sleep deprivation
6.3.1.1	Diversional activity deficit
6.4.1.1	Impaired home maintenance management
6.4.2	Altered health maintenance
6.4.2.1	Delayed surgical recovery
6.4.2.2	Adult failure to thrive
6.5.1	Feeding self-care deficit
6.5.1.1	Impaired swallowing
6.5.1.2	Interrupted breast-feeding
6.5.1.3	Effective breast-feeding
6.5.1.4	Ineffective infant feeding pattern
6.5.2	Bathing or hygiene self-care deficit
6.5.3	Dressing or grooming self-care deficit
6.5.4	Toileting self-care deficit
6.6	Altered growth and development
6.6.1	Risk for altered development
6.6.2	Risk for altered growth
6.7	Relocation stress syndrome
6.8.1	Risk for disorganized infant behavior
6.8.2	Disorganized infant behavior
6.8.3	Potential for enhanced organized infant behavior

Pattern 7: Perceiving

7.1.1	Body image disturbance
7.1.2	Self esteem disturbance
7.1.2.1	Chronic low self-esteem
7.1.2.2	Situational low self-esteem
7.1.3	Personal identity disturbance
7.2	Sensory-perceptual alterations (specify as visual, auditory, kinesthetic, gustatory, tactile, olfactory)
7.2.1.1	Unilateral neglect
7.3.1	Hopelessness
7.3.2	Powerlessness

Pattern 8: Knowing

8.1.1	Knowledge deficit (specify)
8.2.1	Impaired environmental interpretation syndrome
8.2.2	Acute confusion
8.2.3	Chronic confusion
8.3	Altered thought processes
8.3.1	Impaired memory

Pattern 9: Feeling

9.1.1	Pain
9.1.1.1	Chronic pain
9.1.2	Nausea
9.2.1.1	Dysfunctional grieving
9.2.1.2	Anticipatory grieving
9.2.1.3	Chronic sorrow
9.2.2	Risk for violence: Self-directed or directed at others
9.2.2.1	Risk for self-mutilation
9.2.3	Post-trauma syndrome
9.2.3.1	Rape-trauma syndrome

REFERENCES

1. Clarke, D. (1999). Economics of hyperbaric medicine. In E. Kindwall and H.T. Whelan (Ed.), Hyperbaric medicine practice (2nd ed., pp. 144-167). Flagstaff, AZ: Best Publishing Company.
2. Clark, J.M. (1999). Oxygen toxicity. In E. Kindwall and H.T. Whelan (Ed.), Hyperbaric medicine practice (2nd ed., pp. 69-82). Flagstaff, AZ: Best Publishing Company.
3. Cwiklinski, J.M., Messina, V.J., Norkool, D.M., and Weyenberg, G.T. (1999). Hyperbaric nursing. In E. Kindwall and H.T. Whelan (Ed.), Hyperbaric medicine practice (2nd ed., pp. 377-394). Flagstaff, AZ: Best Publishing Company.
4. Hammarlund, C. (1999). The physiology effects of hyperbaric oxygenation. In E. Kindwall and H.T. Whelan (Ed.), Hyperbaric medicine practice (2nd ed., pp. 37-68). Flagstaff, AZ: Best Publishing Company.
5. Joint Commission on Accreditation of Healthcare Organizations (November 4, 2000). Section I, Patient-focused functions, Comprehensive accreditation manual for hospitals: The official handbook, Oakbrook Terrace, IL; Author.
6. Joint Commission on Accreditation of Healthcare Organizations (November 4, 2000). Section II, Organization-focused functions, Comprehensive accreditation manual for hospitals: The official handbook, Oakbrook Terrace, IL; Author.
7. Joint Commission on Accreditation of Healthcare Organizations (November 4, 2000). Section III, Structures with functions, Comprehensive accreditation manual for hospitals: The official handbook, Oakbrook Terrace, IL; Author.
8. Kindwall, E.P. (1999). Management of complications in hyperbaric treatment. In E. Kindwall and H.T. Whelan (Ed.), Hyperbaric medicine practice (2nd ed., pp. 377-394). Flagstaff, AZ: Best Publishing Company.
9. Norkool, D. (1992). Care of the patient receiving hyperbaric oxygen therapy (HBO). In A. Reiner (Ed.), Manual of patient care standards. Gaithersburg, MD: Aspen Publishers, Inc.
10. Springhouse Corporation (1999). Documentation of the nursing process. In, Mastering documentation (2nd ed., pp. 207-264). Springhouse, PA; Author.
11. Springhouse Corporation (1999). Documentation systems. In, Mastering documentation (2nd ed., pp. 61-102). Springhouse, PA; Author.
12. Springhouse Corporation (1999). Legal and ethical implications of documentation. In, Mastering documentation (2nd ed., pp. 17-42). Springhouse, PA; Author.
13. Springhouse Corporation (1999). Nursing documentation and the Medical Record. In, Mastering documentation (2nd ed., pp. 1-16). Springhouse, PA; Author.
14. Springhouse Corporation (1999). Quality Management and Reimbursement. In, Mastering documentation (2nd ed., pp. 43-60). Springhouse, PA; Author.
15. Springhouse Corporation (1999). Documentation Systems. In, Mastering documentation (2nd ed., pp. 61-102). Springhouse, PA; Author.
16. Undersea and Hyperbaric Medical Society (1999). Hyperbaric oxygen therapy: 1999 committee report. Kensington, MD: Author.

CHAPTER II

DOCUMENTATION OF THE NURSING PROCESS AS IT RELATES TO HYPERBARIC OXYGEN THERAPY

H.G. VINCENT

As presented in the chapter on Documentation, the nursing process should be followed to ensure complete and accurate medical records. This process has been divided into five steps: assessment, nursing diagnosis, planning, intervention, and evaluation. Later in this chapter some documentation examples of patient assessments, transcutaneous oxygen summary lists, and hyperbaric oxygen therapy will be reviewed. These form samples, although not endorsed by the Baromedical Nurses Association (BNA), may enlighten new units trying to develop initial documentation formats and existing units in the process of reviewing their own documentation formats.

Following the assessment and nursing diagnosis, planning of patient care must reflect the standards of practice and standards of care established or identified by the facility to be incorporated in patient care. These standards can be established as standardized plans of care or reflected within traditional plans of care utilized by the facility. To assist with this process, the American Nurses Association (ANA) Standards of Nursing Practice and the BNA Guidelines for Standards of Care for the Patient Receiving Hyperbaric Oxygen Therapy are reviewed. (1, 5, 6)

ANA STANDARDS OF NURSING PRACTICE

In 1991, the ANA developed standards of clinical nursing practice that provided guidelines for determining quality nursing care. In updating previous standards, the ANA addressed performance standards and established measurement criteria for evaluating whether nurses met those standards. The standards developed are based on the nursing process and identify both standards of care and standards of professional performance.

STANDARDS OF CARE

STANDARD I: ASSESSMENT

The nurse collects health data about the client, and measurement criteria of these are:

- The nurse bases data collection priorities on the client's immediate health condition and needs.
- The nurse uses appropriate assessment techniques in collecting data.
- Data collection involves the client, significant others, and health-care providers when appropriate.
- The data collection process is systematic and ongoing.
- Relevant data are documented in a retrievable form.

STANDARD II: NURSING DIAGNOSIS

The nurse analyzes the assessment data in order to determine a nursing diagnosis with the following measurement criteria:

- Diagnoses are derived from the assessment data.
- Diagnoses are validated with the client, significant others, and healthcare providers when possible.
- Diagnoses are documented in a manner that facilitates the determination of expected outcomes and plan of care.

STANDARD III: OUTCOME IDENTIFICATION

Expected outcomes are identified by the nurse and individualized to the client by the following measurement criteria:

- Outcomes are derived from the diagnoses.
- Outcomes are documented as measurable goals.
- Outcomes are mutually formulated with the client and healthcare providers when possible.
- Outcomes are realistic and related to the client's present and potential capabilities.
- Outcomes are attainable in relation to resources available to the client.
- Outcomes include a time estimate for attainment.
- Outcomes provide direction for continuity of care.

STANDARD IV: PLANNING

The nurse, with the following measurement criteria, implements identified interventions in the plan of care:

- The plan of care is individualized to the client's condition or needs.
- The plan of care is developed with the client, significant others, and healthcare providers when appropriate.
- The plan of care reflects current nursing practice.
- The plan of care is documented.
- The plan of care provides for continuity of care.

STANDARD V: IMPLEMENTATION

The nurse implements the interventions identified in the plan of care with the following measurement criteria:

- Interventions are consistent with the established plan of care.
- Interventions are implemented in a safe and appropriate manner.
- Interventions are documented.

Standard VI: Evaluation

The client's progress toward attainment of outcomes is evaluated by the nurse against the following measurement criteria:

- Evaluation is systematic and ongoing.
- The client's responses to interventions are documented.
- The effectiveness of interventions are evaluated in relation to outcomes.
- Ongoing assessment data are used to revise diagnoses, outcomes, and the plan of care as needed.
- Revisions in diagnoses, outcomes, and the plan of care are documented.
- The client, significant others, and healthcare providers are involved in the evaluation process when appropriate.

STANDARDS OF PROFESSIONAL PERFORMANCE

Nursing performance standards include guidelines for:

Standard I: Quality of Care

Systematic evaluation of the quality and effectiveness of nursing practice utilizes the following criteria:

- The nurse participates, with the following criteria, in quality-of-care activities as appropriate to the individual's position, education, and practice environment:
- Identification of aspects of care important for quality monitoring,
    - Identification of indicators used to monitor quality and effectiveness of nursing care,
    - Collection of data to monitor quality and effectiveness of nursing care,
    - Analysis of quality data to identify opportunities for improving care,
    - Formulation of recommendations to improve nursing practice or client outcomes,
    - Implementation of activities to enhance the quality of nursing practice,
    - Participation on interdisciplinary teams that evaluate clinical practice or health services, and
    - Development of policies and procedures to improve quality of care.
- The nurse uses the results of quality-of-care activities to initiate changes in practice.
- The nurse uses the results of quality-of-care activities to initiate changes throughout the healthcare delivery system as appropriate.

STANDARD II: PERFORMANCE APPRAISAL

The nurse evaluates nursing practice in relation to professional practice standards and relevant statutes and regulations with the following criteria:

- The nurse engages in performance appraisal on a regular basis, identifying areas of strength as well as areas for professional and practice development.
- The nurse seeks constructive feedback regarding practice.
- The nurse takes action to achieve goals identified during performance appraisal.
- The nurse participates in peer review as appropriate.

STANDARD III: EDUCATION

The nurse acquires and maintains current knowledge in nursing practice utilizing the following measurement criteria:

- The nurse participates in ongoing educational activities related to clinical knowledge and professional issues.
- The nurse seeks experiences to maintain clinical skills.
- The nurse seeks knowledge and skills appropriate to the practice setting.

STANDARD IV: COLLEGIALITY

The professional development of peers, colleagues, and others is contributed to by the nurse and measured against the following criteria:

- The nurse shares knowledge and skills with colleagues and others.
- The nurse provides peers with constructive feedback regarding their practice.
- The nurse contributes to an environment that is conducive to clinical education of nursing students as appropriate.

STANDARD V: ETHICS

Utilizing the following measurement criteria, the nurse's decisions and actions on behalf of clients are determined in an ethical manner:

- The nurse's practice is guided by the standard nurses' code.
- The nurse maintains client confidentiality.
- The nurse acts as a client advocate.
- The nurse delivers care in a nonjudgemental and nondiscriminatory manner that is sensitive to client diversity and that preserves and protects the client's autonomy, dignity, and rights.
- The nurse seeks available resources to help formulate ethical decisions.

STANDARD VI: COLLABORATION

The nurse collaborates with the client, significant others, and healthcare providers in providing client care under the following criteria:

- The nurse communicates with the client, significant others, and healthcare providers regarding client's and nursing's role in the provision of care.
- The nurse consults with healthcare providers for client care as needed.
- The nurse makes referrals, including provisions for continuity of care, as needed.

STANDARD VII: RESEARCH

With the following criteria, the nurse uses research findings in practice:

- The nurse uses interventions substantiated by research as appropriate to the individual's position, education, and practice environment.
- The nurse participates in research activities as appropriate to the individual's position, education, and practice environment. Such activities may include:
    - Identification of clinical problems suitable for nursing research,
    - Participation in data collection,
    - Participation in a unit, organization, or community research committee or program,
    - Sharing of research activities with others,
    - Conducting research,
    - Critiquing research for application to practice, and
    - Using research findings in the development of policies, procedures, and guidelines for client care.

STANDARD VIII: RESOURCE UTILIZATION

The nurse considers factors related to safety, effectiveness, and cost in planning and delivering client care, utilizing the following criteria:

- The nurse evaluates factors related to safety, effectiveness, and cost when two or more practice options would result in the same expected client outcome.
- The nurse assigns tasks or delegates care based on the needs of the client and the knowledge and skill of the provider selected.
- The nurse assists the client and significant others in identifying and securing appropriate services available to address health-related needs.

BAROMEDICAL NURSES ASSOCIATION

Guidelines For: Standards of Care for the Patient Receiving Hyperbaric Oxygen Therapy

In 1988, the first published list of nursing guidelines appeared in a manual directed at patient care standards, and gave the industry a "standardized plan of care" to refer to (see chapter on Documentation). This list not only noted common nursing diagnoses and problems associated with hyperbaric medicine, but also desired outcomes and nursing interventions. The BNA utilized the published plan of care, and with few revisions adopted the following suggested guidelines for hyperbaric nursing in 1998.

1. NURSING DIAGNOSIS/PROBLEM

Anxiety related to knowledge deficit of hyperbaric oxygen therapy and treatment procedures.

Desired Outcomes

Patient and/or family will state:

1. Rationale for hyperbaric oxygen therapy.
2. Goals of therapy.
3. Procedures involved with hyperbaric oxygen therapy.
4. Potential hazards of hyperbaric oxygen therapy.

Nursing Interventions

1. Assess and document patient and/or family's understanding of rationale for and goals of hyperbaric oxygen therapy, and procedures involved with and potential hazards of hyperbaric oxygen therapy.
2. Identify barriers of learning.
3. Include information on the following when identified as a learning need:
    - Purpose and expected outcomes of hyperbaric oxygen therapy,
    - Sequence of treatment procedures and what to expect (i.e., pressure, temperature, noises, wound care),
    - Oxygen delivery systems,
    - Ear clearing techniques,
    - Pulmonary barotrauma, and
    - Prevention of oxygen toxicity.
4. Provide continued opportunities for discussion and instruction.
5. Provide patient and/or family with information brochure on hyperbaric oxygen therapy.

6. Keep patient and/or family informed of all procedures.
7. Document patient/family instruction, using the confirmation of instruction form and the general patient instruction form.

2. NURSING DIAGNOSIS/PROBLEM

Potential for injury related to transferring patient in/out of chamber, explosion of equipment, fire, and/or medical support equipment.

Desired Outcomes

Patient will not experience any injury.

Nursing Interventions

1. Assist patient in and out of the chamber appropriately.
2. Secure equipment inside chamber according to policy and procedure.
3. Monitor equipment and supplies for changes in pressure and volumes.
4. Follow fire prevention procedure per established policy and procedure.
5. Monitor for presence of air in I.V. and invasive pressure line tubing. All air must be removed from tubing, if present.
6. Document that all invasive lines are clear of air prior to chamber pressurization and depressurization.

In a multiple chamber

1. Monitor pressure bags on all pressurized lines. Increase pressure in bags during chamber pressurization and release pressure in bags during depressurization.
2. Re-zero monitors with pressure changes, as appropriate.

3. NURSING DIAGNOSIS/PROBLEM

Potential for barotrauma to ears, sinuses, teeth, and lungs, or cerebral gas embolism related to changes in atmospheric pressure inside hyperbaric oxygen chamber.

Desired Outcomes

Signs and symptoms of barotrauma will be recognized, addressed, and promptly reported.

Nursing Interventions

1. Administer decongestants, per physician orders, prior to hyperbaric oxygen therapy treatment.
2. Prior to treatment instruct the patient in ear equalization techniques, such as swallowing, chewing, yawning, modified Valsalva maneuver, or tilting head.
3. Assess the patient's performance of ear equalization techniques as chamber pressurization occurs.
4. Nursing interventions include:
   - Remind patient to breath normally during pressure changes,
   - Confirm ET/trach cuffs are filled with NS before pressurization, and
   - Notify multiplace chamber operator if the patient is unable to achieve pressure equalization.
5. Document assessments.
6. Continue to monitor the patient during hyperbaric oxygen therapy for signs and symptoms of barotrauma including:
   - Inability to equalize ears, or pain in ears and/or sinuses (especially after initial treatment, and after subsequent treatments),
   - Increases in rate and/or depth of respirations
   - Signs and symptoms of pneumothorax, including:
     - Sudden, sharp chest pain,
     - Difficult, rapid breathing,
     - Abnormal chest movements on the affected side, and
     - Tachycardia and/or anxiety.
7. Follow hyperbaric physician orders for patient management.

4. NURSING DIAGNOSIS/PROBLEM

Potential for oxygen toxicity related to delivery of 100% oxygen at an increased atmospheric pressure.

Desired Outcomes

Signs and symptoms of oxygen toxicity will be recognized and promptly addressed.

Nursing Intervention

1. Report patient assessment outcome to the hyperbaric physician of:
   - Elevated body temperature,
   - History of steroid use,
   - History of oxygen seizures,
   - High dose vitamin C or aspirin use,
   - $FiO_2 > 50\%$, and
   - Other high risk factors as appropriate.

2. Monitor patient during hyperbaric oxygen therapy and document signs and symptoms of central nervous system oxygen toxicity including:
    - Numbness and twitching,
    - Ringing in the ears or other auditory hallucinations,
    - Vertigo,
    - Blurred vision,
    - Restlessness and irritability, and
    - Nausea.

(NOTE: CNS oxygen toxicity can ultimately result in a seizure.)

3. Change 100% oxygen source to air for patient if signs and symptoms appear, and notify the hyperbaric physician.
4. Monitor the patient during hyperbaric oxygen therapy and document signs and symptoms of pulmonary oxygen toxicity, including:
    - Substernal irritation or burning,
    - Tightness in the chest,
    - Dry, hacking cough,
    - Difficulty inhaling a full breath, and
    - Dyspnea on exertion.
5. Notify the hyperbaric physician if signs and symptoms of pulmonary oxygen toxicity appear.

5. NURSING DIAGNOSIS/PROBLEM

Potential for inadequate therapeutic gas delivery related to delivery system and patient's needs/limitations.

Desired Outcomes

Signs and symptoms of inadequate oxygen delivery will be recognized and reported promptly. Assess the patient's condition, needs, and limitations for the best suited gas delivery system:

Nursing Intervention

1. Assess the patient's condition, needs, and limitations for the best-suited gas delivery system.
    - Head hood for children with facial deformities, or per patient preference,
    - Face mask,
    - "T" piece for patients who are intubated or have a tracheostomy, and
    - Ventilator for intubated patients who require ventilation assistance.
2. Monitor the patient's response to the oxygen delivery system, including their ability to tolerate chosen system.

3. Assist the hyperbaric technician with the delivery system, as appropriate.

   Head Hood

   a. Assist patient with application and removal of hood;
   b. After assembly, check for leaks; and
   c. Observe patient for signs and symptoms of CO_2 buildup, including restlessness.

   Face Mask

   a. Assist patient with mask application and removal, and reposition mask as needed; and
   b. Check for leaks and continuity of seal against the patient's face.

   T-Piece

   a. Setup process;
   b. Monitor patient's rate, depth of respirations, and listen to breath sounds;
   c. Notify the hyperbaric physician if patient is experiencing difficulty breathing; and
   d. Suction as needed.

   Ventilator

   a. Document management of ET cuff with NS prior to descent;
   b. Keep suction equipment nearby and ready for use (suction as needed);
   c. Monitor and document patient's tidal volume, respiratory rate, and breath sounds prior to chamber pressurization, after chamber pressurization, then every 30-60 minutes or as ordered;
   d. Monitor patient for respiratory distress, and notify hyperbaric physician if apparent;
   e. Manually oxygenate the patient if necessary (ambu bag);
   f. Monitor $TCPO_2$ levels and ABG PO_2 levels as ordered; and
   g. Notify hyperbaric physician of abnormal readings.

6. NURSING DIAGNOSIS/PROBLEM

Anxiety and fear related to feelings of confinement anxiety associated with hyperbaric oxygen chamber.

Desired Outcomes

Patient will tolerate the hyperbaric oxygen therapy treatment.

Nursing Interventions

1. Assess patient for any history of confinement anxiety, and relay relevant information to the hyperbaric physician.

2. Implement preventative measures as appropriate (i.e., education, chamber tour, medication).
3. During the hyperbaric oxygen therapy treatment, monitor and assess for signs and symptoms of confinement anxiety, including:
   - Restlessness,
   - Inability to tolerate face mask or head hood, and
   - Statements of feeling confined or trapped.
4. Address patient calmly.
5. Establish eye contact with the patient.
6. Reassure patient that he/she is safe.
7. Engage patient in problem-solving his/her feelings of confinement anxiety.
8. Administer anti-anxiety medications per hyperbaric physician's orders and assess effectiveness of medication.
9. Notify hyperbaric physician of patient's response to the anti-anxiety measures and ability to tolerate confinement.
10. Document results of intervention(s).

7. NURSING DIAGNOSIS/PROBLEM

Pain related to associated medical problems.

Desired Outcomes
Patient will state satisfaction with pain management.

Nursing Interventions
1. Assess patient's experience of pain and whether pain is increased during hyperbaric oxygen therapy.
2. Medicate patient for pain before hyperbaric oxygen therapy, as needed, and document efficacy of analgesic.
3. Have analgesic available during hyperbaric oxygen therapy treatment.
4. Reposition patient for comfort.
5. Avoid I.M. medications immediately prior to treatment.

8. NURSING DIAGNOSIS/PROBLEM

Discomfort related to temperature and humidity changes inside hyperbaric chamber.

Desired Outcomes
Patient will tolerate the internal climate of the chamber.

Nursing Interventions

1. Periodically assess patient's comfort with humidity and temperature.
2. Offer the patient comfort measures (i.e., a blanket, hot water bottle, or a cool cloth).

9. NURSING DIAGNOSIS/PROBLEM

Potential for ineffective individual coping related to stresses of illness and/or poor psychosocial support systems.

Desired Outcomes

Patient will be able to comply with hyperbaric oxygen therapy treatment procedures.

Nursing Interventions

1. Provide support and encouragement without exceeding treatment outcome expectations.
2. Discuss patient's ability to cope with other caregivers, and stay informed of progress and helpful approaches.
3. Facilitate communication between patient and/or family and other hyperbaric oxygen therapy staff members.
4. Encourage patient, if able, to discuss concerns and feelings.
5. Document pertinent discussions and assessments.

10. NURSING DIAGNOSIS/PROBLEM

Potential for dysrhythmia related to disease pathology.

Desired Outcomes

Signs and symptoms of dysrhythmia will be recognized and promptly addressed.

Nursing Interventions

1. As ordered, monitor EKG readings while patient is inside the chamber.
2. Monitor and document blood pressure as indicated.
3. Assess and document any signs of hypokalemia in patients with acute necrotizing infections.
4. Maintain I.V. infusions as ordered.
5. Maintain invasive pressure monitoring and record values as indicated.
6. Obtain lab samples as ordered.
7. Notify hyperbaric physician as needed.

11. NURSING DIAGNOSIS/PROBLEM

Potential for fluid volume deficit related to dehydration or fluid shifts.

Desired Outcomes

Signs and symptoms of fluid volume deficit will be recognized and promptly reported.

Nursing Interventions

1. Assess fluid and electrolyte balance and maintain hydration and/or pressure support as per physician order.
2. Monitor patient's I&O as indicated.
3. Monitor patient's vital signs as indicated.

12. NURSING DIAGNOSIS/PROBLEM

Altered cerebral tissue perfusion related to:

- ***Carbon monoxide poisoning***
- ***Decompression sickness***
- ***Acute necrotizing infection***
- ***Gas embolism***
- ***Other***

Desired Outcomes

Signs and symptoms of decreasing neurologic functioning will be recognized and reported promptly.

Nursing Interventions

1. Perform baseline neurological assessment prior to treatment.
2. Monitor and document neurological checks per established condition-specific protocol.
3. Compare ongoing neurological assessments with baseline assessment.
4. Assess and document patient's motor and sensory functioning.
5. Provide reorientation and emotional support as needed.
6. Provide neuro-psychometric testing as ordered.
7. Notify hyperbaric physician of significant changes as indicated.

13. NURSING DIAGNOSIS/PROBLEM

Potential for alteration in comfort, fluid, and electrolyte balance related to nausea and vomiting.

Desired Outcomes

Patient will experience decreased symptoms of nausea and vomiting.

Nursing Interventions

1. Assess and document patient's complaints of nausea.
2. Maintain airway integrity to prevent aspiration.
3. Notify hyperbaric physician of patient's nausea and administer medication as ordered.
4. Place NG tube if ordered.
5. Monitor and document amount of emesis on patient's Intake & Output (I&O) record.

14. NURSING DIAGNOSIS/PROBLEM

Altered health maintenance related to knowledge deficit for:

- ***Management of chronic wound***
- ***Restrictions following decompression sickness***
- ***Symptoms to report after carbon monoxide poisoning***

Desired Outcomes

Patient and/or family will state suggestions, restrictions, and symptoms to report following hyperbaric oxygen therapy.

Nursing Interventions

1. Assess for knowledge deficits related to underlying pathology.
2. Discuss with patient and/or family discharge instructions and needs. Include as appropriate:

Wound Healing

- Basic principles of wound healing and hyperbaric oxygen therapy's effects on healing.
- Effects of smoking on wound healing.
- How a diet adequate in protein, fluids, and vitamin C enhances wound healing.
- Consultation with multidisciplinary health care teams, as indicated.
- Instructions in wound care procedures and supplies.

Decompression Sickness

- Rest, avoid caffeine and alcohol, encourage fluids and adequate diet, avoid strenuous activity, and avoid hot bath or shower for 24 hours after completion of hyperbaric oxygen therapy.
- Contact the hyperbaric department or Divers Alert Network (DAN) if any symptoms return.
- Avoid altitude exposure for 72 hours or under-water diving per physician's recommendations.
- Reinforce importance of follow-up after discharge.

Carbon Monoxide Poisoning

- Instruct the patient and family to report symptoms of behavior changes, lethargy, persistent vomiting, persistent headache, increased memory loss, chest pain, tremor, ataxia, or decreased menstruation.
- Instruct the patient not to use the involved vehicle, furnace, or machinery until it is fully inspected and repaired by a professional serviceman.
- Reinforce importance of discharge follow-up.
- Provide patient and/or family with written discharge instructions.
- Document patient/family teaching and any return demonstrations required.

SOME EXAMPLES OF DOCUMENTATION FORMATS HYPERBARIC MEDICINE

In preparation for writing this textbook, the BNA sought examples of forms utilized in hyperbaric medicine. This is not an endorsement of any one form or sets of forms, but merely shows some types of documentation format and how the nursing process is being met with each. Each step of the nursing process will be identified with associated forms.

ASSESSMENT

A nurse's assessment of a patient begins when the patient is first encountered, and continues throughout the hospitalization as more information is obtained on the changes of condition. The initial nursing assessment can be noted in a number of ways, as described in the chapter Documentation. Most forms analyzed used a combination of closed- and open-ended styles rather than the narrative format. It is interesting to note that with the relatively limited number of professional nurses working in a relatively small field, there are a number of units associated with different hospitals and/or companies who use similar forms. This author's personal experience was that many forms were "borrowed" from other units when initial forms were established for a new unit. When contract companies entered the market, a group of units could be utilizing virtually the same forms.

This first example of assessment documentation is a good, thorough form, but lengthy at four pages. The assessment time period is a very labor- and time-consuming process, but we need to guard against forms that overly increase that labor and time. This "Wound Physical Assessment" may also lend itself to being a good information source for the physician to complete a history and physical, which is a JCAHO requirement.

The next example of documenting the assessment is a two-page form which not only allows documentation of the patient's medical history, but also previous wound care and screening of ears (for hyperbaric medicine). The most notable drawback is the limited area if the patient has more than one wound.

In keeping with JCAHO requirements, the initial assessment must be completed within the allotted time period (established by the facility), and must be signed off by a registered nurse. Check with your facility to ensure compliance.

WOUND PHYSICAL ASSESSMENT | Data Stamp

WOUND INFORMATION:

1. **Location of wound** ______
2. **How did it start?** Injury? [ ] Yes [ ] No ______
   Surgical incision or procedure? [ ] Yes [ ] No
   Appeared gradually over time? [ ] Yes [ ] No ______
3. **When did your wound start?** ______
4. **Has it ever completely healed?** [ ] Yes [ ] No ______
5. **Where have you been treated for your wound?** ______

PERSONAL HABITS:

1. **Tobacco use past:** [ ] Yes [ ] No Date stopped: ______ **Present:** [ ] Yes [ ] No Type: ______
   Amount: ______ Packs Per day for ______ Years
2. **Alcohol use past:** [ ] Yes [ ] No Date stopped: ______ **Present:** [ ] Yes [ ] No Type: ______
   Amount: ______ Drinks per week for ______ Years
3. **Caffeine use past:** [ ] Yes [ ] No Date stopped: ______ **Present:** [ ] Yes [ ] No Type: ______
   Amount: ______ Cups per week for ______ Years
4. **Describe your activities:**
   Able to walk without assistance: ______ Use crutches: ______ Use cane: ______
   Confined to bed or wheelchair: ______ Use brace: ______
5. **Who will help care for you?** ______

Social History:

Circle answer: **Married / Widowed / Single / Divorced** ______

Children [ ] Yes [ ] No If yes, number of children ______ **Do you live alone?** [ ] Yes [ ] No If no, who lives with you? ______

Do you have Home Health Care? [ ] Yes [ ] No If yes, Name of Home Health Agency ______

Telephone number: ______ Address: ______

Past Medical History:

		Month/Year	Describe
Diabetes Mellitus	☐ No ☐ Yes	______	______
Lung Disease	☐ No ☐ Yes	______	______
Heart Disease	☐ No ☐ Yes	______	______
Kidney Problems	☐ No ☐ Yes	______	______
Eye Problems	☐ No ☐ Yes	______	______
Hepatitis/Liver Problems	☐ No ☐ Yes	______	______
Rheumatoid Arthritis	☐ No ☐ Yes	______	______
Cancer	☐ No ☐ Yes	______	______
Chemotherapy	☐ No ☐ Yes	______	______
Radiation Therapy	☐ No ☐ Yes	______	______
Cataracts	☐ No ☐ Yes	If yes, ☐ Left ☐ Right ☐ Both	______
High Blood Pressure	☐ No ☐ Yes	______	______
Any other medical hx?	☐ No ☐ Yes	______	______

______

page 2

DIABETIC INFORMATION:

Do you monitor your glucose regularly? ☐ No ☐ Yes **If no**, would you be willing to have a nurse explain the importance? ☐ No ☐ Yes

It usually runs: Morning ________ Noon ________ Dinner ________ Bedtime ________ Monthly ________

Test blood ______________ times a day/week with: ________________________

Test urine ______________ times a day/week with: ________________________

Do you see an Opthalmologist for yearly eye exams? No Yes

Do you follow a routine diet plan? ☐ No ☐ Yes *(If no, consider a dietitian consult)*

Do you follow a routine exercise plan? ☐ No ☐ Yes *(If no, consider a diabetic nurse clinician consult)*

Would you be interested in learning more about your diabetes, treatment options, complication management, and prevention? ☐ No ☐ Yes

SURGICAL HISTORY:

Type of Surgery		Month/Year	Describe
Kidney Transplant	☐ No ☐ Yes	________	________
Amputation	☐ No ☐ Yes	________	________
Skin Grafts	☐ No ☐ Yes	________	________
Blood Vessel Surgery	☐ No ☐ Yes	________	________

Other Surgeries: ________________________

SYSTEM REVIEW

HEAD, EYES, EARS, NOSE, & THROAT:

			Description
Frequent Headaches	☐ No	☐ Yes	________
Blurred/Double Vision	☐ No	☐ Yes	________
Dizziness	☐ No	☐ Yes	________
Change in Hearing	☐ No	☐ Yes	________
Ringing in Ears	☐ No	☐ Yes	________
Sore Throat	☐ No	☐ Yes	________
Trouble Swallowing	☐ No	☐ Yes	________

NEUROLOGICAL:

Change in memory	☐ No	☐ Yes	________
Trouble with Balance	☐ No	☐ Yes	________
Change in Sensation	☐ No	☐ Yes	________

RESPIRATORY:

Frequent Colds	☐ No	☐ Yes	________
Difficulty Breathing	☐ No	☐ Yes	________
Cough / Dark Phlegm	☐ No	☐ Yes	________
Asthma/Hay Fever	☐ No	☐ Yes	________
Emphysema	☐ No	☐ Yes	________

CARDIOVASCULAR:

Chest Pain	☐ No	☐ Yes	________
Heart Irregular	☐ No	☐ Yes	________
High Blood Pressure	☐ No	☐ Yes	________
Use Oxygen at Home	☐ No	☐ Yes	________
Pacemaker	☐ No	☐ Yes	________
Swelling in Ankles	☐ No	☐ Yes	________

DIGESTIVE:

			Description
Heartburn	☐ No	☐ Yes	
Vomiting	☐ No	☐ Yes	
Constipation	☐ No	☐ Yes	
Diarrhea	☐ No	☐ Yes	
Black Stools	☐ No	☐ Yes	
Blood with Stools	☐ No	☐ Yes	

BLADDER/KIDNEY:

Frequent Urination	☐ No	☐ Yes	
Burning on Urination	☐ No	☐ Yes	
Blood in Urine	☐ No	☐ Yes	
Difficulty with Urination	☐ No	☐ Yes	

MUSCLES/BONES/JOINTS

Leg Pain - at Rest	☐ No	☐ Yes	
- with Walking	☐ No	☐ Yes	
Back Pain	☐ No	☐ Yes	
Joint Aching Pain	☐ No	☐ Yes	
Swelling of Joints	☐ No	☐ Yes	
Difficulty with Joint Motion	☐ No	☐ Yes	

SKIN:

Rash	☐ No	☐ Yes	
New Growths	☐ No	☐ Yes	
Color Change in Moles/Warts	☐ No	☐ Yes	

ALLERGIES TO MEDICATION NKDA YES, LIST BELOW

MEDICATION	REACTION

CURRENT MEDICATION	DOSE	PURPOSE

Completed by: ______________________ Date: __________

Reviewed with: ______________________ Date: __________

page 4

FAMILY HISTORY

Mother: Alive / Deceased ____________________

Father: Alive / Deceased ____________________

Siblings# _______ Alive ____ Deceased: ____ ____________________

PLAN OF CARE

INIT.	DATE	PLAN DESCRIPTION

Initial	Signature/Name printed	Initial	Signature/Name printed

CLIENT ASSESSMENT FORM
CF0002-093097

Name: ______________________, ____________________ ___ **Inpatient Rm #**_______
LAST FIRST MI

□M □**Outpatient** □ **Another Facility:**_______________________ **Rm #**_______

□F □**SNF:** ___________________ **Rm #**_______ □Trans. Co. □Ambulance □P.O.V.

DOB: ___/___/___ **TRANS.:** □Amb. □Crutches □Stretcher □W/C

Chief C/O: ____

Hx of Present Condition: ____________________________________

Patient Hx: (circle appropriate number) **Previous Pressure Exposure:** □HBO □Flying □Scuba

1.	Seizure Disorder	14.	Renal Problems	27.	Smoker (___/day)
2.	COPD	15.	Uncontrolled Fever	28.	ENT Problems:
3.	Respiratory Problems	16.	Optic Neuritis	28.a.	Sinus
4.	Pneumothorax	17.	Sperocytosis	28.b.	Mastoiditis
5.	Recent URI	18.	Diabetes - Type I (Ins. Dep.)	28.c.	Hemotypanium
6.	Thoracic Surgery	19.	Diabetes - Type II (Non Ins.)	28.d.	Otitis Media
7.	Pregnancy-LMP_____	20.	Cardiac Problems	29.	Intercurrent Infection
8.	Cataracts	21.	Thyroid Problems	30.	Claustrophobia (anxiety)
9.	Hypertension	22.	Radiation TX.	31.	Drug Use History
10.	Cancer	23.	ETOH Use	32.	Other:__________
11.	Blood Clot	24.	Bleeding Problem	33.	Allergies:__________
12.	PVD	25.	Osteoporosis		__________
13.	Contractures	26.	Stomach or Bowel Problems: __________		

Comments: ____

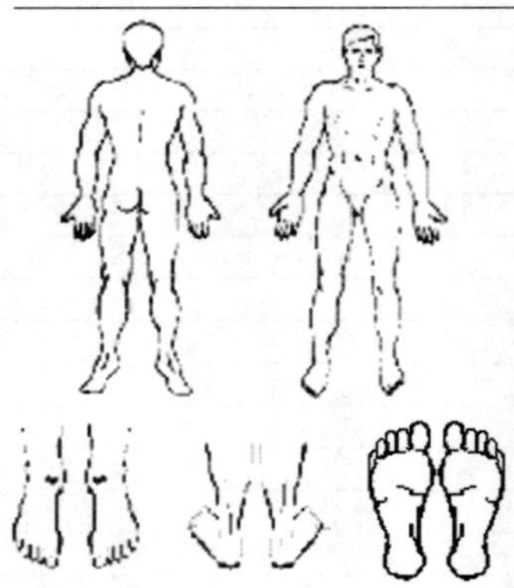

□ **PRESENT WOUND CARE** □**NO WOUND CARE**

Drainage		**Odor**	**Dressing Material**
□None	□Yellow	□Foul	□Alginate
□Small	□Green	□Musty	□Gauze
□Mod.	□Brown	□None	□Non-adherent
□Large	□Clear		□Dressing: ______
	□Purulent	□Serous	______
Other	□Serosanguinous		□N.S. Gauze
□Erythema			Gauze with other:
□Edema			______
□Other: ______			□Hydrocolloid Dsg.

Size: L _____ W _____ D _____

Stage: □0 □1 □2 □3 □4 □5 □Hydrogel Dsg.

(circle system: NPUAP / Wagner)

Comments:______________ □Compression TX:

□**Tympanometry** (□**WNL**, □**Not WNL**) ; **TM's =** □**T-0,** □**T-1,** □**T-2,** □**T-3,** □**T-4,** □**T-5**
Comments: ____

LOC: □**Alert,** □**Oriented,** □**Confused Easily,** □**Disoriented,** □**Sedated,** □**Other:**____________

LUNGS: □**Clear,** □**Wheezes,** □**Crackles,** □**Rhonchi,** □**Other:**____________

Current VS: T:_____**, P:**_____**, R:**_____**, BP:**_____ **Comments:**______________

History/Assessment (cont.)
Previous Tx. for same/similar condition? ___ Yes ___ No
If Yes, dates of RX ______________________
Past Surgeries: ____

Pulses: Rt. Post. Tibial _____ Lt. Post. Tibial _____ Rt. Dor. Ped._____ Lt. Dor. Ped._____

Nutrition Interview: Height_______ Current Weight________ Usual Weight_______
_____ Eats < than 2 meals/day _____ Eats fruit or drinks fruit juice < bid
_____ Eats < 2 servings of vegetables/day _____ Has chewing or swallowing problem
_____ Eats < 2 serving of dairy prod./day _____ Has chronic nausea and/or vomiting
_____ Eats < 6 servings of breads/day _____ Has chronic diarrhea or constipation
(bread, cereal, noodles, pasta, rice, etc.)

High Nutrition Risk: (consult dietician if any are checked)
_____ Significant unintentional weight loss (5% in 1 month, > 5% in 3 mon., or > 10% in 6 mon.)
_____ Infected or heavily draining wound _____ Chronic elevated glucose

Moderate Nutrition Risk: (consult dietician if any checked)
_____ I have had unintentional weight loss and 1 eating habit from Nutrition Interview
_____ I have 2 or more eating habits from Nutrition Interview

Home Care:
Do you currently have or have you used Home Health services? ____ Yes____ No

If yes, which agency? ______________________________
Do you have regular help at home? ____ Yes ____ No, Describe:______________
Do you have a bathroom on the main floor? ____ Yes ____ No.
Do you use any of the following? ___ walker ___ cane ___ wheelchair ___ lift

Education:
Do you have trouble with? ___ sight ___ hearing ___ learning ___ memory
How learns best: ___ talking to ___ demonstrating to ___ reading ___ videos
Circle last grade completed: 1 2 3 4 5 6 7 8 9 10 11 12 13 14 15 16
Others to be included in your teaching:
(name)________________________ (relationship)________ (phone)________
(name)________________________ (relationship)________ (phone)________

Diabetic Patients: (consult diabetic educator if any asterisk {**} item checked)
Do you take an oral agent for your diabetes? ___ Yes ___ No If Yes, then -
name: ____________________, dosage: __________, freq.: ________
Do you take insulin for your diabetes? ___ Yes ___ No If yes, then - type,
dosage, freq.:______________________________________
Do you do self-glucose monitoring? ___ Yes ___ No **
Your usual glucose range? __________, if > than 150 **
Do you have any questions you would like to discuss with a diabetic educator?
___ Yes ** ___ No

Referrals Made: (fill in date on referrals made)
Hyperbaric: ________________ Social Service: ________________
Dietary: ________________ Physical Therapy: ________________
Diab. Educ.: ________________ Orthotist: ________________
H.H. Agency ________________ Other: ________________

(signature) ______________________ Date ______ (signature) ______________________ Date ______

Nursing Diagnosis

According to the facility's policies and procedures, standardized diagnoses should be used or formulated by the nursing staff. The North American Nursing Diagnosis Association (NANDA) Taxonomy list of standard nursing diagnoses (see chapter on Documentation), is a good reference. Many facilities have incorporated this into their documentation processes. None of the forms submitted to the BNA had areas to note the nursing diagnoses. Although this does not mean it is not done, it may be an area that needs to be addressed.

One form that was submitted meets the JCAHO's requirement to have one location in the outpatient medical record, where the diagnoses, current medications, allergies, and significant invasive procedures are listed. This "summary list" is to be kept current at all times (each visit). The author's personal experience has shown this form to be useful for inpatients as well. A separate clinic or treatment area (such as a hyperbaric or wound clinic) is not always informed and kept abreast of the day-to-day, and sometimes hour-to-hour, changes in the care of inpatients. Taking the extra step to ensure that information is correct (especially medications) can save a mountain of problems down the road.

Since this form was only one sided, adding a nursing diagnosis list to the backside would easily solve the question. Another question encountered by the author is whether clinics and outpatient services must adhere to the same documentation requirements of inpatients? A clinic would not be responsible for the total documentation requirements of an inpatient that receives care within it. These are all questions and processes that must be addressed, and the facility standards adhered to.

Additional forms that may help determine the diagnoses or document them would include the documentation of transcutaneous oxygen measurements and photographs of wounds. With the advent of digital photography, it is now fairly common for digital photographs to be incorporated directly to the medical record. Where once Polaroid pictures or 35 mm slides were taken and either stored or married with the medical record, it is now very possible to print directly to the form which documented the care given.

CF0003-082896

HYPERBARIC MEDICINE – SUMMARY LIST

DATE ________ **NAME:** ______________________, ____________ __ ______________
LAST FIRST MI Patient Phone No.

REFERRED BY: ______________________ **PHONE NO.:** ______________

REASON: ____

Appointments		Physicians	A (on Admission) or Date Referred	IN.
APP. DATE: ______________	APP. KEPT ☐			
APP. DATE: ______________	APP. KEPT ☐			
COMMENTS: ______________				

KNOWN ADVERSE AND ALLERGIC DRUG REACTIONS: ______________

Indicate **A (on Admission)** or the **Date Started**; if **Medication**, then **Dose, Route,& D/C Date** (if D/C'd); **Initial ALL Entries; Sign and Inital Signature Block**

	DATE	MEDICATION	D/C	IN
1.				
2.				
3.				
4.				
5.				
6.				
7.				
8.				
9.				
10.				
11.				
12.				
13.				
14.				
15.				

	DATE	SIG. DIAGNOSES & CONDITIONS	IN
1.			
2.			
3.			
4.			
5.			
6.			
7.			

	DATE	SIG. OPERATIVE &/OR INVASIVE PR.	IN
1.			
2.			
3.			
4.			
5.			
6.			
7.			
8.			

IN	STAFF SIGNATURES

	DATE	SIG. NON-INVASIVE PROCEDURES	IN
1.			
2.			
3.			
4.			
5.			
6.			
7.			
8.			

Disposition of Patient: (Initial & Date Entry)

Transcutaneous Oxygen Notes

SITE	Electrode	Room Air	100% O_2 Challenge	MINUTES AT PRESSURE			
				ATA	ATA	ATA	ATA
#	Temp. (Cent.)	$TcPO_2$ mmHg	$TcPO_2$ mmHg	$TcPO_2$ mmHg	$TcPO_2$ mmHg	$TcPO_2$ mmHg	$TcPO_2$ mmHg

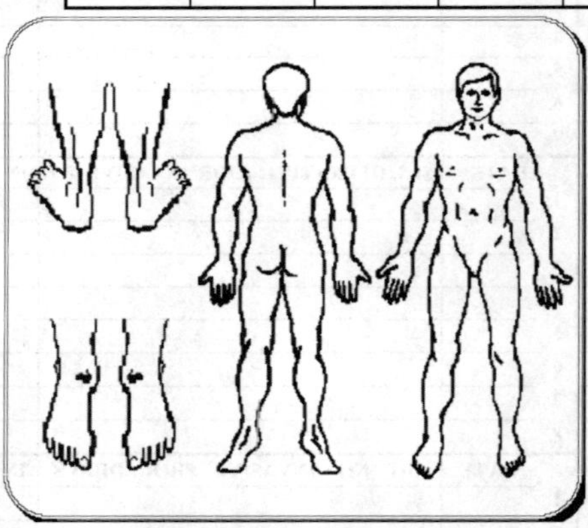

Diagram Electrode Placement

Scale		SITE #	SITE #	SITE #	SITE #
1.0-					
Excellent 0.9-	Room Air				
0.8 -	O_2 Chal.				
Good 0.7 -					
0.6 -	min.				
Fair 0.5 -					
0.4 -	min.				
Poor 0.3 -					
0.2 -	min.				
0.1 -	min.				

Regional Perfusion Index

Comments: ______________________________

______________ (Nurse/Tech) ______________ (Date/Time) ______________

Evaluation: ______________________________

____

____

______________ (Physician) ______________ (Date/Time)

Suggested Sites:
1. Medial and Lateral AKA, BKA, TMA sites
2. Medial and Lateral Supramalleolus

Other Sites:
1. Medical and Lateral Calcaneous
2. Periwound (i.e., proximal and distal)
3. Reference (2nd Intercostal Space)

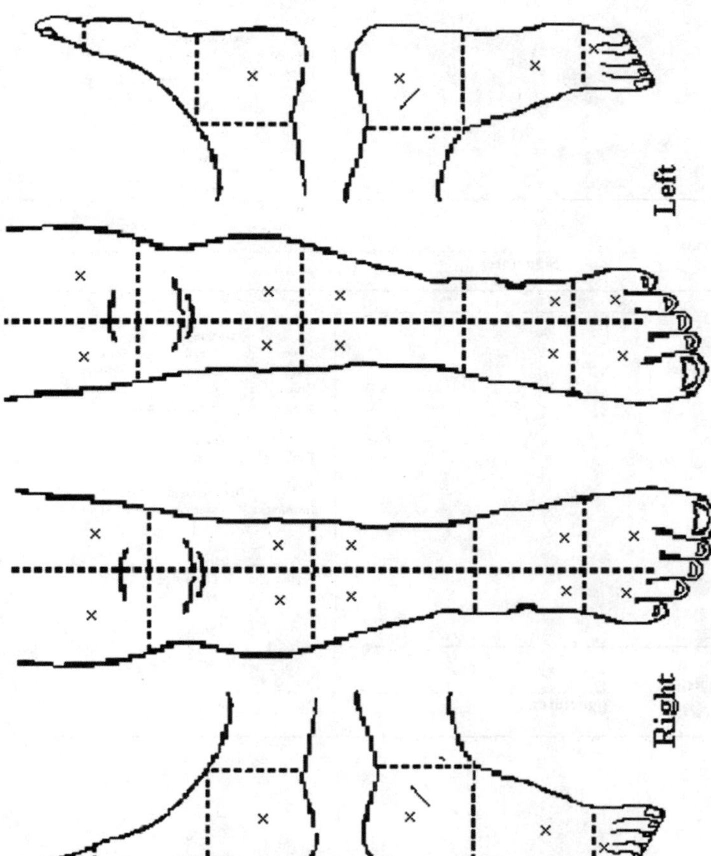

PHOTOGRAPHIC WOUND DOCUMENTATION

Drainage

None Small Mod.
Large Yellow Green
Brown Clear Purulent
Serous Serosanguinous

Odor

Foul Musty None

Debridement

Instrument Mechanical Autolytic
Enzymatic w/: ______________

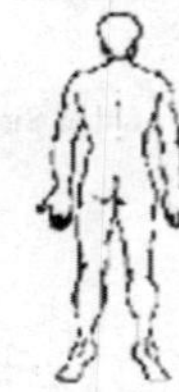

(Circle Wound Location)

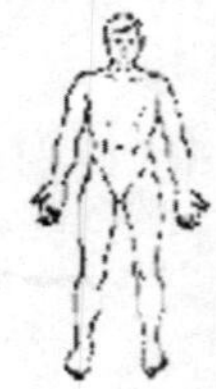

Other

Erythema Edema Other:

Size

L ________ W ________ D ________

Stage

0 1 2 3 4 5

(circle system: NPUAP/Wagner)

Comments: ______________________________

Signature: ______________________________

Drainage

None Small Mod.
Large Yellow Green
Brown Clear Purulent
Serous Serosanguinous

Odor

Foul Musty None

Debridement

Instrument Mechanical Autolytic
Enzymatic w/: ______________

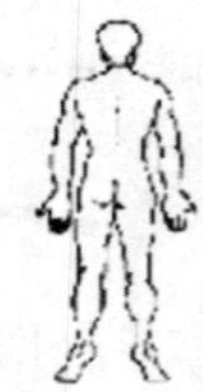

(Circle Wound Location)

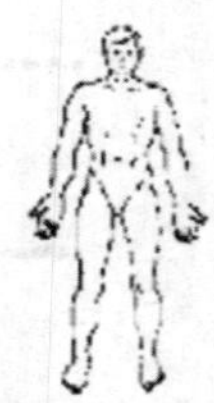

Other

Erythema Edema Other:

Size

L ________ W ________ D ________

Stage

0 1 2 3 4 5

(circle system: NPUAP/Wagner)

Comments: ______________________________

Signature: ______________________________

CF0005D-090496

Planning

There were no documentation forms submitted for this publication which contained planning. This author's experience has included utilizing Kardex forms for the plan of care. Whatever the form utilized within your facility, or whatever you are experienced with, the BNA's "Guidelines For: Standards of Care for the Patient Receiving Hyperbaric Oxygen Therapy" should be your reference source. There are also plenty of wound care reference sources on the market for wound care interventions.

Another method of ensuring reassessment and an ongoing process to maintain the patient plan of care, may include performing "team planning" (see chapter on Documentation). The Undersea and Hyperbaric Medical Society (UHMS) has recommended Utilization Review (UR) periods noted along with each approved diagnosis in their publication *Hyperbaric Oxygen Therapy: 1999 Committee Report.*

Personal experience (the author's) has been to perform UR within the recommended time of the UHMS and include the treatment team. This may include but is not limited to dietary, physical or occupational therapy, respiratory therapy, nursing service (if the hyperbaric department is separate), pharmacy, case managers, and the business office. Such "team planning" could prevent future problems and actually decrease the overall time of admission through multidisciplinary coordination of the plan of care. Areas that may need to be reviewed and updated are: current diagnosis, medications, additional diagnostic work (x-ray, lab, etc.), patient progression (wound size, decrease in infection, etc.), patient goals, patient and/or family education, nutrition, discharge planning, and the expected outcome.

Documentation of "team planning" may be as simple as adding a multidisciplinary progress note divided into subheadings for each area to be noted. Some of the information could be filled in ahead of time to decrease the overall time required of the "team" to review the patient and update the plan of care. Once complete, team members in attendance should be noted on the form, and appropriate orders entered into the medical record to make the plan of care complete.

Intervention

Documenting nursing interventions has long been the standard of practice (see chapter on Documentation). In hyperbaric medicine, treatment documentation has long been focused on reassessment, types of interventions, routine care, and changes in condition. Some examples of these include the documentation of the hyperbaric treatment and clinic visit for wound care.

The first example notes both HBO and wound care, but is limited in that it allows definitive space for only one wound. Additional wounds would need to be included on either additional forms in the narrative provided or in additional narrative space such as a multidisciplinary progress note.

The next form is similar to the first, in having both HBO and wound care documentation and being limited to space for only one wound. The notable portion of the form is the additional space for education and discharge planning. This is an ongoing JCAHO requirement and must be noted. When additional forms are needed to do this, omissions may occur. You may want to adapt your forms to something similar to these. Remember to incorporate as much closed- and open-ended styles of documentation to speed the process of noting interventions and findings.

When looking at a wound care only form, or a wound care portion of the combined treatment note, having definitive area to note more than one wound can be very helpful. The following form includes space for four separate wounds and utilizes mostly closed-ended style of documentation.

Patient education documentation can be combined with other forms (as previously noted) or noted on a separate form dedicated as such. One such example of a separate education is included as the next example.

HYPERBARIC MEDICINE - TREATMENT NOTES
CF0001-110197

TX#____ **Date:** ____ **ATA/Length:** ____/____ **NO HBO**
SNF/IP: Rm. #____ OP: Trans. Co. ____ Ambulance ____ P.O.V. ____

PRE ; POST (type)
T: ____ ; ____
P: ____ ; ____
R: ____ ; ____
BP:____( ) ; ____( )
(A=A-Line, N=NIBP, C=Cuff)

TRANS.
__Amb.
__Crutches
__Stretcher
__W/C

LOC
__Alert
__Oriented
__Easily Confused
__Disoriented
__Sedated

LUNGS
__Clear
__Wheezes
__Crackles
__Rhonchi
__Other ____

TM'S
T-0 T-3
T-1 T-4
T-2 T-5

PATIENT SAFETY / ED.
☐ Safety Restrictions
☐ Voided / Foley Drained
☐ IV Backcheck Valve
☐ IV Hep Lock

MONITORS
☐ EKG
☐ BP (__A, __N)
☐ IV Pump, #____
☐ Ventilator
☐ $TcPO_2$, #____

GLUCOSE
Last Meal @ ____
Pre: ____ @ ____
Pre: ____ @ ____
Pre: ____ @ ____
Post: ____ @ ____

☐ Pre Tx. Meds: ____
L.S.: ____ Rate: ____ R.B.: ____ L.B.: ____ Rate: ____ R.S.: ____
TX. BP's: ____( )@____; ____( )@____; ____( )@____ (A, N)

Tx. Admin. By: ____

☐WOUND CARE ☐NO WOUND CARE PERFORMED

Drainage
☐None ☐Yellow
☐Small ☐Green
☐Mod. ☐Brown
☐Large ☐Clear
☐Purulent
☐Serosanguinous

Odor
☐Foul
☐Musty
☐None
☐Serous

Debridement
☐Instrument
☐Mechanical
☐Autolytic
☐Enzymatic w/: ____

Dressing Material
☐Alginate
☐Gauze
☐Non-adherent Dressing: ____
☐N.S. Gauze
☐Gauze with other: ____
☐Hydrocolloid Dsg. ____
☐Hydrogel Dsg. ____
☐Compression TX: ____
☐ ____
☐ ____

Other
☐Erythema
☐Edema
☐Other: ____

☐Wound Cleansing with: ____

Size: L ____ W ____ D ____
Stage: ☐**0** ☐**1** ☐**2** ☐**3** ☐**4** ☐**5**
(circle system: NPUAP / Wagner)
Comments: ____

Wound Care Admin. By: ____

(Additional Clinician Comments)

PHYSICIAN PROGRESS NOTES: ☐ **Physician Present Throughout Treatment**

Page 1 of 2

Imprint Patient Information

HYPERBARIC OXYGEN TREATMENT NOTES

Outpatient **Inpatient** (room # ______) **Other:** ______________ **Date:** ______________

Mode of Arrival: Ambulatory Wheelchair Stretcher Walker Cane Crutches
Accompanied by: ______________
Condition on Arrival: Awake/Alert Oriented Confused Unresponsive
Vital Signs: BP: ______ HR/Pulse: _____ (Reg/ Irreg.) RR: ______ Temp: ______
Pretreatment blood glucose: ______ Repeat blood glucose: ______
Last Medication/Narcotic/Sedative: None or Time: ______ Medication: ______________
Interval History: *(check if normal, if not explain)*
Visual Change: ______________ SOB: ______________
Headache: ______________ Cough: ______________
Ear Pain: ______________ Chest Pain: ______________
Other: ______________
Safety Check: Discussed with patient/inspection complete Yes No **Patient ground checked:** Yes No

HBO_2 MD: ______________ **Chamber No.** ______ **Patient treatment number:** ______
Diagnosis: ______________ **Treatment table:** ______ ATA/100% O_2 for _____ min.
Other table: ______________
Treatment times: **Physician present for entire treatment**
Compression begun: ______ rate: ______ reached pressure: ______ Decent: ______ minutes
Decompression begun: ______ rate: ______ reached surface: ______ Ascent: ______ minutes
Therapist Notes: ______________

Total Time at Depth: ______________ minutes **Total Treatment Time:** ______________ minutes
Tolerance to treatment: Tolerated well, voiced no complaint See therapist notes

Wound: (location) ______________ Dressing change: Yes, *see back* No N/A
Appearance/Drainage ______________
Equipment in Use: None (or check all appropriate)
EKG Monitor/Interpretation: ______________ Arterial Pressure Line
NG/GT tube PE tubes (R) ____ (L) ____ $TcPO_2$ in Chamber
Foley Catheter Chest Tube (R) ____ (L) ____ Other drains (type): ______________
IV: Location: ______________ IV Solution: ______________ Rate: ______ ml/hr
INTAKE: PO ______ cc IV ______ cc Other ____/____ cc OUTPUT: ____/____ cc

Condition on Discharge: Awake/Alert Oriented Confused Unresponsive
Discharged to: Home Inpatient Nursing Home Ext. Care Fac. Admit to Hospital
Via: Ambulatory Stretcher Wheelchair Walker Private Auto Ambulance Taxi
Therapist Signature/Title: ______________

Physician Examination and Progress Notes
Ear exam: TMís clear PE tubes Other: ______________
Eye exam: WNL Other: ______________
Lungs: Clear Rales Rhonchi Wheezing Diminished Other: ______________
Intervention: ______________

Diagnosis: ______________
Plan: ______________

Physician signature: ______________

Continued on back

Page 2 of 2

Imprint Patient Information

HYPERBARIC OXYGEN TREATMENT NOTES

Progress Notes:

Education

Init.	Date	Describe Teaching	Patient Response/Understanding

Dressings

Init.	Date	Wound Description	Dressing Supplies

Discharge Planning

Init.	Date	Describe

Init.	Signature/Title	Init.	Signature/Title

Visit Date: ____________ patient identification

PATIENT CLINIC VISIT

1.Patient Arrived: Ambulatory Walker Crutches Cane Wheelchair Stretcher

Accompanied by: ______________________________

2.Vital Signs: ______________ T____ HR____ R____ B/P______ Blood Glucose _________

3.Any change in medication, blood transfusions, hospitalization, ancillary service since last visit? yes no NA

(If yes, indicate on patient summary and update form)

Visit # ______ Type of Visit: WCC visit Inpt visit HBO Other: ______________________

WOUND ASSESSMENT

Wd. Location				
Wd. #				
Wd. Width (mm)				
Wd. Length (mm)				
Wd. Depth (mm)				
Undermining (mm)				
Epithelialization	< 100% > 100%	< 100% > 100%	< 100% > 100%	< 100% > 100%
Debridement/Remodel	Yes No	Yes No	Yes No	Yes No
Compliance	Yes No			
Decrease Wound Size	Yes No	Yes No	Yes No	Yes No
Pain Control: NA 4% Lidocaine Local injection(1% / 2%) 2% Lidocaine gel Other:				
If wound Treatment complete, Outcome				
H = Healed **GH** = Graft Healed **S** = Surgical Closure **C** = Converted **GP** = Graft Partial **N** = Non-Healed **Q** = Quit **D** = Died **M** = Moved **K** = Consult **X** = Transferred **Amputations: BK** = Below Knee **AK** = Above Knee **TM** = Transmetatarsal **TR** = Toe/Ray				
Wound/Graft Appearance	Erythema Callous Necrotic Healing	Erythema Callous Necrotic Healing	Erythema Callous Necrotic Healing	Erythema Callous Necrotic Healing
Fibrin Amount	None Mild (1% - 25%) Moderate (26% - 75%) Marked (75% - 100%)	None Mild (1% - 25%) Moderate (26% - 75%) Marked (75% - 100%)	None Mild (1% - 25%) Moderate (26% - 75%) Marked (75% - 100%)	None Mild (1% - 25%) Moderate (26% - 75%) Marked (75% - 100%)
Granulation Tissue Color	Pale/Grey Pink Red None Covered w/Epithelium	Pale/Grey Pink Red None Covered w/Epithelium	Pale/Grey Pink Red None Covered w/Epithelium	Pale/Grey Pink Red None Covered w/Epithelium
Exposed Bone	Yes No	Yes No	Yes No	Yes No
Exp Tendon/Ligament	Yes No	Yes No	Yes No	Yes No
Eschar	Yes No	Yes No	Yes No	Yes No
Odor	Yes No	Yes No	Yes No	Yes No
Drainage amount	None Small Moderate Large	None Small Moderate Large	None Small Moderate Large	None Small Moderate Large
Drainage Color	Clear Serous Serosanguineous Green Yellow Purulent	Clear Serous Serosanguineous Green Yellow Purulent	Clear Serous Serosanguineous Green Yellow Purulent	Clear Serous Serosanguineous Green Yellow Purulent
Periwound Appearance	Maceration Intact Callous Necrotic Erythema	Maceration Intact Callous Necrotic Erythema	Maceration Intact Callous Necrotic Erythema	Maceration Intact Callous Necrotic Erythema
Temp. of Extremity	NA Hot Warm Cool Cold	NA Hot Warm Cool Cold	NA Hot Warm Cool Cold	NA Hot Warm Cool Cold
Skin Intergity	NA Varicosities Pigmentation Edema Dermatitis	NA Varicosities Pigmentation Edema Dermatitis	NA Varicosities Pigmentation Edema Dermatitis	NA Varicosities Pigmentation Edema Dermatitis
Pain (0 = No Pain)	0 1 2 3 4 5 6 7 8 9	0 1 2 3 4 5 6 7 8 9	0 1 2 3 4 5 6 7 8 9	0 1 2 3 4 5 6 7 8 9

patient identification

Progress Notes

Education/Discharge Planning

Dressings

Home Health

Orders Faxed	N/A	Yes	Telephoned:	N/A	Yes If yes, spoke with:

Compression Therapy

N/A Yes If yes, indicate Patient Summary/Update Form

Discharge

Stable	Ambulatory	Wheelchair	Stretcher	Other:
Home	Ext. Care Fac.	Sent to ER	Room (#)	
Admit to Hospital - Location:				
Referred to Primary MD		Other:		
Accompanied by:				
Left via:	Private Auto	Ambulance	Other:	

Signature/Title:	Date:
Signature/Title:	Date:

EDUCATION CHECKLIST

CF0014-110197

(All education is age and education level appropriate) **Teaching - Month/Day/Year** (Mark N/A for items not applicable)

Patient and/or Family Educated On:				
GENERAL - WOUND CARE				
I. Introduction: To staff and Philosophy				
II. Admission and Evaluation Process				
III. Hours of Operation				
IV. Reimbursement: Medicare, Medicaid, Other				
V. Safety and Infection Control				
VI. Nutrition Education: Dietician or staff				
VII. Diabetic Teaching: Diab. Educator or staff				
A. Diet				
B. Insulin Management				
C. Foot Care				
VIII. Chronic Wound Negative Host Factors				
XI. Wound Care Specific to Patient				
X. Compression wraps				
XI. Compression hose				
XII. Other:				
HYPERBARIC				
I. Purpose				
A. Therapy is in conjunction with other treatments.				
B. Increases O_2 levels in affected areas.				
C. Physicians will confer regularly.				
II. Dive Procedure				
A. Preparation of patient - 100% cotton clothing				
B. Safety Restrictions covered.				
C. Descent (pressure increasing within the chamber)				
1. Techniques in clearing (equalizing) ears				
2. Hot and Humid				
D. At Pressure				
1. Most treatments are 90 minutes O_2 at pressure.				
2. May have 5-10 minutes air-breathing during tx.				
E. O_2 is a medication (drug).				
F. Ascent (pressure decreases within the chamber)				
1. Decompression is over a 5-15 minute period.				
2. Inside temperature of the chamber is cooler.				
III. Clearing of Ears				
A. Autoinflation techniques				
B. Tympanometry				

EDUCATION CHECKLIST

CF0014-110197
Page 2

(All education is age and education level appropriate) **Teaching - Month/Day/Year** (Mark N/A for items not applicable)

Patient and/or Family Educated On:			
IV. Effects of Smoking on Healing			
A. Nicotine constricts blood vessels, decreases flow.			
B. Smoking decreases O_2 absorbed by lungs.			
C. Smoking should be stopped during HBO therapy.			
D. Can't stop: No Smoking 2 hr. pre- & 2-4 hrs. post-HBO.			
V. Side Effects of HBO			
A. Visual changes may exist up to 4 months post-HBO.			
B. Cataracts may mature sooner.			
C. Contraindicated in pregnancy unless CO involved.			
D. Barotrauma: ear, sinus, and/or tooth squeeze			
E. Claustrophobia - Confinement Anxiety			
VI. Tell Clinician if Having Cold Symptoms such as: sinusitis, stuffy			
VII. Visitors: Should wait in waiting room if appropriate.			
Clinician Initials: (Signatures and corresponding Initial at bottom)			

Initial	Signature	Initial	Signature
____	____________________	____	____________________
____	____________________	____	____________________

Additional Instruction and Acknowledgement of Teaching with Understanding

Date	

Last, but not the least of intervention, is discharge planning. Discharge planning is an ongoing process that should begin before the actual admission of the patient. Discharge planning can be noted in a number of ways, on a number of different types of forms. This may range from treatment or clinic notes, to education records and progress notes. When the patient is discharged from service or to another service, a single form is commonly used. This example is actually a two-part form. The patient or family member signs and retains one copy, and the original is placed in the medical record.

EVALUATION

The final step of the nursing process may not mean the end of the medical record. Evaluation of the plan of care should be an ongoing process so as to best meet the patient's needs. The previously noted "team planning" and UR would include evaluating the patient's progress up to that point. In addition to these notes, physicians may need to have specific notations regarding procedures or specific interventions such as debridement. Physician Progress Notes as noted previously (see chapter on Documentation) contain the physician's observations and patient progress. When more than one physician is involved with the care of the patient and not specifically included in UR or "team planning," these will be very helpful. One example of physician wound care documentation is noted in this form.

OTHER

We have looked at a number of different formats on how to document the nursing process and reviewed some specific examples. Although no one form is endorsed by the BNA, many of these examples are very useful and have already survived the scrutiny of JCAHO. The last form this author would like to leave you with is not a chart form, but a form for billing. Now that you have updated your forms to optimally document the nursing process for your unit and facility, make sure you are reimbursed for the work done. With all the recent changes from Medicare and the changes that will occur in the future, we as professionals need to stay abreast and ensure that complete documentation includes the billing process. This example is just one of many currently in use, but may generate ideas on how best to meet the needs of your unit and facility. (1, 2, 3, 4, 5, 6, 7, 8)

WOUND CARE AND HYPERBARIC DISCHARGE INSTRUCTORS

Patient Name:______________________________ Date:______________

Mode of Discharge: ☐Amb. ☐Cruches ☐Stretcher ☐W/C

With Whom:______________________________

To Where:______________________________

Restrictions ☐ None

- ☐ No lifting
- ☐ No smoking
- ☐ No weight bearing
- ☐ Elevate extremity
- ☐ Avoid sitting for long intervals
- ☐ As directed by physician
- ☐ Other:______________________

Notify physician (Dr.________________, Office #:______________) should anything of the following occur:

1. Temperature 101° F, or higher for 24 hours.
2. Drainage and or increase of previous drainage from incision or wound.
3. Incision or wound increases, or becomes red and/or swollen.
4. Pain not relieved by medication.

Special Wound Care Instructions given to:

- ☐ Patient
- ☐ Family Family Member Name:______________________
- ☐ Other Other Name:______________________
- ☐ Home Health Agency:______________ Phone #:____________
- ☐ See Attached:______________________

Follow-up:

- ☐ Please return to Department on ______ for follow-up evaluation and photos
- ☐ Contact Department at ____-____-____ or your physician for any questions you may have.
- ☐ Instructions given for the follow-up care of Pressure Equalizing Tubes
  ☐ Yes (see attachment) ☐ No ☐ N/A
- ☐ Review possible visual changes due to prolonged HBO treatments as discussed under consent for HBO.
- ☐ ______________________________

I understand and have received a copy of the above instructions that have been reviewed by the clinician. I have also been encouraged to follow-up with my primary physician.

______________________________ Signature of patient/responsible person

______________________________ Signature of Discharge Nurse

CF0D8-093097 White Copy - Chart Yellow Copy - Patient

PATIENT INFORMATIN

WOUND CARE PHYSICIAN PROGRESS NOTES

DATE:

PATIENT NAME:

Subjective/Objective:

WOUND CARE/DEBRIDEMENT

						Refer. MD contacted?
Debridement	No	Yes, with	scalpel	curette	other	Phone
Wound Care	No	Yes				Letter
Culture/Biopsy	No	Yes				N/A
Other:	No	Yes				

Level of Debridement

Skin, Partial Thickness	Skin, Subcutaneous & Muscle
Skin, Full Thickness	Skin, Subcutaneous, Muscle &Bone
Skin & Subcutaneous Tissue	Other:

Procedure Notes and Plan:

Instructions:

Next visit:

Physician signature:	Date:	Time:

COMPREHENSIVE WOUND HEALING CENTER

Date:____________________________

WOUND CARE DIAGNOSIS CODES (Mark #1 for primary, #2 for Secondary, etc.)
Diagnosis submitted must be substantiated by documentation in medical record

CELLULITIS	
__Foot/Heel (Not Toe)	682.7
__Arm/Shoulder(Not Finger)	682.3
__Leg/Ankle/Back/Hip/Knee/Thigh	682.6
__Buttock	682.5
__Groin/Trunk/Back	682.2
__Toe	681.10
__Head (Not Face)	682.2
__Neck	682.1
__Gangrenous	785.4
__Other Wound Site	____

DIABETES	
__Diabetes, no complication	250.00
__Diabetes, with renal manif.	250.4_
__Diabetes,w/opthamalic manif	250.5_
__Diabetes w/neuropathy	250.6_
__Diabetes w/peripheral disease	250.7_
__Diabetes w/other specif. manif.	250.9_
__Diabetes w/unspecif complic.	250.9_
5th digit required for above codes....	
0 = NIDDM, not stated as controlled	
1 = IDDM, not stated as controlled	
2 = NIDDM = Uncontrolled	
3 = IDDM, Uncontrolled	

OSTEOMYELITIS,REFRACTORY	
__Chronic	730.10
.00 site unspecified	.11 shoulder
.12 upper arm	.13 forearm
.14 hand	.15 pelvic/thigh
.16 lower leg	.17 ankle/foot
.18 other specified sites	.19 multiple sites

OTHER DIAGNOSIS	
__Deformity of toe (Hammer)	735.4
__Dehiscence-Op wound	998.3
__Dermatosclerosis/Sclerdoerma	710.1
__Edema	782.3
__Graft Failure (Prep for graft)	996.52
__Granuloma	686.1
__Meleney s Ulcer	686.09
__Non-Healing Surgical Wound	998.83
__Onychia and Paronycia of Toe	681.11
__Psoriasis	696.1
__Pyoderma Gangrenosa	686.01

ULCERS	
__ Pressure Ulcer/Decubitis	707.0
__Ankle	707.13
__Chest/Face/Groin/Hand/Hip/Neck	707.8
__Skin	707.9
__Calf	707.12
__Foot	707.15
__Heel	707.14
__Knee	707.19
__Lower Extremity w/gangrene	707.10
__Lower Extremity	707.1
__Thigh	707.11
__Toes	707.15

PHYSICIANS SERVICES

OFFICE OUT PATIENT - NEW GW 93.57	
Intermediate	99203____
Extended	99204____
Complex	99205____

ESTABLISHED PATIENT GW 93.57	
Brief	99211____
Limited	99212____
Extended	99213____
Complex	99214____

DEBRIDEMENT GW-86.28/86.22 (DR. D)	
Skin Partial Thickness	11040____
Skin Full Thickness	11041____
Skin-Subcutaneous Tissue	11042____

OTHER SERVICES GW - 93.95	
Hyperbaric Oxygen Treatment	99183____
Transcutaneous Oxygen Single	93922____
Transcutaneous Oxygen Multi	93923____

SECONDARY DIAGNOSIS:

____

OTHER NOTES:

____

____

UNDERLYING CONDITIONS			
__Paraplegia	344.01	__Hidrandentis	705.83
__Neuropathy	355.9	__Venous Statis Ulcer	459.81
__Neuropathy, Lower Limb	355.8	__Peri-stomal Gastrojejunal Ulcer	534.90
__Peripheral Vascular Disease	443.9	__Peri-stomal Gastrojejunal Ulcer	569.61
__Chronic Lymphadema	457.1	__Peri-stomal Urostomy Ulcer	997.5
		__Peri-stomal Ileostomy Ulcer	569.61

REFERENCES

1. Cwiklinski, J.M., Messina, V.J., Norkool, D.M., and Weyenberg, G.T. (1999). Hyperbaric nursing. In E. Kindwall and H.T. Whelan (Ed.), Hyperbaric Medicine Practice (2nd ed., pp. 377-394). Flagstaff, AZ: Best Publishing Company.
2. Joint Commission on Accreditation of Healthcare Organizations (November 4, 2000). Section I, Patient-focused functions, Comprehensive accreditation manual for hospitals: The official handbook, Oakbrook Terrace, IL; Author.
3. Joint Commission on Accreditation of Healthcare Organizations (November 4, 2000). Section II, Organization-focused functions, Comprehensive accreditation manual for hospitals: The official handbook, Oakbrook Terrace, IL; Author.
4. Joint Commission on Accreditation of Healthcare Organizations (November 4, 2000). Section III, Structures with functions, Comprehensive accreditation manual for hospitals: The official handbook, Oakbrook Terrace, IL; Author.
5. Norkool, D. (1992). Care of the patient receiving hyperbaric oxygen therapy (HBO). In A. Reiner (Ed.), Manual of patient care standards. Gaithersburg, MD: Aspen Publishers, Inc.
6. Springhouse Corporation (1999). Documentation of the nursing process. In, Mastering documentation (2nd ed., pp. 207-264). Springhouse, PA; Author.
7. Springhouse Corporation (1999). Documentation Systems. In, Mastering docmentation (2nd ed., pp. 61-102). Springhouse, PA; Author.
8. Undersea and Hyperbaric Medical Society (1999). Hyperbaric oxygen therapy: 1999 committee report. Kensington, MD: Author.

NOTES

CHAPTER I

CARE OF THE PATIENT RECEIVING HYPERBARIC OXYGEN THERAPY

W. McHOWELL

INTRODUCTION

When it comes to treating the diverse nature of patients in the hyperbaric environment, nurses are uniquely qualified to deal with the technology of hyperbaric medicine as well as the physiological and psychological support of the patient. Because patients seen in the hyperbaric unit are from various backgrounds, levels of acuity, and diagnosis, the hyperbaric nurse needs to be experienced in all areas of nursing.

Although there are many healthcare professionals involved in the care of patients in the hyperbaric unit, the skills of nurses are essential to evaluate patients before treatment, during the treatment, and after the treatment. In addition, nurses working in the hyperbaric field also have considerable expertise in dealing with problems involving healing wounds and wound care.

MEDICATIONS

One of the factors a nurse has to consider before treating a patient in the hyperbaric environment is the interaction between hyperbaric oxygen and the patient's medications, both prescription and over-the-counter (OTC). Most medications can be given without complications, but there are some that are contraindicated in the HBO environment and others that require additional monitoring.

The medications considered as absolute contraindications are Doxorubicin (Adriamycin), Bleomycin, Disulfiram (Antabuse), Cis-Platinum, and Mafenide Acetate (Sulfamylon). Any patient taking these medications or having a history of taking these medications needs to be evaluated for potential complications.

Chemotherapeutic agents such as Adriamycin, Bleomycin, and Cis-Platinum are affected by oxygen at pressure in a variety of ways. Adriamycin is thought to become cardiotoxic when treated in HBO, but since it is inactivated and cleared by the system in 24-48 hours it should be safe to treat patients after halting the medication for 2-3 days. HBO has been used to treat tissue damage secondary to Adriamycin extravasation when use has been discontinued.

Bleomycin is an antibiotic used in treating a variety of tumors and lymphomas. Studies have shown that increases of oxygen concentrations to 32% years following Bleomycin therapy can result in severe interstitial pneumonitis and death, and pulmonary toxicity is one of the dose limiting factors.

Cis-Platinum is used in the treatment of a number of types of cancers. It interferes with DNA synthesis that also delays fibroblast production and collagen synthesis. Exposure to HBO appears to exacerbate the cytotoxic effect on the tissue and impede wound healing. In emergency situations (i.e., CO poisoning, necrotizing fasciitis, decompression sickness, etc.) the benefits outweigh the risks of treating the patient.

Antabuse was initially considered a medication that would block both central and pulmonary oxygen toxicity. It was later found that it blocks the production of superoxide dismutase (SOD), which is the body's natural protection against oxygen toxicity. In emergency situations such as carbon monoxide poisoning where there would be a single treatment, the patient should not have problems. The contraindication is in patients that would receive multiple treatments in the HBO environment.

Sulfamylon is a topical antibacterial used extensively in thwarting bacterial infections in burn wounds. It is a carbonic anhydrase inhibitor that causes peripheral vasodilation, and when combined with the central vasoconstriction produced by HBO therapy, causes a negative complication. If a burn patient is to be treated in the HBO chamber, Sulfamylon can be replaced by silvadene (silver sulfadiazene).

The most appropriate routes of medication administration for patients undergoing HBO therapy are oral and intravenous. Due to the vasconstrictive effects, the normal absorption of medications is delayed when administered intramuscularly and subcutaneously.

The two major effects of hyperbaric oxygen on cardiac function are bradycardia and a decrease in conduction velocity. These elements affect a wide variety of cardiac pharmacologic agents, including antiarrythmics. Due to the potential for bradycardia and arrythmias associated with exposure to HBO therapy, any patient taking cardiac medications or having a history of cardiac problems should be monitored during treatments.

In addition, a patient taking medications containing digitalis glycosides should be observed closely for toxicity if the patient complains of fatigue, muscle weakness, depression, diaphoresis, headache, facial neuralgias, dizziness, hypotension, visual disturbances, anorexia, nausea, vomiting, or diarrhea. Since patients with cardiac histories are EKG-monitored, the patient should be monitored for a change in rate (less than 60/minute), rhythm, and developing arrythmias.

Since quite a few of the patients being treated in the chamber are diabetics, dealing with insulin dosages and blood sugar levels is a concern. Treatment in the HBO environment for the insulin-dependent diabetic can cause a hypoglycemic effect and in some cases hypoglycemic seizures. It is assumed that this effect is due to the inhibition of the anti-insulin hormones (somatotropic hormone and glucagon) in the HBO environment. In addition to requiring a blood sugar of at least 120 before treatment, all diabetics should eat and possibly, if indicated, hold their insulin until after the treatment. If the blood sugars continue to be too low, consideration should be taken to adjusting insulin dosages during treatment. This phenomenon is not seen in patients on oral hypoglycemics.

Anticonvulsants are medications used to prevent seizures, but have no protective influence against oxygen toxicity. If a patient has a known seizure history and is on anticonvulsants, drug levels need to be drawn to ascertain that the patient has therapeutic drug levels. In addition, patients need to be observed closely for symptoms of oxygen toxicity during their treatments as the warning signs of pre-seizure activity might not be present.

Central Nervous System stimulants, such as amphetamines, caffeine, etc., interact unfavorably in the HBO environment. It is thought that the patient is predisposed to oxygen toxicity due to the increased metabolic activity. This is also the reason that thyroid replacements act in a similar fashion by increasing the metabolic rate.

Acetazolamide is a carbonic anhydrase inhibitor that increases blood flow by preventing the oxygen-induced vasoconstriction caused by hyperbarics. This predisposes patients to potential oxygen toxicity and should not be used in patients being treated deeper than 2 ATA. In addition, glaucoma eye drops are carbonic anhydrase inhibitors and should be taken into consideration when evaluating a patient's medical history.

Narcotic analgesics are sometimes required when patients in moderate to severe pain are being treated in the chamber. Unfortunately, narcotic drugs generally depress respiration and enhance oxygen toxicity. Reducing the reactivity of medullary centers to CO_2, combined with the depressing effects of HBO on respiration, can lead to a rise in $paCO_2$, which causes the vasodilation and enhances oxygen toxicity. This is the reason that narcotic analgesics should be given in the smallest effective dose for the patient.

Nicorette, nicoderm, and similar prescription medications are alternate sources for the dependent smoker who is withdrawing from smoking. While this is a good idea for the hyperbaric patient as well as patient attempting to heal wounds, consideration must be taken in treating the patient taking nicotine replacements. The first problem is that nicotine causes peripheral vasoconstriction that can potentiate the peripheral vascular vasoconstriction associated with HBO therapy. In some cases a Raynaud's syndrome-type reaction can be noted in the patient upon completion of a treatment.

The second problem deals with another side effect associated with the medication. Nicotine is known to be one of the most toxic of all poisons. Therefore, replacement medications should be used with care. Rapidly chewing multiple pieces of gum or using multiple patches can cause acute nicotine overdose with symptoms of nausea, vomiting, arrhythmias, tachycardia, sialorrhea, headache, dizziness, hypertension, hypotension, seizures, and possible death. It is suggested that patients remove patches or do not take nicotine replacements two hours prior to scheduled treatments.

Steroids have been shown to increase the risk of oxygen toxicity seizures. In addition, steroids increase the healing time of wounds, and since quite a few hyperbaric patients have wounds this is important. If at all possible, find out if decreasing the dosage is an option for the patient.

There is no human data indicating that infusion of lipids during HBO potentiates oxygen toxicity, but animal data suggests that this is a possibility. It is suggested that the lipids infusion be given four hours before HBO treatments.

PHYSICAL ASSESSMENT

The patient needs to have an extensive physical exam that covers all areas affected by exposure to hyperbaric oxygen. Additionally, there are certain specific evaluations needed for certain indications being treated. After developing baseline data, these evaluations are used to evaluate the efficiency of the treatment schedule.

Ear Exam

Physical examination of the ear includes inspection of the auricle, the ear canal, and tympanic membrane. Before using the otoscope, examine the auricle and external canal for signs of deformities, skin lesions, inflammation, swelling, tenderness, crepitation, or malalignment.

After inspecting and palpating the auricles and surrounding tissues, the inner canal and tympanic membrane are visualized using the otoscope.

Using the largest ear speculum that the patient's ear will comfortably accommodate, position the patient's head so you can visualize through the instrument. The ear canal can be straightened by grasping the auricle and pulling gently to the rear with an upward movement slightly away from the head. Hold the otoscope handle with your thumb and fingers, and brace your hand against the patient's face to allow you to follow any movements made during the exam. While inserting the speculum, observe the ear canal for excessive hair, cerumen, redness, or any obstructions of the canal.

The occlusion of the auditory canal with cerumen prevents the visualization of the tympanic membrane and may affect the ability to equalize. Irrigating the canal with a mixture of water and hydrogen peroxide at body temperature will remove the occlusion a majority of the time. In patients with perforation of tympanic membrane or otitis media, irrigation is contraindicated. (See Table I)

TABLE I—EAR IRRIGATION	
1	Collect all equipment: basin, syringe (bulb syringe, rubber bulb syringe, pomeroy syringe), otoscope, towel.
2	Explain procedure to patient.
3	Hold the emesis basin close to his/her head under the affected ear.
4	Clean the auricle and meatus of the auditory canal prior to starting irrigation to prevent introduction of dirt into the canal.
5	Warm irrigating fluid to body temperature.
6	To aid irrigation straighten the auditory canal by pulling upward and backward, straightening out the canal.
7	Place the tip of the irrigating syringe at the opening of the canal, making sure that the the opening isn't occluded and preventing the fluid from running out of the ear.
8	Gently irrigate, directing the flow upward and toward the posterior of the ear canal wall. This allows the cerumen to flow out of the ear and protects the tympanic membrane.
9	Observe the patient for signs of dizziness, pain, nausea, or panic.
10	Maximum of 500 cc's should be used in irrigation.

If the irrigation does not remove the cerumen obstruction it may be necessary to loosen the impaction with medications (cerumenex, debrox, colace, mineral oil) or manually. A small curette or cerumen spoon can be used to scoop out the wax, but should be limited to healthcare professionals with skill doing the procedure due to potential damage to the tympanic membrane.

Barotrauma of the ear is the most common complication of hyperbaric therapy. A classification scale of severity in barotrauma was developed using the appearance of the tympanic membrane by Wallace Teed, M.D. (See Table II)

TABLE II—TEED SCALE	
Teed 1	Erythema or injection around the handle of the malleus.
Teed 2	Erythema or injection of the entire tympanic membrane.
Teed 3	Hemorrhage into the tympanic membrane appearing as bright red patches.
Teed 4	Deep blue/black appearance of the tympanic membrane due to blood filling the middle ear with the possibility of rupture present.

CARDIOPULMONARY

Before the initiation of HBOT, all patients are required to undergo a chest x-ray (CXR) to evaluate pulmonary and cardiac disorders. The posterioanterior and right lateral CXR views are used to detect pulmonary disorders, mediastinal abnormalities, and cardiac disease as well as the presence of pneumonia, atelectasis, pneumothorax, cysts, pleural effusion, fibrosis, silicosis, neoplasms, cor pulmonale, and congestive heart disease. These are all relative contraindications to HBOT and should be further evaluated.

Although not a requirement for therapy, an electrocardiographic (EKG) workup should be performed on any critical care patients, patients with a cardiac history, or patients over 50 years old. In addition to giving hyperbaric staff a baseline view of cardiac status, it helps identify primary conduction abnormalities and determines the need for further diagnostic testing. All patients should be monitored for their first treatment in the chamber, and patients with abnormal EKG results, a history of cardiac disease, or an idiosyncratic response to oxygen at pressure should be monitored during all treatments in the chamber.

In patients who have a history of congestive heart failure (CHF) or have suggestive findings on the CXR or EKG, an echocardiogram is indicated. By evaluating the injection fractions, patients who could potentially develop CHF in response to hyperbaric oxygen are detected. This allows the staff to determine the benefits-to-risk ratio and prepare the patient for therapy with an appropriate medication regimen.

Patients expected to undergo a lengthy treatment regimen should have baseline pulmonary function tests (PFT) done before starting therapy. Repeating treatments at intervals that are inadequate to allow total recovery from the alveolar and interstitial edema, alveolar hemorrhages, and collagen exudates can cause fibrosis and emphysema. The PFT measures Lung Volumes and Lung Capacity. Decreased flows may indicate an obstructive lung disease and decreased volumes indicate a restrictive disease state.

WOUNDS

A baseline assessment of wounds is important when evaluating the healing progress of the wound and the treatment guidelines. The wounds can be classified by color, depth of wound, or by using an ulceration scale (see Table III). The description should include the anatomic location (extremity, bony prominence, or other landmarks); size (length/width/depth); presence of undermining, tunneling, or rimming of wound bed; appearance of the wound bed and surrounding tissue (Table III); drainage (Table IV); presence of foreign objects (sutures, staples, or environmental debris); pain; temperature; and etiology.

The wound should be measured in centimeters at the start of care and then on a weekly basis. Use the head and foot of the patient as a point of reference for measuring length, and measure width hip to hip or 90 degrees to length to allow for continuity of care.

Table III—WOUND CLASSIFICATION

Color	Description
Red	Indicates clean, healthy granulation tissue.
Yellow	Exudate/Slough The presence of an exudate or slough produced by microorganisms and a requirement for cleaning or debridement. The exudate can be whitish yellow to beige in color.
Black	Eschar Indication of necrotic tissue which will slow rate of healing and provide a site for microorganisms to proliferate.
Thickness:	Full Thickness Partial Thickness

TABLE III—WOUND CLASSIFICATION (continued) ULCERATION STAGING SYSTEM	
Stage 1	Non-blanchable erythema of intact skin, with possible discoloration, warmth, or firmness as indicators. These are indications of potential skin ulceration.
Stage 2	Partial thickness skin loss involving the epidermis or dermis. The ulcer is superficial and presents clinically as an abrasion, blister, or shallow crater.
Stage 3	Full thickness skin loss involving damage or necrosis of subcutaneous tissue, which may extend down to, but not through, the underlying fascia. The ulcer presents clinically as a deep crater with or without the undermining of adjacent tissue.
Stage 4	Full thickness skin loss with extensive destruction, tissue necrosis, or damage to muscle, bone, or support structures (for example tendon, ligaments, or joint structures). Tunneling and sinus tracts may also be associated with stage 4 pressure ulcers.

TABLE IV—DRAINAGE DESCRIPTION		
Type	**Description**	
Serous	Clear, watery plasma	
Sanguinous	Bloody/fresh bleeding	
Serosanguinous	Plasma and red blood cells	
Purulent/Pus	Thick, white blood cells and living or dead organisms; yellow, green, or brown; color can suggest the type of infecting organism	
Amount	Absent (dry) Moderate	Minimal Copious
Odor	Absent	Present

TABLE V—DESCRIPTION OF WOUND AND SKIN SURROUNDING		
Surrounding Skin	Erythema	Induration
	Maceration	Denuded
	Excoriated	Ecchymotic
	Edematous	
Wound Edges	Attached	Epithelial Ridge
	Not Attached	Rolled Under

DISTINGUISHING BETWEEN ARTERIAL/VENOUS/DIABETIC ULCERS

ARTERIAL ULCERS

Predisposing Factors- peripheral vascular disease, diabetes, advanced age.

Anatomic Location- between or tips of toes, over phalangeal heads, around lateral malleolus, sites suspected of rubbing of footwear and trauma.

Other Signs & Symptoms- thick, shiny, dry skin, hair loss on ankle and foot, thickened toenails, pallor upon elevation and dependent rubor, cyanosis, decreased temperature, absent or diminished pulses.

VENOUS ULCERS

Predisposing Factors-	valve incompetence in perforating veins, history of deep vein thrombosis (DVT), previous history of ulcers, obesity, advanced age.
Anatomic Location-	on medial lower leg and ankle, on malleolar area.
Other Signs & Symptoms-	firm edema, dilated superficial veins, dry, thin skin, evidence of healed ulcers, periwound and leg hyperpigmentation, possible dermatitis.

DIABETIC ULCERS

Predisposing Factors-	diabetic patient with peripheral neuropath.
Anatomic Location-	on plantar aspect of foot, over metatarsal heads, under heel.
Other Signs & Symptoms-	diminished or absent sensation in foot, foot deformities, palpable pulses, warm foot, subcutaneous fat atrophy, similar assessment to arterial ulcers if the patient has vascular disease.

Wounds being treated should be photographed to establish a base-line evaluation, monitor progress, support the efficacy of reimbursement considerations, assist in medical/legal ramifications, employ in medical education, and provide follow-up for the referring physician. Signed consent is required from the patient/family prior to photographing the wound. Information can be included in the photograph by using a ruler (to establish size of wound) with date and code which identify the patient. Color slide film has been the established standard, but the development of digital photography has made wound photography easier to use and store.

The neurological exam is important in dealing with patients being treated with arterial gas embolism, decompression sickness, and other indications that have a nervous system component. The areas that need to be checked are orientation, memory, level of consciousness, cranial nerves, motor nerves, sensory nerves, coordination, reflexes, or any language problems (Table VI).

TABLE VI—NEUROLOGICAL EXAM	
Orientation	Time Place Person Purpose
Memory	**Immediate**-Test with number series **Recent**-Within last 24 hours **Remote**-Background
Mentation	Test by trail of sevens, subtract 7 from 100, 7 from 93, etc.
Level of Consciousness	Watch for fluctuation
Cranial Nerves	**Olfactory Nerve**-Sense of smell **Optic Nerve**-Sight **Oculomotor/Trochlear/Abducens**- Eye movement, follow finger with eyes (up/down/left/right) **Trigeminal Nerve**-Chewing, can they clench teeth **Facial Nerves**-Mouth, can they smile, do both sides of the lips move **Acoustic Nerves**-Hearing, test one ear at a time **Glossopharyngeal/Vegas Nerves**-Talking, check for gagging and proper enunciation **Spinal Accessory Nerves**-Shoulder muscles, have patient shrug shoulder while you press down on them **Hypoglossal Nerve**-Tongue, can the patient stick out their tongue (not side to side)

TABLE VI—NEUROLOGICAL EXAM (continued)	
Sensory Nerves	Use sharp or dull objects to see if can distinguish between them Test: Back of hand Base of thumb Base of little finger Base of great toe Bottom of feet
Motor Nerves	Muscle strength Range of Motion Muscle Tone-Spastic or flaccid
Coordination	**(Cerebellar function)** **Point in space**-Can patient touch your finger held in front of them **Finger to nose**-Move finger from touching your finger to their nose **Gait**-Walking and tandem (heel to toe) **Rhomberg test for balance**-Standing straight with feet together, arms extended in front with palms down and eyes closed
REFLEXES	**Basic reflexes**-Biceps, triceps, forearm, knee, ankle, Babinski reflex

NUTRITION

An ongoing nutritional assessment is necessary because the visual appearance of the patient is not a reliable indicator of whether the patient is receiving the proper amounts of nutrients. One of the most common causes of delayed healing is malnutrition. Laboratory values such as total protein, serum albumin, pre-albumin, and hematocrit are indicators that must be assessed and monitored regularly. If any of these tests are abnormal, a nutritional assessment by the dietician should be ordered.

ANCILLARY TESTING

Bone scans are generally performed on patients being treated for chronic refractory osteomyelitis in the hyperbaric chamber. Although a bone scan does not distinguish between abnormal and normal bone formation, the results can identify all types of bone malignancy, infection, fractures, and other disorders when viewed in light of the patient's surgical and medical history, x-rays, and other laboratory test results.

When treating chronic lower extremity non-healing wounds, assessment of the peripheral vascular status is a requirement to estimate the benefit of HBOT. The non-invasive tests that evaluate the blood flow in the major arteries and veins of the legs are doppler ultrasonography and transcutaneous oxygen monitoring (TCOM). These measure the oxygen supply in the tissues, and the results determine if further invasive testing (arteriogram) is required or if there is a suitability of adjunctive HBOT.

The laboratory tests needed before the patient is cleared for treatment vary depending on the treatment indication. All patients should have a complete blood count and urine specimen as a basic workup. Other tests can include type and cross match, platelet count, PT, PTT, chemistry profile, wound cultures, arterial blood gases, carboxyhemoglobin level, cardiac enzymes, renal profile, SED rate, protein level, serum albumin, and prealbumin levels.

PHYSICAL EXAM PRIOR TO HBO TREATMENT

Prior to each treatment baseline vital signs should be taken on all patients. This should include temperature, heart rate, blood pressure, lung sounds, otoscopic exam, and blood sugar on all insulin-dependent diabetics. Having a baseline heart rate and blood pressure allows decisions to be made concerning the changes expected on the cardiovascular system from exposure to hyperbaric oxygen.

Since febrile patients have a decreased seizure threshold, it is important to identify them before treatment. Notify the physician if the temperature is greater than 100°F to decide whether the treatment should be given. Interventions prior to treatment for an elevated temperature include administering Tylenol orally or rectally (aspirin is not suggested), ice compresses to axilla and groin, or a tepid water sponge bath. During the treatment the ice compresses to axilla and groin can continue, and the airflow of the chamber can be maximized. I.V. fluids can be cooled prior to infusion. If the patient's temperature is greater than 103°F and does not respond to cooling measures, or if the fever is of unknown origin, the treatment should be held.

While assessing the breath sounds of the patient, evaluate them for signs of cold or flu (cough, fever, sore throat, runny nose, nausea, diarrhea, malaise). These symptoms may be worsened by exposure to HBO and therapy should be postponed until subsided or cleared by the physician. An otoscopic exam will evaluate the ability of the patient to equalize for the treatment.

Auscultation of the lungs allows a hyperbaric nurse to evaluate the functioning of the lungs and discover any obstructions in the system. Breath sounds are caused by the movement of air through the tracheobrocho-alveolar system. These sounds are evaluated according to pitch, intensity, quality, and relative duration of the inspiratory and expiratory phases. Abnormal sounds include rales, rhonchi, and pleural friction rub and will require additional assessment if noted.

Pre-treatment blood sugars in the insulin-dependent diabetic are necessary due to the hypoglycemic effect of HBO. It is assumed that this effect is due to the inhibition of the anti-insulin hormones (somatotropic hormone and glucagon) in the HBO environment. In addition to requiring a blood sugar of at least 120 before treatment, all diabetics should eat and if possible hold their insulin until after the treatment. An ongoing assessment of blood sugar in diabetics is also necessary due to the effects of high blood sugars on wound healing.

Orthopedic injuries are common in the trauma injuries seen in the hyperbaric environment. The ability to do a neurovascular assessment, where vascular integrity, neurologic integrity, and pain level are assessed, is a basic skill. The color (pink, pale, cyanotic, mottled), temperature (warm, cool, cold), capillary refill (rapid, sluggish, absent – measured in seconds), edema (absent, mild, moderate, pitting), pulses (strong, weak, not palpable, audible by doppler, absent), sensation, and pain (constant, intermittent, sharp, dull, burning, aching, with stretching, at rest) are parameters evaluated. Always compare both sides of the body if possible, or use your limbs for comparison.

One of the more common complications treated in the HBO unit is compartment syndrome, or increased pressure within a limited space (muscle compartment) which compromises the circulation and function within that space. In compartment syndrome there is progressive pain that is out of proportion to what is expected in similar injuries. This pain is increased with passive stretch of the muscles in the compartment involved.

The patient being treated for carbon monoxide poisoning is often given the psychometric testing in the form of the Carbon Monoxide Screening Battery. The screening battery was developed to provide improved assessment of patients with carbon monoxide intoxication when there is a contradiction between the carboxyhemaglobin levels and the clinical presentation. It consists of six tests (general orientation, digit span, trail making, digit symbol, aphasia screening, and block design) that have proven to be consistently reliable, reproducible, sensitive, and valid. The screening battery must be used together with other clinical assessment procedures when making appropriate treatment responses. Results may be affected by alcohol or drugs, head injuries, cerebral illness, or mental retardation.

Some units test the patient for visual acuity before the beginning of treatments and then continue on a weekly basis during the therapy. This is due to the potential side effect of transient visual acuity changes noted in patients with myopia and presbyopia. By using a Snellen Eye Chart or Jaeger Card (hand held) it should be easy to get a visual acuity for the patient. If the patient wears glasses or contacts, make sure they are wearing them during the testing.

The "fifth vital sign" – pain – also has to be addressed prior to the commencement of the hyperbaric treatment. Controlling pain prevents suffering; promotes faster healing and strength building; helps patients become more active, sleep, and eat better; increases the patient's sense of well-being; and helps them develop a more positive outlook regarding the therapy. If a patient is in pain, the chances of a complete treatment diminish considerably if the pain is severe.

There are several pain scales that are effective, but you should adhere to one for continuity of patient care. If the patient reports pain you need to document the description (Table VII), location, when it started, does it radiate, and modalities that help relieve the pain. Controlling the pain can be accomplished by medications (opiods, non-steroidal analgesics, antidepressants, anticonvulsants, and steroids) or non-medicinal approaches (breathing/relaxation techniques, distraction, imagery, positioning, etc.). If the patient has not stopped smoking for hyperbaric treatments, point out that smoking decreases the effectiveness of the analgesic medications.

TABLE VII—PAIN DESCRIPTION

Sharp	Burning
Stabbing	Dull
Cramping	Tingling
Throbbing	Crushing
Pressure	Numbness
Shock-like	Radiating
Aching	Spasm
Increases with Movement	Increases with Breathing
Increases at Night	

FINAL PREPARATION BEFORE HBO TREATMENT

After patients have been cleared physically for their treatment in the chamber, they have to be prepared to be safely treated. There are substances and personal items prohibited in the hyperbaric chamber. All substances containing petroleum or alcohol (i.e., cosmetics, hair spray, nail polish, deodorants, lotions, colognes, perfumes, ointments) are prohibited due potentially serving as a fuel in the oxygen environment of the hyperbaric chamber. The patient should remove all jewelry, rings, watches, necklaces, hair combs, etc. before entering the chamber to prevent scratching the acrylic cylinder of the hyperbaric chamber.

Hard contact lenses should be removed before entering the chamber due to the potential formation of bubbles between the lens and the cornea. In addition to blurring vision, there is the possibility of damage to the cornea due to "lens squeeze" during ascent. Hearing aides should be removed due to introduction of electricity into the chamber. All types of prosthetic devices should be removed before treatments (i.e., artificial limbs, hairpieces, etc.). Some units require the patient to remove eye glasses and dentures prior to treatments. In most cases these items can go into the chamber if the nurse determines that the patient is alert enough to prevent compromise of the airway with dentures or not scratch the side of the chamber with eyeglasses.

All clothing and linen used inside the chamber should be 100% cotton to prevent the development of static electricity when rubbed together. The presence of static electricity in an oxygen environment is dangerous due to the possibility of a developing a spark. Since the human body produces electricity on its own, patients should be grounded to the chamber and the chamber itself is grounded. In addition, all Velcro should be eliminated from medical equipment used in the chamber due to the potential development of static electricity when pulled apart.

Premedication of patients before treatments is important to prevent complications and to make the treatment as comfortable as possible. If a problem in equalization has been encountered or expected, premedication with a decongestant (Sudafed) or nasal spray is suggested. Contraindications include hypertension, severe coronary artery disease, patients on MAO inhibitors, and narrow angle glaucoma. Treatment should be used cautiously in patients with hyperthyroidism, diabetes, ischemic heart disease, advanced arteriosclerosis, elevated intraocular pressure, or prostatic hypertrophy as it might aggravate these conditions. Care must be taken with nasal spray due to the potential for rebound congestion or irritation of the throat with long term use.

When confinement anxiety is anticipated, premedication with an anti-anxiety medication (Valium, Ativan) is advised. These medications should be given at least 30 minutes prior to starting treatment so they will start taking effect before treatment. Heavy smoking accelerates the medication's metabolism and decreases the medication's effectiveness. Advise patients that if they are being treated as an outpatient in the hyperbaric unit, they will be required to have transportation as they should not be driving or operating heavy equipment after being medicated.

In patients who have painful indications, premedication with an analgesic should be given prior to the treatment. If the medication is given intramuscularly, it should given at least 30 minutes before scheduled treatment. A complete pain assessment needs to be done on the patient to evaluate the effectiveness of the medication, and as with the anti-anxiety medications, patients medicated with narcotic analgesics should not drive or operate heavy equipment.

Vitamin E is believed to offer some protection against the effects of oxygen toxicity by counteracting the oxygen free radicals. Generally, a daily dose of 400 mg is considered effective.

It may be necessary to restrain unconscious patients or patients with a decreased level of consciousness to protect them from self-injury and the damage of medical equipment during treatments. Any patient with central lines, chest tubes, or endotracheal tubes must be considered for restraint in the chamber. Soft cotton restraints will be applied and secured to the bottom of the gurney tray, with additional restraint obtained by the appropriate use of sheet restraints if needed. Restraints that contain metal or Velcro cannot be used for safety reasons. Although the restraints may be applied at the discretion of the hyperbaric nurse, a physician's order is required to comply with Joint Commission on Accreditation of Healthcare Organizations (JCAHO) standards.

Before the initiation of the hyperbaric treatment, a safety check needs to be completed and documented in the chart. A safety check basically states that the nurse treating the patient has gone through a checklist of safety procedures before treating the patient. It includes checking for ground placement, items prohibited in the chamber, 100% cotton linen and clothing, and the correct application of medical equipment.

Before starting the treatment all medical equipment that is on or going to be attached to the patient needs to checked. This includes intravenous (I.V.) lines, arterial lines, EKG monitor leads, blood pressure cuffs, ventilators, naso-gastric tubes, suction devices, gastrostomy devices, foley catheters, casts, external fixator devices, splints, etc.

For patients requiring continuous intravenous infusions during hyperbaric therapy, a special extension set was developed for the monoplace chamber. It includes a pass-thru and has a back check valve which allows the I.V. fluid to flow in only one direction. It is important that all the connections are tight and there are no leaks in the tubing.

Specialized pumps are used to overcome the pressure inside the chamber and should not be used elsewhere in the hospital to prevent injuries. There should be more than enough I.V. fluid to complete the treatment, transport, and to flush the line.

On all first-time treatments and patients with a cardiac history, the EKG monitor will be used non-invasively to observe the patient. Before placing the patient in the chamber it is a good idea to check the rhythm on the monitor and to check all the leads. With the blood pressure monitor, it is also a good idea to get a baseline reading at ambient pressure to assure proper placement of the cuff.

All suction devices (Jackson Pratt, hemovac, etc.) and drainage devices (nasogastric tubes, gastrostomy, etc.) taken into the chamber must be vented (i.e., a foley drainage bag or opened to ambient pressure). This prevents problems caused by changes in pressure during treatment. All metal parts of the devices should be removed or taped over to prevent scratching the acrylic. During the treatment a sterile glove is placed over the tube to act as a reservoir for drainage.

Foley catheters require no special attention except to avoid kinking in the tubing and to empty the vented tubing bag before treatment. The bag should be placed flat on the gurney between the legs of the patient to aid drainage. The retention balloon of the foley catheter is filled with sterile water and is not affected by changes in pressure. It the patient has an endotracheal tube or tracheostomy with an air-filled cuff, it will be necessary to replace the air in the cuff with sterile water or sterile normal saline. After treatment the sterile fluid needs to be replaced with air to prevent necrosis around the cuff area.

In some units the patient is connected to a transcutaneous oxygen monitor during the hyperbaric treatment. This non-invasive test is generally used to validate the effectiveness of hyperbaric therapy in hyperoxygenating the blood in compromised tissues.

Treating a patient with a chest tube in the hyperbaric unit requires the placement of a Heimlich valve to prevent the progression of the pneumothorax or hemothorax to a tension pneumothorax. After making sure there is a firm airtight connection of the chest tube drainage tubing, the tubing should be taped to the valve to prevent accidental dislodging.

Securely tape a sterile glove to the end of the Heimlich valve to act as a reservoir for any drainage during the treatment. In patients being treated for a hemothorax, there is the potential of a clot forming at the site of the valve, so frequent observations of the site are required. Compression and decompression rates should be slowed to allow adequate pleural venting. Continuous observation of chest tube function and signs of pneumothorax (Table IX) should be monitored, especially on decompression.

Each patient should be asked before starting a hyperbaric treatment whether they have had used the restroom prior to entering the chamber. The need to void or have a bowel movement can cause the early termination of a treatment or acute discomfort in patients during the treatment. Additionally, patients on diuretics might consider changing the time they take the medication until after the treatment.

THE HYPERBARIC TREATMENT

One of the most important nursing tasks during treatment is the observation of the patient for signs and symptoms of barotrauma, oxygen toxicity, and the other complications/side effects encountered in HBOT. Getting to know the patient, his idiosyncrasies, and his family allows noting subtle changes in the patient's behavior or acuity.

After instructing the patient in equalization or auto-inflationary techniques (including yawning, swallowing, chewing gum, and modified Valsalva techniques), begin compression at 1 psig/min in small increments except in conditions that are life threatening (AGE, DCS). Encourage the patient to use the technique or combination of techniques that is most effective or comfortable.

Remind patients to begin the equalization techniques when the chamber door is closed and to continue as long as the pressure increases or decreases. Patients also need to be reminded that the modified Valsalva maneuver is only to be used during decompression and that they need to breathe normally during the treatments (never holding their breath). Forceful Valsalva in an attempt to clear the ears during descent can possibly cause a rupture of the Labyrinth Window inside the ear.

If the patient experiences mild to moderate pain, stop pressurization and decrease to the point of no pain, encouraging the patient to continue equalization techniques. Resume compression when the discomfort subsides. If the patient experiences severe pain, if the mild to moderate pain is not relieved when pressure is held, or if decompression does not help relieve pain, the patient should be removed from the chamber and examined by an Ear/Nose/Throat (ENT) physician.

The use of myringotomy and the placement of myringotomy tubes (MT) can be prophylactic in patients unable to equalize to prevent barotrauma or to treat patients who have developed barotrauma due to complications of HBO therapy. Prophylactic placement of MT should be considered if the patient is comatose or unable to follow instruction in the equalization of the middle ear. The rate of compression with MT should remain the same until the patient has learned to equalize pressure following placement.

There is the possibility of gas expanding in the gastrointestinal tract during ascent that could cause reflux, belching, or discomfort. Actual GI barotrauma is rare and generally inconsequential due to the intestines being surrounded by soft tissue, so the compression and re-expansion are not significant. To prevent GI barotrauma, have the patient breathe normally (don't swallow air) and avoid large meals or gas-producing food or drink before treatments.

Barodontalgia or tooth squeeze occurs when a small pocket of air is collected in a tooth upon compression and expands on decompression. This air space may be from decay, being trapped under a filling, gum infections, recent extractions, fillings, or root canals. Tooth squeeze is uncommon, but prevention is relatively easy. If the patient has had extensive dental work it is generally a good idea to wait 24 hours before treatment in the hyperbaric unit.

Before the beginning of treatment, the patient needs to be assessed for the possibility of confinement anxiety, and the contributing or precipitating factors should be found. Signs and symptoms of confinement anxiety or claustrophobia, an adverse response to HBO therapy, may occur before the treatment, any time during the treatment, and persist after the treatment. To prevent or decrease the effects of confinement anxiety, use premedication, distraction (tv, movies, music, books on tape, relation tapes), or a hyperbaric nurse/family member sitting at the side of the chamber.

Offer support and understanding to the patient's reaction to anxiety. Encourage the patient to ventilate on present feelings, and ask specific questions regarding the cause, if any, of the anxiety reaction. Reinforce that the patient has control over the treatment and that he will be removed from the chamber when requested. Additionally, assure the patient that there will be a nurse present the entire time he is in the chamber.

TABLE VIII—SIGNS AND SYMPTOMS OF CONFINEMENT ANXIETY	
Clenching of Fists	Urgency to Empty Bladder
Flushed Face	Defensive Attitude
Complaint of Nausea or Diarrhea	Hyperventilation
Sudden Complaint of Pain or Discomfort	Profuse Diaphoresis
Feelings of Being Smothered or Suffocated	Flat Affect

Monitor the patient during decompression – especially during emergency decompression – for signs of pneumothorax. If the signs and symptoms (Table IX) develop, recompress the patient if possible and hold decompression when relief is noted. Notify the hyperbaric physician, prepare a thoracentesis tray, have an oxygen mask ready, and order a stat ABG and CXR in preparation of removing the patient from the chamber. Wait for the physician's arrival to resume decompression and be prepared to assist with the insertion of a chest tube.

Observe the patient for signs of arterial gas embolism (AGE) during decompression, especially if the patient is suspected of having a pneumothorax or subcutaneous emphysema. The possibility of a concurrent AGE existing is high. If the signs and symptoms (Table IX) are noted and AGE is suspected, recompress the patient to 3.0 ATA immediately. Do not decompress the patient until the physician is present, unless CPR is required.

TABLE IX—SIGNS AND SYMPTOMS OF BAROTRAUMA		
Pneumothorax	Sudden Dyspnea Tracheal Shifts Symmetrical Chest Movements Increased Respiratory Distress with Decompression	Stabbing Chest Pains
Subcutaneous Emphysema	Crepitus Dysphagia Retrosternal Discomfort Feeling of Fullness in the Throat—Dyspnea	Voice Changes Syncope
Arterial Gas	Loud Groaning Cry Followed by a Jacksonian Seizure Loss of Consciousness Other Neurological Abnormalities	

One of the complications encountered in treating the patient at pressure with 100% oxygen is potential central nervous system or pulmonary oxygen toxicity. Development of CNS oxygen toxicity symptoms can be seen any time during the treatment protocols, but pulmonary toxicity is seen mainly in prolonged treatment protocols. Close monitoring of the patient is to prevent the occurrence of the complications associated with oxygen toxicity.

The pretreatment assessment is one of the major tools in preventing oxygen toxicity. Evaluating patients' temperature (febrile patients have decreased seizure threshold), acidosis levels, and therapeutic drug levels of patients on anticonvulsants help remove some precipitating factors. The treatment protocol can be modified by adding air breaks to help prevent oxygen toxicity seizures. The physical facilities can be modified by using low light in the treatment area and by not using fluorescent lights above the chamber.

Air breaks are used to decrease the potential for oxygen toxicity due to extended treatments or contributing factors being present. This requires the patient to wear a face mask with a tight seal and to breathe medical air for a prescribed period of time. This helps decrease the oxygen level and thereby the potential for oxygen toxicity.

One or more of the signs and symptoms (Table X) of CNS oxygen toxicity can be treated by switching the chamber gas source to air or by removing the patient from the chamber. If the patient progresses to a seizure, observe for cessation of the seizure and decompress at a rate of tolerance. In cases of status epiliticus, decompress during the clonic phase of the seizure. Benzodiazapines may be administered intravenously to control seizure activity.

When the patient is out of the chamber, immediately check the blood sugar if hypoglycemia is suspected. In addition, the patient should be evaluated for potential barotrauma due to emergency ascent to make sure there is not a pneumothorax or other pulmonary trauma. A complete patient workup/history needs to be completed to determine the cause of the oxygen seizure. Resume the treatments only after being cleared by the hyperbaric physician.

TABLE X—SIGNS AND SYMPTOMS OF CNS OXYGEN TOXICITY	
Facial pallor	Sweating
Bradycardia	Palpitations
Depression	Apprehension
Visual Field Constriction	Tinnitus
Auditory Hallucinations	Visual Hallucinations
Vertigo	Inspiratory Predominance
Diaphragmatic Spasms	Nausea
Fibrillation of Lips	Syncope
Twitching of Lips, Cheeks, Nose or Eyelids	Convulsions

Prolonged exposure to oxygen at pressures greater than atmospheric is often associated with impaired pulmonary function. Continued exposure can cause the patient to develop progressive impairment of pulmonary function with the potential of developing adult respiratory distress (ARDS). Monitoring for signs and symptoms (Table X) and comparing to pre-treatment pulmonary function tests (PFT) are important in diagnosis and treating this complication.

TABLE XI—SIGNS AND SYMPTOMS OF PULMONARY TOXICITY	
Substernal Burning	Chest Tightness
Cough	Dyspnea
Dry Hacking Cough	Changes in PFT Results
Difficulty Inhaling a Full Breath	

AFTER HBO TREATMENT

After completing the hyperbaric treatment, the patient should be assessed before being discharged home or returned to the patient care unit. If the patient had any difficulty equalizing during compression or decompression, or the pre-treatment exam was positive for signs of barotrauma, a post-treatment otological exam should be performed. If the patient is an insulin-dependent diabetic and the pre-treatment blood sugars were within expected normal or low levels, a post-treatment blood sugar test should be performed.

Depending on the treatment indication, individualized assessments should be performed. Patients with acute traumatic ischemia, compartment syndromes, crush injuries, and re-implantations should have a neurovascular and a wound assessment. Carbon monoxide patients might require a repeat psychometric exam or repeat carboxyhemoglobin level. Patients being treated for acute retinal artery insufficiency will require an extensive visual workup. Patients being treated for decompression sickness, arterial gas embolism, or cerebral edema should have a neurological assessment.

After the appropriate assessments are completed and the patient is suitably discharged, it is important that all information pertinent to the treatment is documented. This is important not only for medical/legal reasons, but also for the staff who may be treating the patient in the future. It allows them to know the baseline information and what is important to make the treatment as comfortable as possible for the patient.

REFERENCES

1. Collison, L. (1993), Hyperbarics When Pressuring Patients Helps. RN, March, 44-49.
2. Hyperbaric Facility Safety: A Practical Guide. 1999. Workman, W.T., Best Publishing Co., Flagstaff, AZ.
3. Hyperbaric Medical Review for Board Certification Exams. 2000. Bookspan, J., Undersea and Hyperbaric Medical Society. Kensington, MD.
4. Hyperbaric Medicine Practice, Second Ed. 1999, Kindwall, E.P., Whelan, H.T., Best Publishing Co., Flagstaff, AZ.
5. Interaction of Drugs in the Hyperbaric Environment-The 21st Undersea Medical Society Workshop. 1979. Walsh, J.M. Undersea and Hyperbaric Medical Society. Bethesda, MD.
6. King, C. (1982), Checking the Patient's Neurological Status. RN, December, 57-61.
7. King, C. (1982), Examining the Thorax and Respiratory System. RN, August, 55-63.
8. King, C. (1982), A Systemic Plan for Assessing the Head and Face. RN, January, 55-58.
9. Laughlin, R.M. & Clancey, G.J. (1982), Neurovascular Examination of the Injured Extremity. Orthopedic Nursing, Jan/Feb, 43-48.
10. Lewis-Cullinan, C. & Janken, J. (1990). Effect of cerumen removal on the hearing ability of geriatric patients. Journal of Advanced Nursing, 15, 594-600.
11. Malkiewicz, J. (1982), How to Assess the Ears and Test Hearing Acuity. RN, March, 56-63.
12. Mayer, D.M., Torma, L., Byock, I., Norris, K. (2001). Speaking the Language of Pain. American Journal of Nursing, Vol 101, No 2, 44-49.
13. Mechner, F. (1975). Patient Assessment: Examination of the Ear. American Journal of Nursing, March, Vol. 75, No. 3.
14. Merry, J.A. (1988). Take Your Assessment All the Way Down to the Toes. RN, January, 60-63.
15. Monoplace Hyperbaric Chamber Safety Guidelines- Report to the Chamber Safety Committee of the Undersea and Hyperbaric Medical Society. 1991. Ed. Weaver, L.K. & Strauss, M.B. Undersea Hyperbaric Medical Society. Bethesda, MD.
16. O'Hanlon-Nicols, T. Neurologic Assessment (1999). American Journal of Nursing, Vol 99, No 6, 44-49.
17. Singer, A.J. (2001). Dissolving Ear Wax. American Journal of Nursing. Vol. 1, No. 1, 22.
18. Stevens, S.A. & Becker, K.L. 1988. Neurological Assessment-A Simple Step by Step Approach. Nursing 88, September, 53-61.
19. Textbook of Hyperbaric Medicine, 3rd Revised ed. (1999). Jain, K.K. Hogrefe & Huber Publishing, Seattle, WA.

CHAPTER II

STAFF AND PATIENT CARE CONSIDERATIONS IN THE MULTIPLACE ENVIRONMENT

B. BAKER

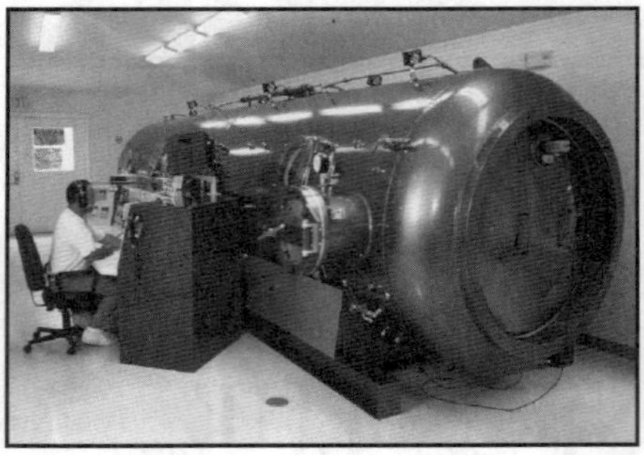

Multiplace Chamber

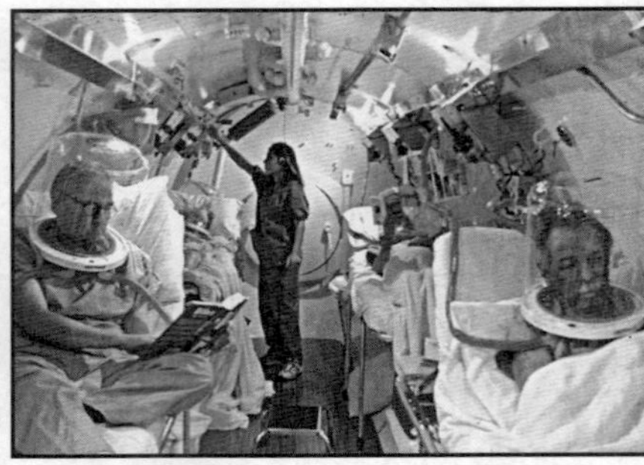

Inside Multiplace Chamber

THE MULTIPLACE SETTING

Multiplace hyperbaric chambers are designed to accommodate multiple patients for hyperbaric oxygen therapy. Some multiplace chambers have space for eighteen or more patients. The multiplace atmosphere contains normal, dry, filtered, compressed air. Patients breathe oxygen through a hood, mask, tracheotomy, or ventilator. Patients can either be seated or on a stretcher. There may be two or more compartments, often called "locks," attached to the main chamber. Additional compartments may be used for patient treatment, or to transfer a person to or from the main chamber without affecting the main chamber's pressure. The National Fire Protection Association (NFPA) in its document NFPA 99 *Guide to Health Care Facilities* designates the multiplace chamber as a Class "A" chamber. Chapter 19 of NFPA 99 is dedicated to hyperbaric facilities and offers an abundance of rules and regulations including design, operations, and maintenance.[1] This document is considered law in many states. All staff members working in the hyperbaric facility should be familiar with its contents.

Multiplace chambers require a support system of personnel and equipment more complex than that of monoplace chambers. During a hyperbaric treatment in a multiplace chamber, the hyperbaric nurse functions either as an inside observer of the patients undergoing HBOT, or as an outside observer. The inside observer is responsible for monitoring and caring for the patients inside the chamber. A chamber console operator is responsible for the safe operation of the hyperbaric chamber and its life support systems, and maintains contact with inside chamber personnel during the treatment. The outside observer works to fill the needs of both the patients and the hyperbaric nurse inside the chamber. The inside and outside observers are often referred to as "tenders," as they tend to the needs of the patients and others actively involved in a treatment. Physician requirements are the same as the monoplace with the exception that the physician may be required to enter the chamber during a treatment.

Multiplace chamber systems are composed of various pieces of equipment that are essential for safety and life support. This includes at minimum, compressors that pump the air that pressurizes the chamber, built-in breathing systems (BIBS) that provide breathing gases for those inside, fire control systems that provide enough water to deluge the chamber in case of fire, backup emergency gases kept on-line in case of fire or loss of pressure, numerous analyzers that monitor the atmosphere inside the chamber, and communications systems that provide a link between outside and inside personnel. Chamber systems are generally maintained and cared for by the chamber's technical staff.

THE USE OF GASES

The multiplace chamber atmosphere is filled with a large volume of compressed air, not oxygen. It would require a great amount of oxygen to fill and compress a multiplace chamber. This would not only be expensive, but would also create a tremendous concern for fire. Therefore, filtered and tested breathing air (78% nitrogen, 21% oxygen, 1% trace gases) is used to "dive" the chamber. One hundred percent oxygen is delivered through built-in breathing devices used for patient therapy and observer decompression.

NITROGEN

There are many considerations required to ensure a safe environment for the patients and inside observers. Since the chamber atmosphere is a compressed-air environment (mainly nitrogen), in-water diving decompression tables must be used for all persons not breathing oxygen while under pressure. Breathing air under pressure, whether in a chamber or on a scuba dive, exposes a person to the potential effects of decompression sickness (the bends). DCS can result in extreme fatigue, mild or serious pain, paralysis, or even death.

Another consideration is the effect nitrogen has when breathed at an increased partial pressure. This is Dalton's Law of partial pressure. Commonly referred to as the "martini law," it is said that nitrogen breathed at one atmosphere has the same effect of drinking one martini at the surface. Two atmospheres equal two martinis; three atmospheres equal three martinis, etc. In other words: "the deeper you go, the better it feels." Nitrogen narcosis can prove challenging for the inside observer when treating patients at greater pressures (i.e., 165 fsw for a USN treatment table 6A). Narcosis can cause impairment and inside personnel may be unable to provide necessary patient care. Hyperbaric facilities that offer such treatment tables frequently perform training dives to deeper "depths" in order to evaluate employee performance while under the effects of nitrogen narcosis.

Oxygen

The same standards used with monoplace chambers for safely handling and breathing 100% oxygen are also applied in the multiplace environment. Not only must patients be monitored for the effects of oxygen induced seizures, the oxygen in the chamber's atmosphere must also be closely monitored in order to avoid an increased risk of fire.

The volume of space inside a multiplace chamber is much greater than that of a monoplace chamber. A build-up of oxygen inside the chamber's atmosphere can create the potential for catastrophe. Items that may not burn well at the surface may, when enclosed in a pressurized environment. Requirements set by the U.S. Navy and the National Fire Protection Association require that the chamber atmosphere be kept below 25% oxygen with audible alarms signaling the chamber operator if oxygen exceeds 23.5%.[2, 3] Electronic as well as manual sampling tubes (Dräger tubes) are used to analyze oxygen percentages. It is the chamber operator's duty to control the environment inside the chamber and to notify inside personnel if oxygen leaks are detected. Inside observers are frequently called upon to "snoop" (check for leaks) using some type of portable oxygen analyzer. Increased ventilation, or even discontinuing oxygen delivery (depending on patient condition) may be required to bring oxygen in the chamber atmosphere down to a safe level. A rule of thumb for fire safety is to treat the multiplace environment as if it contained 100% oxygen, just like the monoplace. There may be some exceptions as to the amount of materials and types of equipment; however, all items should be approved by the unit's Safety Director prior to being allowed inside the chamber.[4] The inside tender and all other staff participating in a treatment should be aware of and familiar with all items going inside the chamber during a treatment. All materials and equipment used inside the chamber should be in compliance with NFPA regulations.[5]

The physiological effects of breathing oxygen under pressure are equally a concern. Giving air breaks is common for multiplace chambers in structuring patient breathing schedules. However, oxygen-induced seizures still occur. The ability of the inside attendant to provide hands-on care in this situation is a definite advantage in the multiplace setting. Most multiplace hyperbaric chambers are capable of reaching pressures equal to 6 atmospheres or greater. Due to the central nervous system effects of breathing oxygen at high partial pressures, it is important to remember that 100% oxygen should never be breathed below 3 ATA.

Carbon Dioxide

Sealing multiple persons in a pressurized container filled with air can significantly raise the level of carbon dioxide in the atmosphere. The U.S. Navy's recommended limit for breathing carbon dioxide (CO_2) is 1.5% surface equivalent volume (SEV).[6] Others suggest more conservative values such as .5%. Breathing a SEV of 10% carbon dioxide can cause a person to lose consciousness, while a SEV of 15% CO_2 can cause muscular spasms and rigidity.[7] Some multiplace chambers contain CO_2 scrubbers, which remove carbon dioxide from the chamber. For chambers without CO_2 scrubbers, the chamber operator must provide adequate ventilation into the chamber to keep CO_2 levels in control. Chamber ventilation is provided by using a continuous or intermittent flow of air through the chamber, while maintaining the desired treatment pressure. Hand pumps with CO_2 detector tubes (available from Draeger) and/or electronic CO_2 monitors provide atmospheric analysis of carbon dioxide inside the chamber. The chamber operator must make any necessary adjustments in ventilation to ensure a safe chamber environment.

Excess amounts of carbon dioxide can also lower the threshold for oxygen-induced seizures. If a patient is wearing an oxygen hood, somewhat similar to wearing a diving helmet with an overboard exhaust, the same principle should apply in keeping CO_2 levels in control. CO_2 levels inside the hood can be decreased by increasing the flow of oxygen into the hood, and by reducing over-inflation of the hood. Some hyperbaric facilities analyze the gases inside a patient's hood during treatment and document the exact gas percentages and flow rates.

In Table 1, CO_2 percentage values at various depths are given equal to the relative surface equivalent volume of carbon dioxide. This table can be used as a guideline for monitoring carbon dioxide percentages in the chamber atmosphere and in the patient's breathing device, i.e., oxygen hood.

Table 1

DEPTH	1.5% CO_2 SEV	1.0% CO_2 SEV	0.5% CO_2 SEV
45 fsw	0.64	0.42	0.22
60 fsw	0.54	0.36	0.18
66 fsw	0.50	0.33	0.17
165 fsw	0.25	0.17	0.08

WORKING UNDER PRESSURE

The primary role of the inside tender is to safely administer hyperbaric oxygen to those patients for which it has been prescribed. The inside tender must be able to ensure patient compliance during HBOT, while being constantly aware of the hazards and physiological effects of the environment in which the work is being performed.

The first achievement during the actual multiplace treatment is getting the patients (and inside tender) to the desired treatment pressure without causing barotrauma. Oxygen delivery devices are generally not applied until reaching this point. During the actual pressurization of the chamber, and any time the chamber is "traveling" (i.e., descending/ascending), the inside tender's eyes should be constantly focused on the patients. Patients must be instructed to use proper equalization techniques during the descent (i.e., drink water, Valsalva). Oftentimes the tender must "talk" a patient through the entire descent, demonstrating and reinforcing correct methods of equalization. Despite thorough pre-treatment patient teaching, middle ear barotrauma remains the most common reported side effect of HBOT.[8]

Once the chamber has reached the desired treatment pressure, the inside tender may begin the process of administering hyperbaric oxygen. Before applying the patient's oxygen delivery device, generally an oxygen hood or mask, the inside tender should reconfirm that the patient has equalized properly and is not experiencing any problems. Once the administration of oxygen has begun, the inside tender should assure the delivery device is tightly sealed and does not leak oxygen into the atmosphere. Oxygen hoods may require some manipulation to achieve proper inflation. Flow meters are attached to oxygen delivery panels dedicated to each individual patient. A balance must be achieved between the supply of oxygen going into the hood, and the exhaust of oxygen exiting the hood. If the hood is over-inflated, carbon dioxide levels may increase. Hoods should not be inflated to the point that they rise and fall with each breath. A neutral or balanced flow will keep the hood somewhat resting on the patient's shoulders. The "shrink wrap" effect happens when gas flow is discontinued, or inadequate to keep a patient's hood inflated. This can significantly raise the level of anxiety in patients, interrupt their breathing, and should be corrected immediately. If a patient's oxygen supply tubing becomes disconnected, oxygen will flow directly into the chamber and raise the ambient percentage of O_2. Inside tenders must be constantly alert to prevent oxygen leaks, and to ensure that patients receive adequate ventilation during oxygen breathing periods.

AMRON OXYGEN TREATMENT HOOD

The dose/time of oxygen delivery periods is dictated by the type of treatment table being used and by the hyperbaric physician. During oxygen breathing periods, tenders should encourage patients to relax, assume a non-constrictive position, avoid conversation, and concentrate on breathing. Patients are in the chamber to receive therapy through the systemic effect of breathing 100% oxygen. Proper breathing techniques (i.e., long, slow inhalations and exhalations) will help ensure patients receive adequate and effective oxygen administration.

The inside tender should monitor all patients closely during oxygen breathing periods, being constantly alert for changes in a patient's condition and signs that may indicate a patient is experiencing the onset of oxygen toxicity. If signs indicating a potential seizure are noticed soon enough, and if oxygen breathing is immediately discontinued, it may be possible to avoid a full grand mal episode. If, however, the signs of oxygen toxicity are ignored or symptoms not reported by the patient, it is likely a seizure will occur. All chamber facilities should have a written protocol for this type of emergency. When critically ill patients are being treated, inside tenders will spend much of the treatment caring for those patients. Monitoring intravenous lines, blood pressure, and other pertinent patient needs will require tenders to spend much of the treatment on their feet. The amount of physical exertion performed while under pressure should be considered when developing decompression schedules for those working inside the chamber.

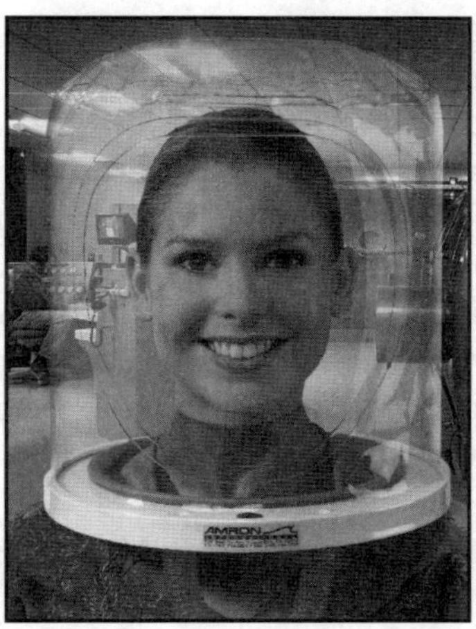

Amron Oxygen Treatment Hood

Air breaks are given to patients during a treatment to help reduce the hazardous effects of oxygen toxicity. These breaks are normally five to fifteen minutes in duration. The number of air breaks depends primarily on the time/amount and partial pressure of the oxygen being breathed by the patients. Generally, it is the chamber operator's duty to notify the inside tender when it is time for an air break. When appropriate, the tender turns off the patient's oxygen supply and removes the delivery device. Tenders should be careful not to let residual oxygen enter the chamber atmosphere. During the air break(s), tenders often distribute water or juice to the patients. This may help in keeping the patients hydrated due to the drying effects of breathing oxygen. It is both professional and reassuring if tenders use this time to inquire about changes in a patient's condition, or offer words of encouragement concerning their therapy. Giving air breaks can be the most demanding task a tender performs during a treatment. Taking oxygen hoods off of sometimes six or more patients, distributing something to drink to each patient, smiling, and being prepared to reapply the oxygen delivery device, all in sometimes a five-minute period can be most challenging. A common joke among multiplace chamber facilities is, "if a tender quits working in hyperbarics, they can always get a job as a flight attendant."

Toward the end of the last oxygen breathing period, it is a common practice for the inside tender to breathe oxygen in order to help reduce the risk of manifesting decompression illness. Perhaps the most important tool used to combat the incidence of inside observer decompression sickness is the use of 100% oxygen. Breathing oxygen at the end of a treatment table, during a slow ascent, and during any decompression "air stop times" may significantly reduce the risk of DCS for inside observers. Tenders most commonly use the aviator-style mask for their oxygen breathing requirements. When used by the tender for oxygen breathing, specific safety concerns should be considered. Firstly, tenders must ensure the mask is held tightly, creating a seal around the face. A tight seal will help ensure that 100% oxygen is being breathed, not the compressed air in the chamber atmosphere. A loose fit during inhalation will allow the chamber air to filter in around the seal. Also, tenders should never strap or permanently affix a mask to their face. A mask securely strapped to the tender's face could prevent the immediate removal of oxygen should the tender begin to experience symptoms of an oxygen-induced seizure. Tenders also often alternate the arms holding the mask in order to help reduce constriction of vessels. If a tender must communicate verbally while breathing from a mask, words should be spoken during exhalation. Inhalations should be taken from the mask, not the chamber atmosphere.

At completion of all oxygen breathing periods, the inside tender turns off the patient's oxygen supply and removes the oxygen delivery device. In a typical oxygen hood setup, the device is composed of two pieces, a hood and a neck seal. Hoods are generally removed prior to ascent, but the neck seal is left attached to the patient until the chamber reaches the "surface." All occupants inside the chamber must have a breathing apparatus available at all times.[9] Should the chamber atmosphere become contaminated, and not fit to breathe, the tender should quickly reapply the hood giving the patient a mechanism for adequate breathing. Prior to leaving bottom, the inside tender should ensure that all sealed containers used at pressure are vented to allow expanding gas to escape. Intravenous lines and pumps should be monitored throughout ascent. Most multiplace chamber operators utilize a "prior to leaving bottom" checklist that is communicated with the inside tender in order to confirm the chamber is safely ready to ascend.

The ascent/decompression of the chamber is a critical point in the hyperbaric treatment. As with the descent/compression of the chamber, pressure changes demand proper equalization of all air spaces. During "travel" tenders should put all other tasks aside, carefully monitoring the patients and any equipment being used. Tenders often remind patients to breathe normally during ascent, and to allow the expanding pressure in the ears to escape on its own, not attempting to pinch the nose, hold the breath, and blow. Gas trapping in the lungs during ascent can cause a pneumothorax, embolism, and/or death. If a patient begins to cough or experience breathing problems while the chamber is decompressing, the inside tender should inform the chamber operator to stop the ascent. Once the patient is stabilized, the ascent may continue.

Depending on the amount of time the tender spends at pressure breathing air, decompression stops may be required prior to the chamber reaching the surface. Task loads should be minimized so that tenders can concentrate on using proper techniques for effective decompression, (i.e., not talking while breathing oxygen, ensuring a tight seal when breathing from a mask, assuming a non-constrictive position). Often during decompression stops, decompression times based on breathing air are used; however, the tender breathes 100% oxygen instead of air. This added safety feature may help in reducing the risk of manifesting decompression sickness for inside personnel. Another technique used to decrease the risk of DCS, if sufficient staff is available, is exchanging inside tenders during a treatment. This technique can be used in order to keep personnel from pushing the limits of nitrogen uptake. Inside observers should be aware of their exposure times at pressure and understand the effects of nitrogen loading and decompression sickness. An excellent chapter written by Paul Sheffield and Christy Pirone in Workman's *Hyperbaric Facility: A Practical Guide,* provides statistics concerning the incidence of DCS for inside observers, along with actual case reports and other useful information for anyone going in the multiplace chamber.[10]

CHAMBER COMMUNICATIONS

Safely treating patients in either the monoplace or multiplace chamber involves continuous monitoring of the patient both verbally and visually. Chamber communications systems provide the means to do so.

Most monoplace chambers are constructed of a clear acrylic tube where the patient reclines or lays during treatment. Chamber personnel are able to clearly see the patient and have the ability to converse with the patient through an intercom system. In comparison, multiplace hyperbaric chambers are constructed of metal, generally steel. Round acrylic windows (view ports) are fitted along side the chamber to allow visual contact. The longer the chamber, the more view ports they may contain. In most clinical multiplace hyperbaric facilities, a video camera is positioned to peer inside the chamber which displays a continuous view on a video monitor. The video monitor is located outside the chamber where the chamber operator and other outside personnel can view the patients and inside personnel. Audible or visual communication between the console operator and inside personnel must be maintained at all times.[11] This is accomplished by using standard headsets, and/or speaker boxes equipped with microphones. For redundancy purposes, sound-powered phones provide backup support.

During the treatment, conversation in and around the chamber area should be kept to pertinent treatment information only. The sense of hearing plays an important role in multiplace chamber safety. Changes in the normal sounds associated with multiplace chamber operations may indicate a potential equipment problem. This could include anything from an air compressor failure to a malfunction in the patient's oxygen delivery system (i.e., oxygen tubing becoming disconnected). Often, when two people strap on headphones with microphones, they tend to forget that others (patients included) may hear what they are saying and become involved in inappropriate discussions. Outside and inside chamber personnel may get into deep personal conversation, causing distraction from their primary roles of monitoring the chamber and the patients. It only takes a second for an equipment failure to occur, or for a patient to begin to experience a problem. Becoming involved in private, soul-bearing, turgid personal conversations over communications systems while treatments are being performed may exemplify a disregard for others, and can lead to interpersonnel problems. Save it for after the treatment!

LIFE SUPPORT REQUIREMENTS

A big advantage of treating patients in the multiplace hyperbaric chamber is the ability to provide "hands-on" patient care. With the availability of qualified staff, and the proper life support equipment, any patient should be able to be treated in the chamber without decreasing the standard of care they may be receiving in any area of the hospital. This means that no matter how critically ill the patient might be, if hyperbaric therapy is indicated, that patient can be treated.

The use of any piece of equipment in a hyperbaric environment, whether 21% oxygen or 100% oxygen, requires special considerations.[12] Equipment that may be hazardous under hyperbaric conditions is not allowed inside the chamber.[13] The chamber atmosphere must be free from toxic fumes and items that could cause combustion. The Navy's Experimental Diving Unit established a Clinical Hyperbaric Evaluation and Testing (CHET) program to evaluate the performance and safety of equipment used inside the chamber. Testing was created to ensure any item entering a clinical hyperbaric chamber is not: toxic, explosive, flammable, or pressure intolerant, and is compatible with oxygen.[14] In addition to the Navy's efforts in evaluating equipment, it is also helpful to consult established hyperbaric facilities for information on their experience and recommendations. The unit's Safety Director is in charge of all equipment used inside the chamber, and must ensure that it is safe and its performance is accurate prior to being used in the multiplace environment.[15]

One of the most common pieces of patient/life support equipment used in hyperbaric chambers is an infusion pump for the administration of intravenous fluids. There are many types used in various hyperbaric settings. I.V. pumps used with monoplace chambers are located outside the chamber. The I.V. tubing is inserted into the chamber through a penetrator, and is attached to the patient prior to entering the chamber. It is imperative that fluid administration sites be well secured since there is no one inside the chamber with the patient to provide I.V. management. If the line becomes disconnected from the patient during the treatment, fluid administration must be stopped.

In the multiplace setting infusion pumps can be located outside or inside the chamber. Using an approved and tested pump outside the chamber works in the same fashion as with the monoplace. Pumps used inside the chamber must be tested for gas trapping, potential fire risk, and accurate delivery of fluids. The presence of an inside attendant allows "hands-on" care of patients receiving I.V. therapy. If the line becomes disconnected in this type of chamber, the inside attendant can start a new line or reattach to the site and continue fluid flow.

For those patients requiring breathing assistance, there are several types of ventilators that can be used in the multiplace environment. Commonly, these ventilators go inside the chamber with the patient. Some are more popular than others. Perhaps the most convenient is a portable type that attaches to the patient's gurney. This allows the patient to be transported to and from the chamber without the need for manual ventilation. Ventilators designed for monoplace chambers may also be adapted to use with the multiplace chamber. As with any piece of equipment going inside the chamber, ventilators must be checked for potential gas trapping, sparking, and accurate function at pressure.

Aspiration of patients in the multiplace chamber can be accomplished by using the vacuum created by the pressure differential between ambient pressure at depth and surface pressure. A regulator is used to control flow while a standard suction canister collects fluids. If aspiration is needed while the chamber is at surface pressure, a motorized vacuum pump may be used.

For cardiac monitoring and pressure monitoring, standard monitoring devices may be used outside the chamber or specific systems used inside the chamber. Outside monitors use through-the-hull penetrators to gain patient connection. Monitoring equipment inside the chamber must be tested and approved by the unit's Safety Director. Multiplace facilities may choose not to allow any electrical devices or receptacles inside the chamber. However, others may decide to do so, some even having defibrillation capabilities inside the chamber. Written protocols should be followed for using any piece of equipment. Fire safety should be paramount in the use of any device in the hyperbaric environment. An open line of communication between hyperbaric facilities gives all units the opportunity to research and decide what equipment is optimally functional for their facility. Any electrical equipment used inside the chamber should be in compliance with the guidelines set by the NFPA.[16]

EMERGENCY PREPAREDNESS

The hyperbaric environment is a volatile environment. Patients and working personnel have lost their lives in the administration of hyperbaric oxygen therapy. Each time a patient or staff member goes inside a hyperbaric chamber, they assume an acceptable risk of injury or death.

Safe and successful daily treatment operations require a team effort. From the moment a patient is consulted, a well designed treatment plan should be followed. Patient teaching is the first step in patient safety compliance. Chamber personnel must diligently perform pre-treatment safety checks, equipment checks, and patient evaluations. Pre-treatment patient checklists provide a method of ensuring that patients have been medically evaluated and screened for items not compatible in the hyperbaric environment prior to being allowed in the chamber. Chamber start-up checklists provide a method for chamber operators to confirm all chamber systems are operating correctly prior to beginning a treatment. There are also "at depth" and "prior to leaving bottom" checklists communicated between the inside observer and chamber operator to help ensure that proper procedures are being followed.

For the inside tender, the time spent at pressure can seem long and sometimes boring. During the patient's oxygen breathing periods, tenders should assume a comfortable non-restrictive position in the chamber and relax. Some tenders may choose to lightly read during a treatment; however, constant awareness must be given to the patients and the surrounding environment. As evidenced in previous hyperbaric mishaps, it takes only a second for a patient to produce an unsafe item that could cause injury or death.[17] The majority of treatments flow smoothly and are trouble-free. It may be easy for some to become complacent from what might seem monotonous work. However, complacency can kill. When things go wrong under pressure, they usually do so very quickly. Early recognition of potential problems is a vital safety concern for both patients and tenders. Treatments need to be performed with consistency. The safest, most proven treatment methods should be used everyday by everyone.

Safe operations are not the result of chance. Safe operations are the result of being knowledgeable and confident in how to act – not react – should an emergency occur. An old saying goes "hope for the best, prepare for the worst." Being prepared involves training. The NFPA requires that all chamber personnel be familiar with emergency equipment and its use.[18] All facilities should participate in a regular safety program that includes hyperbaric, related knowledge reviews, emergency procedures, and NFPA-required fire training drills.[19]

The following is a list of some potential emergencies for which all multiplace hyperbaric facilities should have written policies and procedures:

- Oxygen-Induced Seizures
- Gas Embolism
- Loss of Pressure
- Pneumothorax
- Respiratory/Cardiac Arrest
- Fire Suppression
- Gas Narcosis
- Ear/Sinus Barotrauma
- Claustrophobia
- Loss of Primary Oxygen Supply
- Decompression Sickness of Inside Observer
- Omitted Decompression

STAFFING

Multiplace hyperbaric treatments often involve more than ten patients simultaneously undergoing therapy. It is evident that these operations require more staff than their monoplace counterparts. A typical staff for a routine multiplace treatment includes an attendant for inside the chamber, a chamber operator at the console, and an attendant outside the chamber. Often, there is a qualified backup staff member available for the chamber operator as well. It is common for multiplace facilities to use "two techs and two nurses" as a minimum staff scenario. The presence of a hyperbaric physician depends on the individual unit's policy in compliance with medical regulations.

Each hyperbaric facility must decide on its requirements for staffing. The staff-to-patient ratio should depend on the medical condition of the patients being treated and the treatment table being used. For example, if there are four to six stable patients, all ambulatory, all outpatients, all without any serious medical complications or additional needs other than HBOT, most likely one inside attendant should be able to provide patient care. However, if one of those patients is on a ventilator, receiving multiple doses of I.V. fluids, and combative, then the unit may decide to provide an additional inside attendant, giving one-on-one care for that particular patient. Staffing considerations should also include dive planning procedures in order to help reduce the risk of inside observer incidence of decompression sickness.[20]

Personnel qualifications should be such that patients receive the same standard of care as would be available in an equal medical setting. It is recommended that at least one staff member with advanced cardiac life support certification be present anytime the chamber is pressurized.[21] For the role of inside and/or outside observer, most multiplace chambers use registered nurses, often only those with experience in critical care. Certified paramedics are also sometimes used as tenders, most often working in conjunction with a hyperbaric nurse. Chamber operators commonly have extensive training in chamber life support systems and chamber operations. Chamber operators may be required to have at minimum, certification in basic cardiac life support skills. Every facility should strive to have employees certified in hyperbaric nursing and/or hyperbaric technology (CHRN, CHT). It is also important that employees have some degree of cross training. The NFPA requires all chamber personnel to be able to safely decompress the chamber and its occupants should electrical power be lost during a treatment.[22]

Being exposed to hyperbaric conditions requires specific health concerns. For potential employees wishing to be a part of a multiplace hyperbaric team, a thorough fitness-to-dive examination should be completed prior to being qualified to work inside the chamber.[23] Health issues such as age, extreme fatigue, dehydration, colds, and pregnancy should be considered when employees are required to perform as inside observers. Regular employee audiograms are often required as noise levels inside the multiplace chamber can exceed OSHA standards.[24] Using hearing protection should be considered for all chamber occupants. Recommendations for flying after diving should also be followed for staff members exposed to the hyperbaric environment.

PATIENT ISSUES

The prevention and spread of infection is a concern in any medical setting. The majority of patients referred for HBOT possess some type of wound. Infection control in the multiplace chamber depends on the quality of care provided. The hyperbaric atmosphere does not create a greater hazard in the spread of infection; however, having multiple patients together in essentially the same "room" requires that universal precautions be closely followed. A thorough chamber cleaning as part of a regular chamber maintenance program must be diligently performed. Patients in "contact isolation" status are often treated in the chamber with other patients. Wounds should be covered and careful attention used in order to prevent the spread of infection when dealing with patients in contact isolation.

The consumption of food inside the chamber must be in accordance with the unit's policies and procedures. The by-products of consuming food in the chamber (i.e., liquid spills, crumbs, oil, grease) may present hazards and maintenance issues. Most medical facilities do not allow employees to bring food into patient care areas. The hyperbaric chamber is a patient care area, sometimes present with infected open wounds.

Patient rights and responsibilities are equal to those required for monoplace operations. Safety is the chief concern in daily treatments. Effective patient teaching and daily reinforcement of safety issues is imperative.

Oftentimes the multiplace chamber is filled with a variety of patients and personalities. Not always do the occupants get along with each other or the staff members going in the chamber with them. Personality conflicts and personnel preferences have to be taken into consideration. Some patients constantly evaluate the performance of various inside tenders used during treatments and form quick decisions on whom they like and whom they do not. A critically ill patient being treated in the chamber with stable outpatients may cause anxiety among the other occupants. The presence of bodily odors due to wounds and/or hygiene can also cause patient discomfort during treatments. Therefore, the selection of tenders and the placement of patients inside the chamber must be considered. If a patient is dissatisfied with the way treatments are performed or has a conflict with another patient, that patient may become non-compliant with the course of therapy and never return. The majority of the time, patients are friendly and the treatments actually enjoyable. However, for some patients, being in a multiplace chamber for two hours is like being on a trip to nowhere, stuck in a car with people they do not like. In a perfect world, all people would be considerate and tolerant of others, especially those in medical need. The multiplace environment is quite often not a perfect world!

The need for privacy while multiple patients are being treated inside a multiplace chamber can be quite challenging. Digestive bodily functions are due to occur while patients are in the chamber at pressure. Unless covered and lying on a stretcher where urinals and bedpans can be used, relief is often achieved while the inside tender drapes a sheet around the patient. If tenders experience such needs themselves, another qualified staff member may be substituted, or as sometimes has been done, the outer lock pressurized and used for privacy. If the inside tender must briefly step into the outer lock, it is best done when patients are on an air break, not while breathing oxygen. Audible or visual contact is always maintained between the chamber operator and the inside observer. Visual contact of patients may be kept by outside personnel should the inside tender be "occupied." For the inside tender this is a skillful and somewhat risky task, as one must be able to "stop mid-stream" and respond without delay should a patient require immediate attention. Most tenders choose to wait.

SUMMARY

Working under pressure involves acceptable risks beyond what is experienced by most medical personnel. Thus, the multiplace chamber setting can be a demanding environment for the hyperbaric nurse. Perhaps more so than any other area, nurses are actually exposed to and physically participate in the therapy a patient receives. Patient safety, as well as personal safety, are chief concerns in successful daily operations. Those that meet the challenges are rewarded with an increased knowledge of and appreciation for the application of hyperbaric oxygen therapy.

REFERENCES

1. NFPA 99 Health Care Facilities Chapter 19, 19-1.4.2
2. U.S. Navy Diving Manual 8-15.5.5
3. NFPA 99, 19-2 8.5.2
4. NFPA 99, 19-3 1.3.2
5. NFPA 99, 19-3 2.1
6. U.S. Navy Diving Manual, Sections 3-4.6, 8-15.5.5
7. U.S. Navy Diving Manual, Section 3-15
8. Textbook of Hyperbaric Medicine, Jain, K.K. 1996 Hogrefe & Huber Publishers, Inc. p.100
9. NFPA 99, 19-2.4.1.4
10. Hyperbaric Facility Safety: A Practical Guide, Workman, Wilbur T. Chapter 2 Decompression Sickness of Inside Attendants, Sheffield, P. and Pirone, C. pp. 643-661, Best Publishing Company, Flagstaff, AZ.
11. NFPA 99, 19-3.1.4.7
12. NFPA 99, 19-3.2.1
13. NFPA 99, 19-2.7.3
14. Hyperbaric Facility Safety: A Practical Guide. Evaluating Equipment and Materials, Chimiak, J. Section VI, Chapter 4, p.679, Best Publishing Company, Flagstaff, AZ.
15. NFPA 99, 19-3.1.3.2
16. NFPA 19-2.7.3.5
17. Hyperbaric Facility Safety: A Practical Guide, Section V Chapter 3, Chamber Accidents: A Morbidity/Mortality Survey of Chamber Accidents Over the Past 75 Years, Desautels, David, Best Publishing Company, Flagstaff, AZ.
18. NFPA 99, 19-3.1.4.4
19. NFPA 99, 19-3.1.4.6
20. Hyperbaric Facility Safety: A Practical Guide, pp. 643-661
21. Hyperbaric Facility Safety: A Practical Guide, p. 233
22. NFPA 99, 19-3.1.4.4
23. Hyperbaric Facility Safety: A Practical Guide p.660
24. UCSD Survey referred to in UHMS 2001 Annual Meeting abstract 143, p.77

NOTES

CHAPTER III

AGE-SPECIFIC CONSIDERATIONS

H. NORVELL AND C. LAND

INTRODUCTION

The Joint Commission on Accreditation of Healthcare Organizations has made age-specific competency a focal point during the survey process. The requirements are in the Management of Human Resources chapter in the Comprehensive Accreditation Manual for Hospitals: The Official Handbook (CAMH). Healthcare employees need to be trained on how the age of each patient can impact evaluation, mode of care, and health education needs for the patient. As a hyperbaric nurse, we come in contact with people from all stages of life, from infants to older adults. Each stage in life has certain elements and needs that are shared, and by understanding these, we provide better, more suitable care at each stage. Staff age-specific competencies should address the different requirements hyperbaric patients have at different ages. By incorporating age-specific considerations with your patient, you identify and provide care that meets the individual needs of your patient at that time of life. This also makes the patient an active partner in health decisions. (8)

COMMUNICATION

Communication is "the transmission of a message, thought, or idea from one person to another, using spoken or written words, symbols, pictures, tone of voice, facial expressions, gestures, touch, or behaviors." (9) How we communicate to our patients has the power to create both positive or negative outcomes in care. Being able to understand the patient's needs requires an understanding of age-specific communication skills.

TYPES OF COMMUNICATION

Verbal. Ask the patient or caregiver questions by speaking clearly and slowly enough to be understood. Use eye contact to confirm that the patient is listening and understanding what you are communicating. Assess their level of understanding. Listen carefully to what your patient verbalizes. Always ask for clarification when you need to better understand what is said. (9)

Written. In a hospital setting, we constantly communicate with written communication, as evidenced by the patient chart. Written communication may also be needed when a patient is entubated but still conscious. Drawing pictures is another form of written communication when there is a language barrier or when working with a child. The computer is increasingly becoming a mode of written communication for the patient as well as the healthcare provider.

Nonverbal. Nonverbal communication is always present, provided you observe it. Body language can say volumes especially when paired with conflicting verbal communication. Body language includes hand gestures, facial expressions, eye contact, and body posturing. Watch your own nonverbal communication as well when with a patient. It should express a sense of caring and openness. (9)

Barriers

Any age can have communication barriers. You may not be able to eliminate all barriers you find, but become aware of them and try to minimize them. First, assess the patient's primary language and whether communication might be improved with a translator. Second, determine if there are any speech, sight, or hearing impairments, any apparent learning disabilities, and if the person appears to understand instructions at an age-appropriate level. Establish if the patient is feeling stress about how treatment decisions might affect their schooling, job, or family. Be aware of cultural differences when communicating and try to not offend. Asian cultures, for example, are less comfortable with being touched than other cultures. Make an effort to understand a patient's family structure and support system, and incorporate family caregivers into the treatment plan. (9)

Failure to fully listen to the patient or caregiver can be the greatest barrier to effective communication. Treat the patient as you would want you or your loved one treated. Show respect and self-control with every patient, even the most difficult.

Age-Specific Competency

Competency of staff for age-specific care is essential to quality patient care. A nurse who is not competent can affect hospital or department costs by extending overall treatment or causing patient dissatisfaction with care received. Assessment of staff competency should occur on a periodic and ongoing basis. Through training and education opportunities, staff can maintain competence. (10)

HYPERBARIC AGE-SPECIFIC SKILLS

Pediatric Care

Children have reportedly been treated in hyperbaric oxygen therapy throughout the history of hyperbaric medicine. However, there continues to be some hesitancy on the part of pediatricians and physicians of hyperbaric medicine to use hyperbaric oxygen therapy for the pediatric patient. There are many reports in Russian literature where protocols have been established for examination of hyperbaric oxygen in pediatric disease states ranging from newborn hemolytic disease to ischemic conditions following pediatric surgical procedures. (5) Although in the United States this may not be feasible, there are certainly many conditions which afflict children that fit into the currently accepted indications for hyperbaric treatment which go unreferred. A reciprocal educational relationship between physicians who see children in the emergency room, hospitals, or as outpatients, and the hyperbaric physician should be established to benefit the child patient. "Treating a pediatric patient in need of adjunctive hyperbaric oxygen therapy can be not only therapeutically efficacious but also immensely gratifying and enjoyable for the hyperbaric staff." (5)

The pediatric patient is unique when compared to an adult or aging patient in that both growth and development are dominant occurrences. From the newly born infant through adolescence, there is continuous change in cell proliferation and maturation. Intermittent hyperoxygenation potentiates the protein extracellular growth factors. The action of vascular endothelial growth factor in stimulating capillary proliferation is enhanced by hyperbaric oxygen exposure. Also, fibroblastic replication is increased by hyperbaric oxygen. The specific mechanism by which hyperbaric oxygen accomplishes this is not clear, although it is suggested that growth factors play a role. The levels and distribution of growth factors decrease with age. With abundant growth factors, the younger patients are in an optimal position, compared to adults, for a favorable clinical response to hyperbaric oxygen therapy in situations where cellular proliferation is important. Fewer hyperbaric treatments may be required for significant clinical outcome. (1)

Side effects and morbidity are not statistically different in treating children with hyperbaric oxygen therapy compared to adults. (1)

ORIENTATION

The orientation to hyperbaric oxygen therapy depends on the patient's age and his or her physiological and psychological levels of maturity. In non-emergency situations with children preschool-aged or older, examining the facility and equipment prior to treatment with a parent present makes the environment less stress producing. Orientation to the hyperbaric unit with pictures, dolls, models, and child-oriented stories provides facts and dispels reservations. It is helpful for the staff member completing the orientation to also be there for the first treatment, either as the inside tender in multiplace operations or as the operator in monoplace chambers. Staff consistency for the treatment will reduce anxiety until the child has had a chance to meet everyone involved with patient care. The parents are oriented thoroughly by the physician and nursing staff. Parents of young children should be allowed to stay close to the patient or in sight to help the staff control and treat the child. The child's pediatrician is included in the hyperbaric care team to assist with long term planning.

SIDE EFFECTS IN CHILDREN

The incidence of side effects and complications in children is approximately the same as it is for adults (1.7%). Middle ear barotrauma was the most frequently seen problem (6.0%), and showed a higher frequency in patients between eleven and sixteen years old than in younger patients. Central nervous system oxygen toxicity (0.7%) occurred only in critically ill patients who were unconscious and ventilator-dependent. In children, as in adults, reducing the incidence of otic barotrauma seems to depend both on patient education and screening for Eustachian tube dysfunction (common in children). Undiagnosed, congenital malformations of the lung can lead to air-trapping and pulmonary over-inflation, resulting in pneumothorax and potential air embolism. A chest x-ray should be obtained in infants and children prior to treatment, as clinical presentation of the underlying malformation may be delayed.

Three special risks should be addressed when considering the use of hyperbaric oxygen therapy in pre-term infants or neonates. (1)

Exposure to elevated partial pressures of oxygen has been loosely associated with retrolental fibroplasia. Recent studies have shown that other risk factors are important, and indeed, retrolental fibroplasia has occurred in term infants and in preterm infants not exposed to elevated partial pressures of oxygen. A careful exam of the retina to ascertain the degree of vascular maturity may be helpful in assessing risk.

Bronchopulmonary dysplasia is a common and serious sequelae of barotrauma associated with the use of mechanical ventilation and elevated inspired partial pressures of oxygen in the treatment of respiratory distress syndrome. The mechanisms are not completely clear, but may include some, if not all, of the mechanisms of pulmonary oxygen toxicity in adults. (1) The addition of hyperbaric oxygen therapy to the care regimen of a pre-term infant already receiving assisted ventilation with high partial pressures of oxygen is likely to accelerate this process.

Oxygen is a potent stimulus for closure of the ductus arteriosus. Studies on pregnant ewes have shown that the ductal flow was significantly reduced during hyperbaric oxygen therapy. Total aortic flow was preserved due to increased transpulmonic flow, and this transitional type of circulation disappeared promptly post hyperbaric oxygen therapy. This does not represent a problem for hyperbaric oxygen in pregnancy, but it does represent a potential problem for ductal-dependent congenital heart disorders. In the setting of severe congenital pulmonic outflow obstruction, the flow of blood to the systemic circulation may depend on persistent ductal patency. The increase in blood oxygen tension with hyperbaric oxygen therapy could result in a sudden and catastrophic decrease in cardiac output due to ductal constriction. This is a rare event, but should be kept in mind if treating an infant with complex congenital heart disease. This risk is excluded by an adequate physical examination, chest x-ray, and, if indicated, echocardiography. (1)

BAROTRAUMA PREVENTION

Children may be taught the same ear-clearing techniques taught to adults. Assessment of the child's ability to understand directions and cooperate with the hyperbaric staff is needed to induce a child to clear his ears. Middle ear barotrauma may take longer to resolve in children, and is more likely to lead to bacterial otitis media. Eustachian tube dysfunction is much more common in children. While ear pain in an adult can be rationalized by the adult as necessary for the treatment, children with severe or mild ear pain may be more resistant to further treatment. (1)

Crying children swallow air and have a greater risk for gastric barotrauma, regurgitation, and aspiration. At times, depending on the status and age of the child, a medically qualified attendant may enter the monoplace chamber during the treatment. This allows for hands-on intervention for maintenance of the airway, prevention of aspiration, and maintaining patency of I.V. fluid sites. The attendant may carry a bulb syringe and/or an Ambu bag into the chamber if airway maintenance is in question. Infants may suck on a pacifier. If an infant is stable enough to suck on a bottle during compression to equalize the ears, the attendant needs to be certain to burp the infant before decompression. This allows any gas that has been accumulated in the stomach during the therapy to be expelled. If this does not occur, the gas may expand, possibly causing the regurgitation of stomach contents. A nasogastric tube may be used to vent gastric distention. (5)

ANXIETY

Children have an active imagination. This may be advantageous or it may increase the child's anxiety, i.e., Spock's casket, rocket, submarine, or Snow White's glass casket. Initial teaching and orientation is very important. Examples of a child-focused approach include puppets for role-play and desensitization to the unit by visiting the unit first. Older children may have more anxiety.

During infancy and childhood, the parent controls the treatment regimen of the child, making it essential to work effectively with parents. You must establish rapport with both parents and child and assess their readiness and ability to learn. It is important to determine what type of relationship exists between parents and child and between both the parents. Assess the child's ability to understand concepts, cognitive ability, and emotional maturity. Parents who are very anxious may increase the anxiety of the child. Carefully orient parents to hyperbaric oxygen therapy and pay attention to their concerns to alleviate as much apprehension as possible. Establishing trust is another method of decreasing anxiety. The staff should be careful to always follow through with what the patient has been told will happen.

Distraction during the treatment is another method for making the hyperbaric environment less different and intimidating. In elective as well as emergent situations, distraction during treatment is a valuable tool for stress avoidance. Televisions and VCRs work as excellent distractions in the monoplace chamber. Two rules must be kept in mind when selecting methods of distraction:

- Items used in a multiplace chamber must not represent a safety hazard – common sense will need to be the guide, as few things are labeled "intrinsically safe." Most toys would **NOT** be allowed in a monoplace unit.

- Items must be age-appropriate to be effective – the child's parents are excellent sources of information.

PRACTICAL CONSIDERATIONS IN THE TREATMENT OF CHILDREN

Hypothermia

The ratio of body surface to mass increases with decreasing age, resulting in a greater relative heat loss for infants. Core temperature maintenance is a biological priority and calories will be diverted to preserve it. If the infant's temperature starts to drop, calories will be diverted to preserve it because a sick infant cannot afford to lose calories. Also, the body's ability to generate heat is limited. Adiabatic cooling on chamber decompression further increases convective and conductive losses. Ventilation of the chamber imposes an added stress by increasing evaporative heat loss. Hypothermia is therefore a real concern in the treatment of infants. Special attention must be directed to detection and prevention of heat loss. "Physical assessment of the skin, looking for piloerection, shivering, cool skin, or mottling, identifies the problem when it is already present and potentially harmful." (1) The use of blankets can decrease evaporative losses by preventing exposure of the skin to air currents, as well as limiting convective and conductive losses through their insulating effects. By the time a child has developed language skills sufficient to express the concept of being cold, the body mass to surface area is usually no longer a problem leading to rapid heat losses.

PATIENT RESTRAINT

Physical restraint is often required in the practice of pediatric medicine to prevent the removal of needed medical devices such as I.V. access, nasogastric or endotracheal tubes. Sedation may make the restraints more bearable to the child.

Although detailed studies have defined the safe limits of exposure to hyperbaric oxygen therapy for adults, no such studies have been done to define safe limits for all age groups. Based on case reports in the literature, they do not appear to be at an increased risk for developing pulmonary or CNS oxygen toxicity.

CULTURAL CONSIDERATIONS

Culture has great influence on people in many ways. Child-rearing practices are unique from one culture to another. Customs and values taught by parents and/or extended families influence how patients interpret their illness and how they will interact with a healthcare provider. It is important to know the cultural considerations when treating any age patient. If you get a wide variety of cultures represented in your hospital or facility, it is suggested to have resource material available for reference. A suggested book, but not the only one available, is *Mosby's Pocket Guide* Series: Cultural Assessment, 2nd Edition 1998 by Elaine M. Giessler.

GROUPS DEFINED

Defining age groups can be tricky. Your hospital or organization should determine the different age groups according to the patient population served. They can be grouped by chronological age, functional age, or life stage, the most common type of grouping.(10) The following are groupings by life stage which are summarized for important issues in the hyperbaric environment. There are several great books and articles that define different age groups very well. The references at the end of this chapter would be a good place to start if you are looking for help in that area.

THE CRITICALLY ILL CHILD

With the availability of monitoring hemodynamic parameters in the monoplace chamber, and the ability to maintain multiple intravascular access routes during hyperbaric oxygen therapy, the management of the critical pediatric patient in the chamber does not differ from the management in a pediatric intensive care unit. (5)

Infancy—Birth to 12 Months

Stimulation and consistency are important for developing trust. This stage of life is one of total dependency. Always handle an infant in a gentle, comforting, and soothing manner. Speak in a soft, comforting voice.(8) Embracing and talking to the child and using stimulating toys like mobiles, is important.(6) However, avoid over-stimulation. Be aware of "stranger anxiety" and try to limit the number of staff workers assigned to the infant. An infant has immature heat regulation and needs to be kept warm. Support and protect the infant's head since he or she is still developing muscle strength, and in the neonate, the fontanels of the head are still soft and not completely closed. Keep a safe environment. Children's initial reflex is to place things in their mouths. Hand-washing is very important to remember with children because of their tendency to catch colds when exposed to other children, as they do in day-care environments.(8)

Treatment protocols for infants are 2 ATA for 45 or 60 minutes QD or BID for a chronic condition and 2 ATA for 30 or 45 minutes up to QID emergently.(7) Hyperoxia possibly inducing retrolental fibroplasia is of concern only in pre-term infants during the first weeks of life.

Toddler—1 to 3 Years

These children are rapidly growing and acquiring language skills. Their efforts to communicate shift from crying and gibberish into using simple words and short sentences. It is important to talk to and listen to children. Their world is explored through direct sensory contact, such as tasting, touching, looking, listening, and smelling. They are still very dependent, but start to develop a separate self. Safety is still a key focus because of toddlers' growing independence with mobility and their need to explore. Establish rapport with a toddler by being warm and matter-of-fact. Remember that the toddler does not reason well and may take what is said literally. Use simple, accurate terms when talking to a toddler about hyperbaric therapy. (6)

Typical protocols for a toddler are 2 ATA for 60 minutes QD or BID for a chronic condition and 2 ATA for 45-60 minutes up to QID for an acute condition. (7)

Preschool—3 to 6 Years

Children in this age group, although still identifying with the parent, are developing their own identity and independence. In this stage of life, growth slows a little but motor skills increase, and children begin to learn many new skills such as dressing themselves and toilet training. Cooperative play begins and imaginary friends are common. Explain topics clearly and reassure the child. Injury and disease can be very upsetting to children. Young children tend to create fantasies, so a minor wound may translate that they will loose the entire affected limb. It is appropriate to include both the child and parents in teaching about procedures at this stage and allow them to make some reasonable choices, but remember that he may not be able to recognize another's point of view. Explanations should be simple and matter-of-fact, and always before you start the procedure, toys and games can provide great teaching aids. Preschoolers have many fears and open expressions of these should be dealt with and encouraged. Use distractions to divert attention from frightening procedures. (6,8)

Protocols for this age group are 2 ATA for 60 minutes QD or BID for chronic and 2 ATA for 45-60 minutes up to QID for acute conditions. (7)

Late Childhood—6 to 12 Years

Growth continues slowly until there is a spurt at puberty. Children at this age are developing their own self-concept. They develop a sense of responsibility and reliability and their own set of values. While they are developing a greater sense of self, there is also a great need to fit in. The school-age child is capable of logical reasoning, although some magical thinking may persist. They often still prefer rituals. The child should be included in teaching at this stage. Explain procedures in uncomplicated terms, using correct terminology. Also explain why things are done in a logical, confident, and optimistic manner. (6) Allow the child to explore the chamber and equipment ahead of time. Set aside extra time for training and teaching sessions. Provide privacy when necessary. (8)

Chronic treatment protocols are 2 ATA for 75 minutes QD or BID and acute treatment protocols are 2 ATA for 60 minutes up to QID. (7)

Adolescent—13 to 20 Years

In this stage, growth spurts increase and the body transforms into an adult, sexually mature body, and physical appearance becomes increasingly important. At this age adolescents are able to entertain complex moral thinking, and begin to make up their own minds and choose their own values. Develop a relationship directly with the child. The adolescent can understand explanations and abstract concepts. While the parent should still be included in education, focus mainly on the child. Talk directly to the adolescent, not through the parents. The adolescent is moving away from the parent toward his/her own identity and may resist authority. This is a stress-filled age. He/she is preoccupied with changes in the body and appearance and is making sexual adjustments. The adolescent can't imagine that he/she could be sick or injured, so risk-taking and poor compliance with healthcare recommendations that he/she feels interfere with peer support and acceptance is common. Encourage questions about their fears. It is important to respect the adolescent's modesty and privacy. They respond better to guidance than lectures. Realistic limits that still foster independence are needed. (6) Always explain why something is being done. Respect any expressed or implied religious or cultural beliefs. (8)

Treatment protocols are the same as for adults.

Young Adult—21 to 39 Years

Young adults are still attaining the new skills that will assist them at home and at work. During this period, a person forms long-term relationships and adjusts his/her lifestyle to live with another person. He/she is establishing and managing a home and an occupation, and is beginning a family. All of these milestones are stressful. A person's responsibilities may be barriers to compliance that need to be dealt with. Finances, family responsibilities, and work schedule may make it difficult to follow health recommendations. Explore the impact of hospitalization or illness on the patient's job or family. Health promotion, dealing with stress, risk factors, and identification of resources are all important issues during this stage. (6)

Midlife—40 to 64 Years

Patients at this stage are generally at the peak of their career. Adults of this age have had tremendous life experiences and continue to use them to learn and create and solve problems. This is a time of re-examination of goals, values, and achievements. The individual may be in the process of modifying those parts of his/her life that he/she sees as unsatisfactory. Children are leaving the home, but the individual's parents are now adding new responsibilities for him/her to deal with. While adapting to new roles, the patient is increasingly aware of his/her own mortality. This group needs to be made aware of age-related changes in their senses, such as reduced visual and auditory acuteness and slower reflexes, and how this may affect activities such as driving. This can also be a time of mid-life crisis when some people begin to doubt themselves and their contributions and they need encouragement. Be sure to acknowledge their abilities and contributions throughout life. (6,8)

Geriatric—65 to Death

There is no reason to think a person at this stage is in mental decline. Many patients at this stage are dealing with chronic diseases. The patient is dealing with many losses, decreased independence, and loss of self-esteem and personal satisfaction. Treat these patients with interest and respect, using first names only when invited to do so. In presenting information, stand close to the patient and speak slowly and concisely – not necessarily loudly. In addition to the specific illness, the patient may wish to discuss sexuality and aging, exercise and aging, or nutrition. Be realistic, hopeful, and optimistic in dealing with older patients. Avoid clichés.

Identify barriers to independence and make the most of the patient's abilities. Consider individual needs and provide information about available community resources. Understand that noncompliance in this group may be the result of misunderstanding, physical limitations, or financial barriers. (6) Provide for warmth in the chamber environment because of the possibility of decreased heat regulation. Make the environment safer, such as removing any obstacles or hazards that would interfere or impede with mobility. Offer contacts to support services. Safety grips and similar aids may become crucial at this age. Many people at this age begin to accept that the end of their life is approaching and begin to prepare for it. Major emotional issues for older adults are to remain respected, prevent isolation, encourage expression of feelings and thoughts, encourage humor, and stay positive to help prevent depression. It is important to avoid treating an older adult like a child. (8)

CONCLUSION

There are many distinct differences in people as they pass through each stage of life. As nurses, we need many skills and abilities to meet our customers' needs. Knowledge of the age-related differences in physical, developmental, cognitive, and psychosocial areas makes us even better equipped to take care of our patients.

APPENDICES

Competency Assessment Form Examples

Age-Specific Care Competency

The following is not necessarily the best example, but it is a sample that I adopted from several examples I found in the references listed at the end, using my hospital's age-specific information.

Physical Factors Motor/Sensory Adaptation Cognitive Psychosocial Infancy: Birth to One Year

- Fontanels are open and soft for one month
- Experiences rapid weight gain
- Holds head erect and steady by three months
- Can grasp objects placed in hands for short time
- Responds to human voices by turning to sound at four months
- Startled by sounds unfamiliar or harsh
- Communicates needs through crying, i.e., discomfort or hunger
- Learns by imitation
- Recognizes bright objects and progresses to recognizing familiar objects and persons
- Begins mouthing words by six to nine months
- Explores world through direct sensory contact
- Completely dependent on caregivers
- Develops a sense of trust and security if needs are met consistently

Interventions

- Involve parents in education and planning
- Involve parents in procedure and education of procedures whenever possible
- Keep parents in infant's line of vision
- Provide a protective environment, especially the head of a neonate
- Medication preparations are based on weight
- Ensure infant warmth due to immature heat regulation
- Provide comfort measures such as cuddling and hugs
- Speak softly to infant
- Increase trust by meeting the infant's needs
- Give familiar objects to infant
- Consider safety when performing all procedures

Physical Factors Motor/Sensory Adaptation Cognitive Psychosocial Pediatric: 1 to 12 Years

(Can make this group more defined into Toddler, Preschooler and School-Age, especially if you have a pediatric department)

- Arms and legs lengthen from ossification and long bone growth
- Hearing has fully developed at age three

- First permanent teeth erupt between ages four and five
- Visual acuity 20/20 by age four
- Age six, dexterity increases, child very active
- Sensory fully developed by age six. Can maneuver up and down stairs alone by placing both feet on a step before moving to the next
- At 15 months, feeds self with little difficulty
- Catches and throws ball well
- Age seven, repeats activities to become proficient at them
- Begins imitating parents
- By three, has a 900-word vocabulary and uses short sentences
- Asks meaning of new words
- Capable of producing all sounds in native language
- Parents are key figures
- Tolerates some separation from mother
- Age four, very independent and aggressive, shows off and tattles on others
- May have imaginary playmate
- May become highly self-critical

Interventions

- Keep parents nearby and involved in the child's care
- Explain procedure to child and parent before you start
- Allow choice when possible
- Explain procedures using correct terminology that the child will understand, such as what child will see, feel, hear, and smell
- Allow for longer teaching sessions
- Give one direction at a time
- If child has imaginary friend, listen closely as the child may be conveying his/her feelings or fears
- Offer reassurance, often very critical of how they do things or what happens to them
- Use a firm direct approach when needed
- Use distraction techniques
- Provide for privacy
- Offer bathroom breaks if potty trained
- Provide a safe environment, do not leave unattended
- Medication preparation is based on weight of child
- Oxygen delivery using appropriate size equipment
- Identify motor and social skills to determine types of food that may help meet dietary requirements
- Allow for religious and cultural beliefs as expressed by parents

Physical Factors Motor/Sensory Adaptation Cognitive Psychosocial Adolescent: 13 to 17 Years

- Rapid growth
- Hormonal changes, secondary sexual characteristics develop

- Sensory is fully developed early, the adolescent is clumsy as he/she adapts to body changes
- Need for sleep increases to meet growth demands
- Communication becomes fully developed
- Can handle hypothetical situations or thought
- Begins to think about future occupation
- Has peer groups and is looking into freedom
- Own identity is very important
- Often critical of own features and concerned with physical appearance
- Reluctant to accept advice or criticism

Interventions

- Explain procedure to adolescent directly, with parents present, using correct terminology
- Provide time away from family for expression of questions and unease
- Explain "whys" of procedures
- Provide privacy
- Encourage questions regarding "fears"
- Involve adolescent in decision-making and planning
- Allow adolescent to maintain control, realize there may be some resistance
- Allow for religious and cultural beliefs in providing care
- Medication preparation is based on weight as appropriate for adolescent
- Maintain confidentiality

PHYSICAL FACTORS MOTOR/SENSORY ADAPTATION COGNITIVE PSYCHOSOCIAL ADULT: 18 TO 70 YEARS (Can divide this into Young Adult-18-25, Adulthood-26-38, and Middle Adult-39-69)

- Physical development complete
- Aging begins in late 20s and early 30s
- After age 38, physiologic functions start to gradually slow
- Motor, sensory, and communication skills fully developed
- At 45, starts to have prolonged response to stress, slowing of reflexes, visual changes, and hearing loss
- Muscles and joints respond slower with aging
- Finally viewed as adult
- Learning commitment and making decisions which impact life
- Worries increase if ill or hospitalized because of job or family
- May feel loss because of inability to control what is happening
- Young adult has desire to assume adult commitments
- Adult has strong commitment to goals
- Middle adult often faces mid-life crisis associated with role changes, children leaving home

Interventions

- Listen to needs and respect feelings
- Involve patient in decision-making and control of plan for treatment and care
- Provide education to patient and/or significant others
- Education is based on learning ability identified by assessment
- Explain equipment use and procedures
- Allow for elimination needs
- Allow for religious and cultural beliefs in providing care
- Provide mobility assistance as needed

PHYSICAL FACTORS MOTOR/SENSORY ADAPTATION COGNITIVE PSYCHOSOCIAL GERIATRIC: 70 TO DEATH

- Decrease in visual and hearing acuity
- Taste buds and sense of smell decreases
- Decreased activity level
- Gradual decrease related to physiologic changes related to vision, hearing, taste, and smell
- Decreased pain tolerance
- With decreased sensory, communication may be affected
- Mental functions and memory decreases
- Health problems become an increasing concern
- May feel increased sense of loss as one retires, looses friends/spouse through death, watch for signs of depression

Interventions

- Speak distinctly due to loss of ability to discriminate sounds
- Be a listener
- Provide education based on learning ability identified by assessment
- Use teaching with larger print
- Utilize proper lighting
- Provide frequent breaks due to fatigue and decreased muscle tone
- Assist with position changes slowly due to possible hemodynamic changes

REFERENCES

1. P. Thoms; R. Borer, Jr.; and F. Martorano, "Hyperbaric Medicine in Pediatric Practice." Hyperbaric Medicine Practice 2nd Edition, E. Kindwall and H. Whelan, Editors. Best Publishing Company. Flagstaff, AZ. 1999, (pp. 340-351).
2. Kindwall, E., Hyperbaric Medicine Practice 2nd Edition. E. Kindwall and H. Whelan, Editors. Best Publishing Company. Flagstaff, AZ, 1999, (pp. 340-351).
3. Oriani, G.; Marroni, A.; and Wattel, F. (editors), Handbook on Hyperbaric Medicine. Springer – Verlag, Berlin, Germany. 1996. (pp. 207-210, 325-326).
4. Davis, J.C. and Hunt, T.K. (editors), Hyperbaric Oxygen Therapy. Undersea and Hyperbaric Medical Society, Bethesda, Maryland. 1977. pp. 329-341.
5. Martorano, F.J. and Hoover, D., "The Child Hyperbaric Patient." Rocky Mountain Regional Baromedical Center, Porter Memorial Hospital, Denver, Colorado. (Handout from presentation).
6. Patient Education and Age Appropriate Information used with permission from Curative Health Services and adapted from Falvo, D., Effective Patient Education: A Guide to Increased Compliance. Aspen Publishers, Maryland. 1994.
7. Dose Schedules for Pediatrics came from Handout from Long Beach Memorial Hyperbaric Unit.
8. Age Specific Care, Gateway Medical Staffing, Inc., St. Louis, MO 2000.
9. Wolgin, F., Advanced Skills and Competency Assessment for Care Givers with Age Specific Considerations, vol. II, Prentice-Hall Inc. Upper Saddle River, NJ, 1999.
10. Topics in Clinical Care Improvement: Age-Specific Competence, Joint Commission on Accreditation of Healthcare Organizations, Oakbrook Terrace, IL 1998.
11. Hall, J.L., "Developing Meaningful Age-Appropriate Competencies for Clinical Services," Journal for Nurses in Staff Development, 1999, Vol. 15, No. 6, pp. 241-251.
12. Burke, A., "Age Specific Competency Throughout the Life Span," www.nursingceu.com
13. Luckmann, J. Ed., Saunders Manual of Nursing Care, W.B. Saunders Co., Philadelphia, PA, 1997.
14. 2001 Hospital Accreditation Standards, Joint Commission on Accreditation of Healthcare Organizations, Oakbrook Terrace, IL.

NOTES

1. [illegible] Hyperbaric Medicine [illegible] Hyperbaric Medicine Practice, 2nd Edition, [illegible] and H.T. Whelan, editors. Best Publishing Company, Flagstaff, AZ. [illegible]

2. [illegible] Hyperbaric Medicine Practice, 2nd [illegible] Best Publishing Company, Flagstaff, AZ, [illegible]

3. Oriani G, Marroni A, and Wattel F, [illegible] Handbook on Hyperbaric Medicine. Springer-Verlag, Berlin, Germany, [illegible]

4. Davis JC and Hunt TK, [illegible] Hyperbaric Oxygen Therapy. [illegible] Hyperbaric Medical Society, Bethesda, Maryland. [illegible]

5. [illegible] and Hoover, [illegible] "The Critical Hyperbaric Patient" [illegible] Porter Memorial Hospital, Denver, Colorado. [illegible] presentation.

6. Patient Education and Age-appropriate [illegible] Centura Health Services and adopted [illegible] Patient Education [illegible] Guide to Increased Compliance. Aspen Publishers, [illegible]

7. [illegible] Hyperbaric Unit.

8. [illegible]

9. [illegible] Skills and competency [illegible] Age-Specific [illegible]

10. [illegible]

11. Hill [illegible] Development [illegible] Age-appropriate competencies [illegible] Journal of Nurses in Staff Development [illegible]

12. [illegible]

13. [illegible] Manual of Nursing [illegible] Philadelphia, PA 1997.

14. [illegible] Hospital Accreditation Standards [illegible]

CHAPTER IV

INDICATIONS FOR HYPERBARIC OXYGEN THERAPY

D. CRITZ

INTRODUCTION

Hyperbaric oxygen therapy is defined as a treatment by which the entire person is exposed to greater than 1.2 atmospheres absolute (ATA) while breathing 100% oxygen. This treatment can be provided in a monoplace (single person) chamber or a multiplace chamber. There are currently thirteen disease categories for which the Undersea and Hyperbaric Medical Society (UHMS) recommends the use of hyperbaric oxygen therapy.

In 1976, the Executive Committee of the Undersea and Hyperbaric Committee established the Hyperbaric Oxygen Therapy Committee. The Committee has the responsibility of reviewing research and clinical information as it relates to the efficacy of the use of hyperbaric oxygen therapy in the treatment of specific diseases. The data for disease treatment is reviewed every two years and a new Oxygen Therapy Committee Report is published.

Proposed new indications are reviewed on an annual basis during the UHMS Scientific meeting. A position paper on the proposed indication is presented to the Oxygen Therapy Committee. Two committee members are then assigned to review data and present it to the Committee. For an indication to be accepted, there must be a consensus of the Hyperbaric Oxygen Therapy Committee.

HYPERBARIC TREATMENT INDICATIONS: APPROVED USES

DECOMPRESSION SICKNESS (DCS)

Actions of HBO:
- Hyperoxygenate hypoxic tissues
- Hasten elimination of inert gas
- Reduce edema
- Overcome intravascular and other free gases

Decompression sickness arises from the formation of gas bubbles in tissue or blood in volumes sufficient enough to interfere with the function of an organ or to cause alteration in sensation. Rapid decompression during ascent from diving, flying, and working in a compressed air tunnel or in a hyperbaric/ hypobaric chamber may cause DCS. Bubbles usually form within the venous system and are carried by the blood to the right side of the heart and eventually lodge in the lungs. When bubbles reach the arterial system, which normally doesn't occur, the symptoms escalate. Effects of the bubbles can be either from mechanical obstruction or surface activity found at the blood/gas interface. The blood-gas interface can activate the complement system, result in platelet aggregation, and activate the Hagemen factor.

Two types of DCS may occur: Type I (musculoskeletal pain) and Type II. Aching pain in a limb after diving is the most classic and common symptom of DCS. Type II DCS can occur alone or in combination with musculoskeletal pain. The three principle targets of Type II are pulmonary, vestibular, and nervous systems. Multiple symptoms can be present and vary depending on the systems affected.

Treatment of choice for decompression illness is recompression with 100% oxygen in a hyperbaric chamber to wash out inert nitrogen and to replace it with oxygen that is metabolized. The result is immediate reduction in the volume of bubbles (Boyle's Law), eliminating symptoms, and restoring tissue oxygenation. Beneficial effects in cerebral blood flow result in a reduction of edema and an increase in oxygen diffusion distance, resulting in less cell destruction.

Several reference guides are available for detailed information on symptoms and treatment guidelines. Divers Alert Network (DAN) is available twenty-four hours/day for consultation.

ACUTE CARBON MONOXIDE POISONING (CO)
(including smoke inhalation and cyanide poisoning)

Actions of HBO:

- Hasten the elimination of carbon monoxide from hemoglobin and other tissues
- Hyperoxygenate hypoxic tissues
- Antagonize brain lipid peroxidation

Carbon Monoxide (CO), a colorless, odorless, non-irritating gas, is the leading cause of death from a poisonous gas in the United States.

CO attaches itself to hemoglobin with an affinity 200-250 times that of oxygen and blocks oxygen transport to vital tissues. CO acts as a tissue toxin, disrupting cellular metabolism and preventing oxygen's release to the tissues and vital organs. The oxygen dissociation curve shifts to the left, keeping oxygen bound to the hemoglobin and causing tissue hypoxia and eventually death with high exposures.

Toxicity causes hypoxia, impaired tissue perfusion, hypotension induced by hypoxia, and CO binding to cardiac myoglobin, which depresses myocardium. Cellular toxicity secondary to cytochrome malfunction demonstrates cytochrome oxidase binding to CO. Mitochondrial (energy of our cells) malfunctioning is the reason patients may remain comatose when carboxyhemoglobin levels have decreased to zero. Persistent mitochondrial malfunction explains manifestations of toxicity that occur days after the exposure. Brain lipid peroxidation may provide a link between hypoxia and cellular toxicity related to clinical symptoms and CO levels. Research has noted that by preventing lipid peroxidation in the brain, side effects associated with exposure to carbon monoxide may be decreased.

Flu-like symptoms are often associated with CO poisoning. Headache, drowsiness, fatigue, nausea, vomiting, weakness, and dizziness can cause a delay in diagnosing the patient. Significant neurological deficits such as alterations in thinking, concentration, recall, and short-term memory loss can result from exposure to non-fatal levels of carbon monoxide.

Sources of CO occur anywhere fossil fuels are burned, such as furnaces, automobile exhaust, hot water heaters, gas stoves, space heaters, charcoal grills, gasoline engines, etc.

The first line of treatment for carbon monoxide is 100% oxygen with a non-rebreather mask. Patients who manifest signs of serious intoxication (i.e., alteration of mental status or neurological signs, unconsciousness, cardiovascular dysfunction, pulmonary edema, or severe acidosis) should be referred for hyperbaric oxygen therapy within six hours of exposure.

Acute or chronic exposures may cause a variety of neurological side effects or sequelae. These vary from cognitive and personality changes, psychic akinesia, parkinsonism, psychotic encephalopathy, amnesia, apathy, dementia, mutism, irritable distractibility, urinary and fecal incontinence, gait disturbance, muscle weakness, and symptoms resembling those of multiple sclerosis. These symptoms may be present in 2-30% of patients.

Gas Embolism ("Arterial Gas Embolism" or AGE)

Actions of HBO:

- Oxygenate ischemic/hypoxic tissues
- Reduce edema
- Reduces volume of gas bubbles
- Increases diffusion gradient of gas embolism

Air or gas embolism occurs when gases enter the venous or arterial vasculature causing varying degrees of ischemia in the affected areas. Symptoms may range from being undetectable to producing immediate and rapid death. When air enters the venous side, it is usually reabsorbed in the body or filtered by the pulmonary system. When air enters the arterial side, the result is frequently cerebral air embolism or coronary. As little as 0.4 cc of blood-air delivered to the right place in the medulla can be fatal.

Gas embolism can result from sudden decompression during diving and altitude exposure, cardiovascular surgery, angioplasty, trauma, invasive line insertions, mechanical positive pressure ventilation, pneumothorax, invasive procedures, and various pelvic, thoracic, vascular, and neuro surgeries. Rare causes may be from faulty abortion and orogenital sex during pregnancy.

Manifestations of AGE can include loss of consciousness, focal neurological deficits, seizures, cardiac arrest, arrhythmias, or ischemia. Venous embolism may exhibit symptoms of hypotension, tachypnea, or pulmonary edema.

Hyperbaric therapy reduces the bubble size (Boyle's Law). At 6 ATA bubble size can be reduced to one-sixth its size. At 3 ATA bubble size can be reduced to less than half the size, thus allowing more oxygen to the area and reversing tissue hypoxia. In conjunction with pressure, 100% oxygen will wash out any inert gas, leaving metabolizable oxygen.

Patients with less serious symptoms should have 100% oxygen on and be placed in the supine position. Oxygen reduces the size of the air bubble by depleting the nitrogen and reverses hypoxia and ischemia in the brain tissue or affected area.

GAS GANGRENE (CLOSTRIDIAL)

Actions of HBO:

- Halt production of alpha toxin
- Limit bacterial proliferation
- Hyperoxygenate ischemic/hypoxic tissues
- Improve host defenses

Clostridial myositis and myonecrosis (gas gangrene) is an acute, rapidly progressive intoxication of the muscle by the clostridial organism.

This is an anaerobic, spore-forming, gram-positive encapsulated bacilli of the genus clostridium. The most common is *C. perfringens*, which occurs in 80-90% of wounds.

C.oedematiens occurs in 40%, with *C.septicum* in 20% and *C.histolyticum, bifermentons,* and *fallux* in the other 10%. *C.perfringens* is a normal flora of the GI tract and is not a strict anaerobe. It may grow freely in oxygen tensions of 30 mmHg with restricted growth in oxygen tensions up to 70 mmHg. (Kindwall, 1995, p. 374)

The disease process ensues from elaboration of exotoxins by the organisms and may be better described as intoxication rather than an infection. Seven of over 20 exotoxins, produced by the 6 species of clostridial organisms are capable of producing gas gangrene as a lethal toxin in the body. Alpha toxin is the lecithinase C that is a rapidly spreading liquification necrosis.

Clinical data is supported by demonstration of gram positive rods from the fluids of the involved tissue as well as absence of leukocytes.

Two things must happen in the wound for development of gas gangrene:

1. clostridial contamination
2. decreased oxidation reduction potential in the wound

Clostridial contamination is a common event, but when circulatory failure in the local area renders the wound ischemic and hypoxic, this is the precipitating factor in clostridial gas gangrene causing necrosis to the muscles.

Forms of Necrotizing Clostridial Disease

- *Clostridial Myonecrosis with Toxicity:*
  diffuse, rapid spreading of the toxicity from the initial site (true gas gangrene), acute onset following incubation from 4 hours to 2-3 days
- *Localized Clostridial Myonecrosis:*
  seen following non-sterile injections of drugs, usually remains localized
- *Clostridial Cellulitis without Toxicity:*
  involves subcutaneous tissue without invasion of muscle, usually incision and drainage for treatment
- *Clostridial Cellulitis with Toxicity:*
  same clinical picture as spreading clostridial myonecrosis, appears to be more localized

Signs and symptoms usually occur one–six hours after injury. Sudden and severe pain may develop in the infected area.

Early phases:

- skin may appear taut and shiny
- progresses to dusky bronze discoloration
- can advance quickly (several inches in one hour)
- hemorragic bullae or vesicles may also be noted
- excudate with sweet odor
- swelling and edema are pronounced
- muscles appear dark red to black or greenish

The patient should be treated as soon as possible with antibiotics, surgery, and if possible treated in the hyperbaric chamber at 3 ATA, 3 times in the first 24 hours and BID until it is felt the clostridial organism is controlled. Then the patient may be moved into a wound-healing protocol.

Treatment composed of a combination of surgery, antibiotics, and adjunctive hyperbaric oxygen therapy has been shown to decrease mortality. Hyperbaric oxygen therapy stops alpha-toxin production by increasing tissue oxygenation greater than 250 mmHg and inhibits bacterial growth, thus enabling the body to utilize its own host defense mechanisms.

EXCEPTIONAL BLOOD LOSS

Actions of HBO:
- Temporally improve oxygenation to hypoxic/ischemic tissues
- Increase dissolved oxygen concentrations

Exceptional blood loss anemia is a loss of red blood cells in which the body's ability to deliver oxygen to vital tissues is compromised as a result of trauma, surgery, medical, or religious reasons.

Red blood cells carry oxygen throughout the body via oxygen pick-up in the lungs. If the amount of red blood cells decreases, the amount of oxygen delivered to the tissues has decreased. This causes ischemia and hypoxic conditions in the body, resulting in death in severe cases. The brain and heart are our biggest oxygen users and quickly have irreversible damage.

Replacement of red blood cells in acute conditions is emergent. However, there are other alternatives, which include fluorocarbons or stroma-free hemoglobin, or other volume expanders. Due to medical reasons, such as incompatibility in type and cross-match, idiopathic autoimmune hemolytic anemia, or patient refusal due to religious beliefs, blood transfusions may not be the option.

Signs and symptoms:
- *Cardiovascular:* chest discomfort, neck pain, angina, arrhythmia, increase heart rate, increased blood pressure, and acute myocardial infarction
- *Central nervous system (brain):* confusion, agitation, decreased cognition
- *Metabolic:* ischemic bowel symptoms
- *Biochemical:* lactic acidosis, respiratory alkalosis

Treatment with supplemental oxygen is essential, and if conditions become critical, hyperbaric oxygen therapy is added. The problem with both therapies is the toxic effect of oxygen. The prime reason for using hyperbaric oxygen therapy is to dissolve enough oxygen in plasma (Henry's Law) in the severely anemic patient to support tissue survival and reverse tissue hypoxia.

Hyperbaric oxygen therapy should be given intermittently every two-four hours or until the RBCs have been replaced and signs and symptoms of tissue hypoxia have been alleviated.

Osteoradionecrosis (Mandible) and Soft Tissue Radiation Necrosis

Actions of HBO:

- Enhance neovascularization in irradiated and other hypoxic tissues
- Reduce tissue fibrosis when used prophylatically

Hyperbaric oxygen (HBO) is used as an adjunct in the treatment of radiation injury at many sites, including the mandible, larynx, chest wall, bladder, and rectum. Radiation injury may occur 6 months or years after the radiation therapy. Delayed radiation tissue injury is characterized by endarteritis, tissue hypoxia, and fibrosis. Caution should be taken regarding surgery on a client with a history of past radiation.

Hyperbaric oxygen's primary indication in the treatment of radiation necrosis is to increase the oxygen gradient in the irradiated tissue or bone, thus initiating angiogenesis. Oxygen levels in the irradiated area are very low, not allowing the body to recognize that an injury has occurred. Tissue oxygen gradients decrease over time in an irradiated area, causing the wound or irradiated area to worsen.

In the normal wound, oxygen gradients may be low in the center of the wound with the gradient of oxygen around the wound at a normal level, around 50-60 mmHg. This allows for the body's natural wound healing phases to occur. In the irradiated wound, the oxygen gradient is very low in the center of the wound and may be low far beyond the wound bed.

During hyperbaric oxygen therapy, the oxygen levels increase to 1500-2200 mmHg, causing an increase of oxygen in the wound bed and surrounding the wound. While oxygen is increased, the gradient remains. This stimulates neovascularization.

Protocols for treatment have been based on research by Drs. Robert Marx and Robert Johnson and are widely published.

Crush Injuries, Acute Traumatic Peripheral Ischemia (ATPI)

Actions of HBO:

- Increase oxygenation to ischemic/hypoxic tissues
- Reduce edema
- Optimize limb salvage

These injuries, if severe, place life and limb of the patient at risk. ATPIs include: crush injuries, compartment syndrome, thermal burns, frost bite injuries, compromised skin grafts and flaps, degloving injuries, and threatened reattachments.

Hyperbaric oxygen should be administered within four–six hours of the injury to assist in protection of the tissues from reperfusion injury. Reperfusion injury will block the capillaries, causing venous congestion and stopping blood flow and oxygen from getting to vital tissues. The physiology of reperfusion injury and hyperbaric therapy is that HBO antagonizes lipid peroxidation of the cell, blocks the sequestration of neutrophils on post-capillary venules, antagonizes the beta 2 integrin system, and generates oxygen radical scavengers. In simple terms, HBO decreases venous congestion, allowing a greater flow of oxygen and blood to the tissues.

Hyperoxygenation of the hypoxic tissue with HBO allows the host to respond to infection and reduces ischemic injury to tissue. HBO will dissolve oxygen in the plasma, allowing oxygen to reach levels of 2200 mmHg.

A secondary effect of tissue hyperoxygenation is edema reduction. Vasoconstriction induced by hyperbaric oxygen therapy reduces inflow by approximately 20% while maintaining outflow, and thus reduces edema by reabsorption of tissue fluids.

Compromised Skin Grafts/Flaps

Actions of HBO:

- Improve oxygenation in marginally perfused tissue
- Improve angiogenesis
- Improve host response

Hyperbaric oxygen therapy is not recommended for the uncompromised wound. Wounds with past irradiation and poor microcirculation may benefit from hyperbaric oxygen therapy.

Compromised skin grafts and flaps need to be treated within 4-6 hours of application to increase the chances of survival with adjunctive hyperbaric therapy. Hypoxic insult to the wound can cause the capillaries to have reperfusion injury, which further decreases oxygen supply. Oxygen of at least 30-40 mmHg is essential for fibroblasts to synthesize collagen matrix for capillary budding in avascular areas. (Camporesi, Baker, 1991, p. 153)

It generally takes two to three days for capillary invasion to take place when a new graft has been placed on the compromised wound bed. During this time period, the freshly applied skin graft may become hypoxic and risk for failure in the compromised wound bed markedly increases.

Hyperbaric oxygen stimulates the capillary proliferation, improves angiogenesis, improves the host response, and intermittently increases oxygenation to the graft site, therefore reducing reperfusion injury to the graft/flap.

Hyperbaric therapy should be initiated as soon as the patient has recovered from anesthesia and is given BID for at least three days, then QD until the graft is assessed and determined to be stable. If the graft/flap has failed and more surgery is planned, hyperbaric therapy can be given on a daily basis to prepare the wound bed for repeated grafting.

Refractory Osteomyelitis

Actions of HBO:

- Elevate oxygen tensions in infected bone
- Augment antibiotic therapy
- Stimulate neoangiogenesis within compromised vasculature of chronically infected bone

Refractory osteomyelitis is a chronic infection of the bone that has persisted for an extended period of time, despite I.V. antibiotics and surgical debridement. Chronic refractory osteomyelitis is usually the result of low oxygen levels at the wound site, foreign objects, hypo-perfusion, inflammation, poor nutrition, ineffective wound care, and antibiotic resistance organisms. Other factors can be poor patient compliance and overall health-related conditions.

Oxygen levels in infected bone, according to studies, are too low to support the wound healing phases. It has also been demonstrated that when adding hyperbaric oxygen therapy to the treatment protocol after conventional therapy has failed to show signs of improvement, oxygen tensions are shown to increase, improving the ability of the phagocytes to kill bacteria. *Staphylococcus epidermid, Pseudomonas aeruginosa, Escherchia coli* and *Staph aureus* in hypoxic conditions are not effectively destroyed by phagocytes. With oxygen tensions greater than 100 mmHg, phagocytes are more successful in killing bacteria.

Hyperbaric oxygen therapy assists in the promotion of fibroblast activity. Fibroblasts cannot synthesize collagen or migrate to the affected area when oxygen tensions are less than 30 mmHg. Intermittent HBO can assist the body in returning to normal fibroblastic activity. In addition, osteoclast function is oxygen-dependent and HBO is able to provide an optimum environment for the osteoclast to remove necrotic bone.

The Cierny-Mader classification of osteomyelitis can be used as a reference in determining what classification of osteomyelitis would benefit from hyperbaric oxygen therapy. (Hampson, 1999, p. 48)

PROGRESSIVE NECROTIZING INFECTIONS (NECROTIZING FASCIITIS, MELENEY ULCER)

Actions of HBO:

- Demarcate potentially viable from non-viable tissue
- Improve wound-healing responses
- Improve oxygen ischemic/hypoxic tissue beds

Necrotizing soft tissue infections are usually polymicrobial in nature; either anaerobic or aerobic. These infections usually occur after trauma, around foreign objects, and post surgery. There is generally a compromising condition, such as diabetes, causing some type of hypoxic conditions to occur and allowing the host to become compromised.

Primary treatment of choice is surgical debridement and the administration of systemic antibiotics. Hyperbaric therapy has been added to assist in the bactericidal effects that oxygen has on anaerobic bacterial growth. Clinical symptoms are tissue necrosis, putrid discharge, gas production, and gross undermining or tunneling of the infection without apparent involvement of the skin. These infections may be difficult to differentiate from the more serious clostridial infections until culture results are available.

FORMS OF NECROTIZING SOFT TISSUE INFECTIONS

1. Crepitant Anaerobic Cellulitis
    - Acute anaerobic infection of soft tissue
    - Gas abscess (sometimes know as clostridial cellulitis)
    - Not a clostridial toxin-induced disease
    - Deep fascia is not involved
    - Inflammation of the subcutaneous tissues
    - Two–five day onset
        - Pain milder than necrotizing fasciitis
        - Foul odor of wound

In the client with non-complicating conditions, surgery and antibiotic therapy is sufficient. In the client that is markedly compromised or if the infection is advanced when diagnosis is made, HBO may be added.

2. Progressive Bacterial Gangrene
    - Subacute chronic dermal ulcer
    - Usually found on the abdomen or thoracic wall
    - May appear around a colostomy or ileostomy site or in a chronic skin lesion

- Major symptoms are extreme pain and tenderness
- Lesion usually appears first or second week after surgery
- Little systemic reaction
- Wound is initially red, swollen, indurated in several days then becomes purplish color
- If progression occurs there are changes to dirty gray-brown or yellow green with a leathery appearance
- Deep fascia is not involved

Etiology is classically the combination of a microaerophilic or obligately anaerobic nonhemolytic *Streptococcus* and *Staphylococcus aureus* or in some cases a *Proteus* species found primarily in the zone of gangrene. (Hampson, 1999, p. 42)

3. Meleney's Ulcer—essentially the same as progressive bacterial gangrene except:
   - Has burrowing necrotic tracks extending through tissue planes and emerging at distant skin sites
   - Usually seen following lymph node surgery in the axilla, groin, neck
   - May be seen after operation of the large bowel or female genital tract

4. Necrotizing Fasciitis—precipitating factors diabetics, alcoholism, parenteral drug abuse, obesity, underlying vascular disease, poor nutrition
   - Severe deep infection, involves the superficial and deep fascia
   - Rapid spread of necrosis along fascial planes with subsequent undermining and necrosis of skin
   - Most commonly affects the extremities
   - Other sites may be abdominal wall, perianal and groin area, post-op wounds
   - Entry of the infection is usually the site of the trauma
   - Acute sudden onset of pain
   - Considerable phlegmon may be present with erythema and cellulitis
   - Fever and chills may or may not be present
   - Blue or brown ecchymotic skin discoloration
   - Onset one–four days
   - Profuse serosanguinous foul excudate
   - Extensive undermining of the skin and subcutaneous tissue occur with the skin becoming blue/black
   - Gas may be present
   - Moderate to marked toxemia

5. Fournier's Gangrene—necrotizing fasciitis
    - Seen in male or female patients, begins with genital pain in the scrotal or vulvar area
    - Essentially the same symptoms as stated in the necrotizing fasciitis category

Acute Thermal Burns

Actions of HBO:
- Limit tissue fluid losses
- Support marginally perfused subjacent tissue
- Limit conversion of second degree burns to third degree
- Promote wound closure
- Minimize edema

Burns should be treated in the hyperbaric chamber within the first 24 hours of injury for optimal outcome. The goal of hyperbaric therapy is to prevent reperfusion injury, reduce fluid resuscitation, decrease the extension of the burn injury, decrease the need for multiple surgery for debridement, decrease hospital stay, and has been shown to decrease the scarring associated with burn injuries.

Transport over distances is not recommended. In order to treat the patient in a hyperbaric chamber, the chamber should be located within the burn facility.

Problem Wounds

It is well established that hypoxia and infection characterize most problem wounds that have failed to respond to established medical and surgical management. HBO therapy specifically addresses both of these factors. The use of transcutaneous oximetry during a problem wound evaluation allows assessment of hypoxin and identification of those who are most likely to respond to HBO. The most common disease process associated with problem wounds is diabetes, which affects 12 million Americans. Diabetics account for 50 to 70% of all nontraumatic amputations in this country. Fortunately, HBO is helping to reduce this number. In a prospective and controlled clinical trail, Baroni (Diabetes Care, 1987) studied the effects of HBO therapy in the management of problem wounds of the lower extremity in a group of diabetics. Using HBO, the amputation rate dropped from 40% to 11%. A subsequent study by Oriani (J of Hyperbaric Medicine, 1992) looked at the role of HBO in diabetic gangrene of the foot. In the HBO group, 95% of the patients healed, and only 4.8% required amputation. In the non-HBO group, 33% required amputation ($p<0.001$). The most recent study by Faglia was prospective and randomized, with surgical blinding. Sixty-eight diabetic patients were consecutively admitted into the study. Only three (8.6%) patients in the hyperbaric group and eleven (33%)

patients in the non-hyperbaric group received major amputation: seven below the knee and four above the knee. The difference was significant at a p-value of 0.016. (Faglia E., et al. Diabetes Care 1996; 19: 1338-43) The adjunctive use of hyperbaric oxygen can restore a favorable cellular millieu in which the healing process and host antimicrobial mechanisms are enhanced.

This section on problem wounds is respectfully submitted with the permission of Dr. Terrance O. Kurtz, D.O., Infectious Disease and Hyperbaric Medicine.

Intracranial Abscess (ICA)

With improved mortality rates in this area, there is a general trend toward a more conservative approach in the management of the ICA patient.

Patients with multiple abscesses in a deep or dominate location, immune compromise, and no response or further deterioration in spite of standard surgical and antibiotic treatment pose major therapeutic problems.

Adjunctive hyperbaric therapy may have additional therapeutic benefit:

- Elevated oxygen concentrations may inhibit the flora found in ICA (anaerobic)
- Hyperbaric oxygen therapy can cause a reduction in perifocal brain swelling
- Enhancement of host's defense mechanisms
- May be of benefit in cases of concomitant skull osteomyelitis

Consider hyperbaric oxygen therapy under the following conditions:

- Multiple abscesses
- Abscesses in a deep or dominant location
- Compromised host
- Situations where surgery is contraindicated or where the patient is a poor surgical risk
- No response or further deterioration in spite of standard surgical (i.e., 1-2 needle aspirates) and antibiotic treatment

Hyperbaric treatment may be given once or twice per day. Coarse of treatment is based upon the patient's clinical response as well as radiological findings. The average number of treatments has been 13 to 20.

REFERENCES

1. Barker, A., Camporesi, E. (1991). Hyperbaric Oxygen Therapy: A Critical Review. Bethesda, MD: Undersea and Hyperbaric Medical Society.
2. Bove A.A., Davis J.C. (1990). Diving Medicine W.B. Saunders Co., Philadelphia, PA.
3. Hampson, N. (1999). Hyperbaric Oxygen Therapy: 1999 Committee Report. Kensington, MD: Undersea and Hyperbaric Medical Society.
4. Jain, K. (1996). Textbook of Hyperbaric Medicine: 2nd Revised Edition. Hogrefe & Huber Publishers.
5. Kindwall, E. (1995). Hyperbaric Medicine Practice: Flagstaff, AZ: Best Publishing Company.
6. Kindwall, E., Goldmann, R. (1995). Hyperbaric Medicine Procedures: St. Luke's, WI: St. Luke's Medical Center.

NOTES

CHAPTER V

ASSESSING THE CRITICALLY ILL HYPERBARIC MEDICINE PATIENT

V. LARSON-LOHR AND J. GARCIA

INTRODUCTION

The nursing care of critically ill patients can be challenging in a well-equipped intensive care unit or emergency department. In a monoplace hyperbaric oxygen environment, the nurse has the added challenge of physiologic changes related to increase in pressure, increase in oxygenation, and the restriction of not being able to provide "hands-on" care for what may be up to several hours. While critically ill patients had been treated in multiplace chambers since the late 1960s, it was not until the mid-1980s that the same patients were treated in monoplace hyperbaric chambers. Lindell Weaver, M.D., in Salt Lake City, Utah, pioneered the way and developed the tools and techniques used to treat extremely ill patients in the monoplace hyperbaric chamber. Many of the methods of treating critically ill patients discussed in this chapter are based on Dr. Weaver's research.

NEUROLOGICAL

Neurological Assessment

The assessment of neurological status is dependent on the presentation of the symptomology and on the diagnosis. You can integrate your neurological examination with other parts of your physical examination. Assess some of the cranial nerves as you examine the head and neck, and inspect the arms and legs for neurological abnormalities as you are inspecting the musculoskeletal system.[1] Organize your thinking into five categories: (1) mental status and speech, (2) cranial nerves, (3) the motor system, (4) the sensory system, and (5) reflexes.

Mental Status

The assessment of the mental status of patient in the hyperbaric setting can be crucial in the overall plan of care for that patient. Will the patient be able to follow instructions for Valsalva techniques? Will the patient be able understand directions as far as safety issues are concerned? What risk is the suicidal patient to self and your staff? These are some of the questions which the hyperbaric nurse must assess in a quick, thorough, and timely manner to ensure the proper management of the patient.

The assessment by the nurse begins immediately upon contact with patient. Begin with the most notable feature, the level of consciousness (LOC). Is the patient alert and aware of his/her surroundings? Is he/she oriented to person, place, time, and self? These determinations come into play when assessing every patient, but particularly the carbon monoxide (CO) poisoned patient and the injured SCUBA diver with decompression illness (DCI). The nurse should utilize a standard recognized qualitative format for the documentation of the patient LOC and cognitive function. The Glascow coma scale and the mini mind-set exam are examples of these measures (Appendix). The form provided has combined both measures for a quick assessment tool by the nurse when indicated. A deficit in either of these measures should immediately be brought to the attention of the attending physician for appropriate intervention and documentation. The mini mind-set can be used to document cognitive impairment for such disorders as CO poisoning and DCI type II. It can also be related to the ability to understand teaching, and the need for Pressure Equalization (PE) tubes in the impaired patient. This will eliminate the patient from having to experience any unnecessary middle ear barotraumas.

Speech needs to be assessed for hoarseness or nasal quality of tone. The hoarseness can be due to paralysis of the vocal cords, while a nasal voice can indicate a paralysis of the palate.[2]

Table 1: Function and Evaluation of Cranial Nerves

Name	Function	Evaluation
Olfactory (N1)	Sensory: Smell	Volatile oils, coffee (each nostril should be tested separately)
Optic (N2)	Sensory: Vision	Visual acuity, visual fields (examine fundus to rule out papilledema, vessel integrity, consensual reaction)
Oculomotor (N3)	Motor: movement of eye upward and inward, elevation of eyelid, constriction of pupil (primary responsibility for consensual reactions)	Consensual reaction, pupil size, dollê eye maneuver, accommodation
Trochlear (N 4)	Motor: movement of eye down and out	Observation
Trigeminal (N5)	Motor and sensory: motor to masticatory muscles; sensory to face	Clenching of the jaw, corneal reflex, sensitivity to pinprick and temperature
Abducens (N6)	Motor: movement to lateral rectus of eye	Observation
Facial (N7)	Motor and sensory: motor to muscles of facial expression and stapedius muscle; sensory to anterior two-thirds of tongue (taste); salivary and lacrimal secretions	Uniformity of facial expression; tase (ancillary tongue); normal tearing
Acoustic (N8)	Sensory: hearing and equilibrium	Hearing acuity, nystagmus, tuning fork on mastoid
Glossopharyngeal (N9)	Motor and sensory: motor to pharynx, salivary and parotid glands; sensory to pharynx, posterior one-third of tongue (taste); carotid sinus	Gag reflex, taste (posterior tongue), carotid sinus reflex
Vagus (N10)	Sensory and motor: lung, bronchi, heart, gastrointestinal tract, great vessels, esophagus, palate, pharynx, larynx	Gag reflex, symmetrical uvula movement when patient says çahé
Spinal accessory (N11)	Motor: trapezius and sternocleidomastoid muscle movement	Shrugging of shoulders
Hypoglossal (N12)	Motor: tongue	Observation of tongue for deviation, tremor, atrophy

Cranial Nerves

The assessment of the 12 cranial nerves can be very extensive. One should try to limit these to a quick screen when possible, unless there is a serious indication of possible impairment. Table 1 describes the function and evaluation of the 12 cranial nerves.[3]

Motor System

The examination of the nervous and motor systems do not come into play for most hyperbaric patients, but they are extremely important in the diagnosis of DCI. Assessment of the motor system can reveal deficits, which can aid in the diagnosis of DCI. The following are examples of a few of the more common screening tests that are used.[4]

Gait and Legs

The heel-to-toe: A gait that lacks coordination, with reeling and instability, is called ataxic. Ataxia may be due to cerebellar disease, loss of position sense, or intoxication. Tandem walking may reveal an ataxia not previously noted.

Walk on the toes, then on the heels: These are sensitive tests respectively for plantar flexion and dorsiflexion of the ankles, as well as balance. Walking on the toes then on the heels may reveal distal muscular weakness in the legs. Further, weak dorsiflexion is a sensitive test for upper motor neuron weakness.

This particular series of screens can be somewhat strenuous on the patient. Utilize your judgment on the selection of screens as related to the patient's physical ability to perform the required actions.

Hop in place on each foot: The test requires a good sense of positioning and normal cerebellar function. Difficulty in hopping may be due to weakness, lack of position sense, or cerebellar dysfunction.

Shallow knee bend: Difficulty here suggests proximal weakness (extensors of the hip), weakness of the quadriceps (the extensor of the knee), or both. Supporting the patient's elbow lightly may be helpful. Alternately, you can have the patient rise from a chair or stool without the use of arm support. This can be useful for patients who are older or less robust.

Romberg Test: This is a functional test of position sense. The patient should first stand with feet together and eyes open, and then close both eyes for 20-30 seconds without support. Note the patient's ability to maintain an upright posture, and be sure not to allow a fall. Normally only minimal swaying occurs.

Arms, Shoulders, and Hands

Check for pronator drift: Usually this test can be combined with the Romberg test. Ask the patient to hold both arms straightforward, palms up, and then close eyes, and maintain this position for 20-30 seconds. The tendency of one forearm to pronate suggests a mild hemiparesis. A sideward or upward drift, sometimes with searching, writhing movements of the hands, suggests loss of position sense. At this point you want to tap the arms briskly downward. The arms normally return smoothly to the horizontal position. This response requires muscular strength, coordination, and a good sense of position. When the position sense is lacking, the patient may not recognize the displacement and, if told to correct it, does so poorly.

Check Grip Strength

Ask the patient to squeeze two of your fingers as hard as possibl and not to let them go. (Cross your fingers, middle finger over the index finger to prevent getting hurt by hard squeezes.) You normally should have difficulty removing your fingers from the patient's grip. A weak grip may be due to either upper or lower motor neuron disease.

Lower Extremities

Grading for muscle strength should be evaluated on a uniform basis. The following is a grading scale for the muscle strength.

Muscle strength is graded on a 0 to 5 scale

0 – No muscular contraction
1 – A barely detectable flicker or trace of contraction
2 – Active movement of the body part with gravity eliminated
3 – Active movement against gravity
4 – Active movement against gravity and some resistance
5 – Active movement against full resistance without evidence of fatigue. This is normal muscle strength.

Additional muscle tone and strength can also be checked in the following areas for deficits:

- Test flexion and extension at elbows
- Test finger abduction
- Test opposition of the thumb
- Test flexion at the hip
- Test abduction and adduction of the hip
- Test flexion and extension of the knee
- Test dorsiflexion and plantar flexion of the foot

To complete a neurological examination, the only remaining recommended requirements are deep tendon reflex testing. Note the speed, force, and amplitude of the reflex response. Comparative testing should always be done.

Reflexes are usually graded on a 0 to 4+ scale

0 No response
1+ Somewhat diminished; low normal
2+ Average; normal
3+ Brisker than average; possibly but not necessarily indicative of disease
4+ Very brisk, hyperactive; often indicative of disease; often associated with clonus (rhythmic oscillations between flexionand extension)

Reflex response depends partly on the force of the stimulus provided. Normally use only the amount of force required to illicit a response. It is easier to note deficits with contra-lateral testing than with symmetrical. Symmetrically diminished or even absent reflexes may be found in normal people.[5]

Some of the sites for deep tendon reflexes are as follows:

- Biceps reflex (C5, C6)
- Triceps reflex (C6, C7)
- Brachio-radialis reflex (C5, C6)
- Abdominal reflexes (T8, T9, T10)
- Knee reflex (L2, L3, L4)
- Ankle reflex (S1)
- Plantar response (Babinski response) (L5, S1)

SENSORY EVALUATION

Many times sensory impairment is obvious in the DCI patient. Some of the more common symptoms are: pain (sharp or dull), numbness or tingling, hot or cold sensations, and/or a heavy feeling in an extremity. When interviewing the patient, it is important to ask if the sensation feels normal, versus if they feel the stimulus. The following are examples of differential stimuli for the assessment of sensory impairment.[6]

- Light touch – Drag the fingertips lightly over the front and back of the arms, trunk and legs with particular attention to the fingers, toes, palms, and soles of feet. Touch the hairs of the arms and legs lightly. Compare contra-lateral sides.

- Sharp and dull – Using the point and head of a safety pin or the eraser and tip of a sharp pencil, press on the skin and ask the patient to identify sharp versus dull. Always compare to contra-lateral sides.

PULMONARY

A complete and accurate pulmonary assessment is essential to avoid or prevent gas expansion problems. Many of the critically ill patients treated with HBO will have some degree of pulmonary dysfunction that requires supple-mental oxygen. A number will also be intubated, requiring mechanical ventilator support.

Assessing the patient for a significant pulmonary history is a key starting point. Is there a history of asthma, chronic obstructive pulmonary dysfunction (COPD), fibrosis, spontaneous pneumothorax, or chest trauma? Has a patient developed adult respiratory distress syndrome (ARDS) due to his/her illness? Each of these conditions will impact patient preparation, the method of compression, and particularly decompression of the patient. In patients with reactive airways, COPD, or with decreased pulmonary compliance, extra time for the exhalation period needs to be allowed. If a patient is not intubated, a slow decompression (1 psig/minute) is used. The same rate of ascent is used with a patient on mechanical ventilation and in addition to an adjustment of the ventilator to allow the exhalation time to be twice the inhalation time.

If there is chest trauma, has any pneumothorax been treated? A patient with a small-untreated pneumothorax can develop a tension pneumothorax on ascent from HBO treatment.[7] Chest tubes can safely be placed in both monoplace and multiplace chambers. Adjustments will have to be made if the chest tube will be placed in a monoplace chamber. The use of a Heimlich valve (Figure 1) attached to the chest tube will allow the escape of air or fluid from the chest cavity and prevent air from entering the chest cavity. If there is drainage, a foley catheter bag or other small container may be attached to collect the drainage.

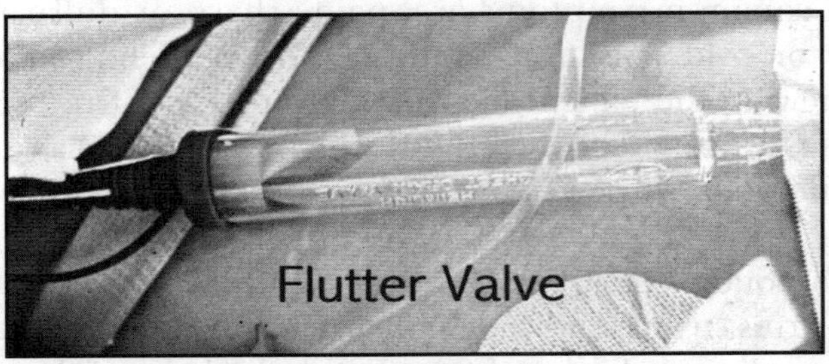

FIGURE 1. Heimlich Valve (Flutter Valve)

Physical assessment of the patient is the next step. Prior to each treatment, the lungs should be auscultated. If wheezing is present, an inhaled bronchodilator prior to treatment is recommended. Response of the patient to the bronchodilator needs to be assessed prior to placing the patient in the chamber. If there is not relief of bronchospasm, the risk/benefit to the patient needs to be weighed prior to placing the patient in the chamber. Patients with rales present prior to treatment should not be placed flat on the stretcher. The stretcher head will need to be elevated 30-45 degrees depending on patient tolerance. Patients who are experiencing congestive heart failure (CHF) or dialysis patients with fluid overload should be carefully watched during the hyperbaric treatment. The effect of vasoconstriction from HBO may further exacerbate CHF or fluid overload.

If the patient is intubated and requires ventilator support, special attention to several key areas is required. The size of the endotrachial (ET) tube is important due to the change in gas density at pressure.[8] A size 8 mm tube is ideal for an adult. If this is not possible, then the largest one that will fit the patient should be used. Adult ET tubes will have cuffs that are inflated with air. Prior to being placed in a hyperbaric chamber, the air needs to be removed and replaced with saline. This is done to prevent the compression of the air (Boyle's Gas Law) during HBO treatment. If the air is left in the cuff during HBO, the air will compress and the patient will develop an air leak, making ventilation difficult if not impossible. At completion of the HBO, the saline will need to be removed and replaced with air. If the saline is left in, there will be a risk of tracheal erosion from increase in pressure at the cuff contact points.

ET tube position should be confirmed with a chest radiograph. The ET tube is well-secured and distance noted at the teeth position. Observe the tube for any possible areas of pressure or erosion to the skin and make adjustments. Observe chest movement and position of trachea.

The degree of ventilator support is important as to whether or not that can be managed in a hyperbaric environment. Key factors are minute ventilation (Ve), fraction of inspired oxygen (FiO_2), and positive end expiratory pressure (PEEP). The ventilators used in the monoplace hyperbaric chamber are limited in the ability to deliver high Ve.[9] Ways to maximize the HBO ventilator will be discussed later in the chapter concerning equipment.

In patients with pulmonary dysfunction that require supplemental oxygen, it may be difficult to elevate their PaO_2 to what may be considered hyperbarically oxygenated. While a PaO_2 level has not been defined, it would be possible to consider the effects of hyperbaric oxygen and at what PaO_2 level are these effects activated.[10] Generally speaking, if a patient requires >60% oxygen, it may be difficult to elevate his/her PaO_2 to the point of receiving benefit from HBO. This must be part of the risk/benefit equation in determining whether the patient should receive HBO.

PEEP can be added to the ventilator by placing PEEP valves in the expiratory circuit. Whenever PEEP is added the patient should be carefully monitored. Auto PEEP can occur and cause cardiovascular compromise. If this should happen, expiratory time can be lengthened with a shortening of inspiratory time. While auto PEEP can be reversed with this maneuver, it can also result in hypoventilation of the patient.

One of the challenges of treating the critically ill patient with HBO is how to monitor level of oxygenation. While techniques have been developed for use with monoplace chambers[11] to sample arterial blood and accurately perform the test, this is not without risk and can be labor intensive. A simpler method is the use of a dual clark electrode connected to a TINA 3 (Radiometer, USA) transcutaneous monitor. A detailed discussion of the use of a transcutaneous monitor for this purpose will occur under the monitoring section of this chapter.

CARDIOVASCULAR

The cardiovascular assessment of a critical care patient receiving hyperbaric oxygen therapy is similar to the cardiovascular assessment of any critical care patient. Cardiac rhythm should be assessed and monitored during the treatment. If the patient experiences a cardiac emergency during HBO treatment, the staff should be trained to handle such an emergency. It is important to remember that a patient at depth is well oxygenated and will remain so for 5-8 minutes.[12] The safest way to bring a patient to the surface who has had a cardiac arrest is to bring him/her up at 5 psig (fastest rate on a monoplace chamber) while staff prepares to deliver emergency care. To do a rapid ascent using the emergency ascent button on monoplace chambers places the person at grave risk for air embolism due to expansion injuries. Once the patient has surfaced, move them to the point farthest away from the open chamber, remove the hyperoxygenated clothing, and, if appropriate, defibrillate. Cold oxygen will fall to the floor and dissipate in 30 seconds[13] and should not place the area at an increased fire risk with the use of a debrillator. The staff needs to be able to respond quickly and appropr iately to such an emergency, so it is our recommendation that the staff be Advanced Cardiac Life Support (ACLS) certified.

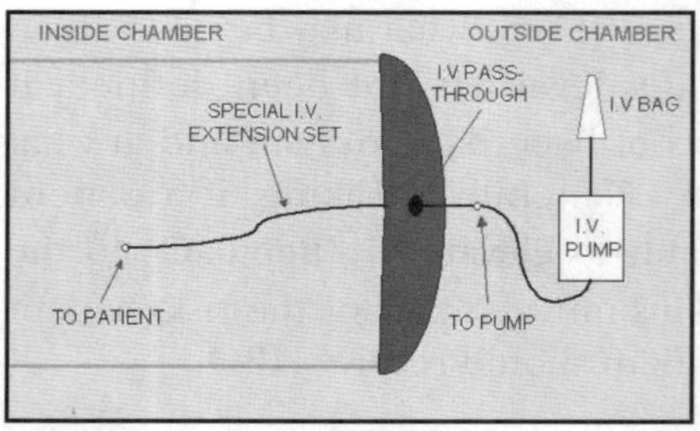

FIGURE 2. I.V. Administration

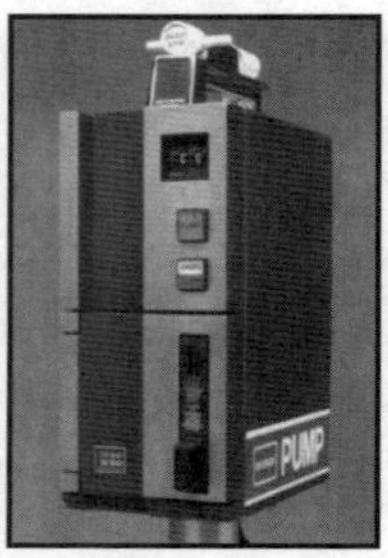

FIGURE 3.
IVAC 530 I.V. Pump

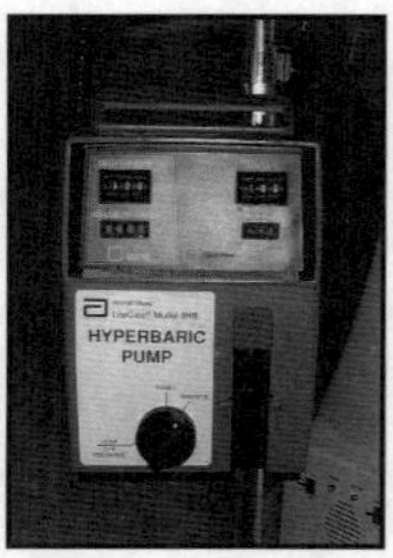

FIGURE 4.
Abbot Pump

A wide range of intravenous therapy (Figure 2) can be managed during HBO treatments. Blood products, vasoactive drugs, parental feedings, antibiotics, and simple crystalloids can be administered. Enteral feedings may also be administered if the feeding tube is placed in the small bowel such as the Miller-Frederick Feeding Tube. Gastric feeding during HBO therapy should be avoided. Vasoactive drugs can be safely managed and delivered to the patient through specially designed infusion pumps. There are currently two pumps that are designed to be used with a monoplace chamber and are capable of pumping against increased atmospheric pressure. The two pumps are IVAC 530 (IVAC Corp., San Diego, CA) (Figure 3) and the Abbott Hyperbaric Pump (Abbott Laboratories, North Chicago, IL) (Figure 4). Both pumps will have inaccuracies at very low and high infusion rates, particularly if they are pumping against greater than 2.0 atmospheres absolute.[14, 15] Adjustments will need to be made by the nurse to the drug infusion rate to hold the blood pressure or cardiac function stable during the HBO treatment. If a vasoactive drug is being administered, cardiac rhythm as well as blood pressure should be monitored throughout the treatment. Overall, the blood pressure should be stable if supported by vasoactive medications before the patient is placed in the chamber. The blood pressure may fluctuate if on a support medication during compression and decompression. Before an adjustment is made in the medication during compression and decompression, it is recommended to observe the blood pressure for a brief period to determine if it will go back to an acceptable range once movement through pressure is complete. (See Figures 8 and 9.)

GASTROINTESTINAL

Gastrointestinal Assessment

The management of the critical care patient in the hyperbaric setting always provides unique challenges. One must take into consideration any gastrointestinal involvement during the treatment regimen. Does the patient have a P.E.G. tube that may leak gastric content onto the skin and cause excoriation? Does the patient have a nasogastric tube, which requires suction, or can it be clamped during treatment?

Inspection of the Abdomen

Note the four quadrants for any obvious abnormalities, such as pulsating masses or bulging organs. Auscultation of the right lower quadrant is usually sufficient in that persistalic bowel sounds transmit easily within the abdominal cavity. In the patient with suspect lower peripheral vascular disease, bruits can be heard above the iliac and femoral arteries.[16] Take note of hyperactive bowel sounds, and ask the patient about recent bowel habits. Nothing would be more embarrassing than an “accident” while in the chamber. A distended bowel from gas formation will actually be eased of pain at 2 ATA while breathing oxygen.[17]

Tubes

The attending nurse should take note of any presence of tubes, i.e., nasogastric (NG). If the patient does have a nasal gastric tube, one should note the amount of drainage from the nursing report prior to transport. Determine if it can be clamped during treatment and obtain a physician order, or if intermittent low pressure suction will be required if the chamber is so equipped. Tube patency and placement should be assessed prior to entering into the chamber.[18] PEG tubes need to be secured to the skin to prevent pulling, and reinforce the dressing to prevent leakage onto the underlying tissue.

GENITOURINARY

ASSESSMENT OF GENITOURINARY SYSTEM

There really is no required examination of the genitourinary system, but there may be situations that must be accounted for. The most common is the need for some type of urinal device for the elderly patient who is taking a diuretic. It would be greatly preferred if the patient can time his/her dosage so that the medication does not peak while the patient is in treatment. Another consideration is the congestive heart failure patient. If this patient and physician decide to withhold the diuretic until after treatment, the patient will be at increased risk for pulmonary edema during the course of the treatment. Monitor breath sounds and saturation levels closely on these patients pre and post treatment.

One of the goals in the treatment of DCI is re-hydration of the patient. Most divers are commonly dehydrated to some degree. During the course a USN treatment table 6, while pushing fluids either orally or intravenously, the need for a urinal is bound to arise. Be sure and have the forethought to have one in the chamber prior to initiating treatment.

FOLEY CATHETERS

Empty the reservoir bag prior to treatment. Ensure that the retention balloon is filled and secure. Place the reservoir bag between the patient's legs in a dependent position. Inspect the catheter for any kinks or leakage. No other special attention is required with a foley catheter except to ensure that it does not get pulled or dislodged upon entry into the chamber.[19]

SPECIAL CONSIDERATIONS

The suicidal patient presents with unique considerations. The opportunity for injury within the hyperbaric environment still exists. The patient must be thoroughly examined for any ignition sources before entering the chamber. Also, note respiration patterns during any change of pressures to ensure no possibility of pulmonary barotraumas. Patient safety must always be in the forefront of our minds, even if it is not in theirs.

RESTRAINTS

If there is a need for the use of restraints with the hyperbaric patient, some issues need to be considered. In our facility, we employ the use of the *Sigma II Perry Baromedical Dual-Place Chamber.* In actuality, this is a large monoplace chamber that has the capability of a separate entry lock for tenders and is air-compressed. The patients are delivered oxygen through a "built-in-breathing system" (BIBS). When we are treating a critical care patient who is ventilator-dependent, the use of chemical intervention is usually required. Also during this same scenario, soft wrist restraints are utilized to prevent the potential for patient injury to self. As always in any setting in healthcare, ensure that the proper documentation is in place. JCAHO standards require a physician order for the restraints, the purpose, and duration of application. Capillary refill times should be noted distal to the application sites, and should be less than three seconds. In addition, with the use of chemical restraints, special attention must be paid to the eyes. Provide a lubricant to both eyes and secure them with a small eye dressing or tape them shut. This will prevent the cornea from being injured during the absence of a blink reflex.

MONITORING

Arterial Oxygenation

In specific patients undergoing hyperbaric oxygen therapy, there can be a need to monitor arterial oxygenation and carbon dioxide levels. In patients on mechanical ventilation, it is necessary to evaluate the effectiveness of the minute ventilation being delivered. Potentially, if the CO_2 is allowed to become elevated, the patient is at greater risk for an oxygen toxic seizure to occur. In patients with pulmonary dysfunction who require supplemental oxygen or other methods of ventilatory support, hyperbaric oxygen can be dosed in order to achieve the desired PaO_2 level. In work done by Weaver[20] it was found that in patients with abnormal pulmonary function, it might be reasonable to treat this group of patients with higher chamber pressures than those patients with normal pulmonary function. It was also noted in their abstract that no decrement in pulmonary function occurred due to hyperbaric oxygen therapy.

There are two methods by which to monitor arterial oxygenation during monoplace hyperbaric oxygen therapy: arterial blood gas sampling and transcutaneous oxygen monitoring. In order to sample arterial blood gases during HBO treatments, a special setup is required[9] and immediate access to a blood gas analyzer is necessary. Any blood sample obtained by this method must be held under pressure and analyzed in less than two minutes. The only blood gas analyzer that has demonstrated the ability to measure hyperbaric oxygen tensions is the ABL 330 (Radiometer, Copenhagen, Denmark). This method of determining hyperbaric oxygen and carbon dioxide levels is only recommend for staff with experience in this area and support equipment readily available.

Determining oxygenation and carbon dioxide levels with the use of a transcutaneous monitor is much simpler and has demonstrated good correlation with arterial PaO_2 and PcO_2.[21] In order to monitor both carbon dioxide and oxygen levels, a dual clark electrode in required. In a monoplace environment, a TINA 3 (Radiometer, Copenhagen, Denmark) or a Perimed (Stockholm, Sweden) monitor may used. The electrode should be placed in a central area that does not have scar tissue present or had previously been irradiated. Traditionally, midclavular, third intercostal space has been used for monitoring core oxygenation. There is no correlation found between PaO_2/PcO_2 and tcom readings from a lower extremity.

EQUIPMENT

Monoplace Chamber Ventilator

Currently the only FDA approved ventilator for use in the monoplace hyperbaric environment is the Sechrist 500A (Figure 5). This is a pneumatic time-cycled ventilator with the controls located outside the hull and the ventilator circuit and block located inside the hull. The ventilator operates only in control mode with adjustments for flow, inspiratory time, and expiratory time. An oxygen driving pressure of 65-85 psig is required for adequate flow through the ventilator.[22] Oxygen flows through a single hose from the controller, passing through the ventilator pass-through in the hull of the chamber and connecting to the inlet hose of the ventilator block. Tidal volume is measured inside the chamber with a spirometer connected to the limb of the ventilator circuit. Airway pressure is measured in the ventilator block with manometer, not at the proximal airway. Positive End Expiratory Pressure (PEEP) can be added by placing a PEEP valve or Emerson Water Column in the expiratory circuit. The ventilator will deliver 100% oxygen, or, with modifications, 21% oxygen.[23] You cannot blend to obtain other oxygen concentrations.

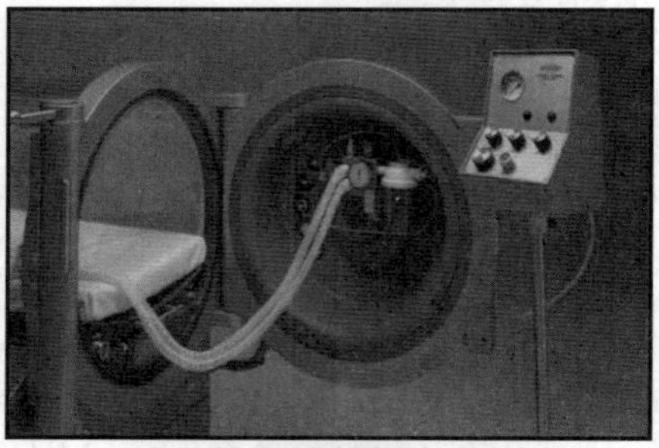

FIGURE 5. Sechrist 500A Ventilator

Whenever a patient is mechanically ventilated, the greatest risk of harm is from pulmonary barotrauma. The patient should be well sedated, if not on a neuromuscular blocking agent, to prevent this complication. If the patient is not sedated, asynchronous respirations with this control ventilator could occur, resulting in air-trapping or increasing auto-PEEP that could lead to a gas expansion injury.

Close monitoring and adjustment of ventilator settings to maintain the required tidal volume is required during compression and decompression. In testing of the 500A ventilator done by Weaver,[24] it was found to have significant variability of tidal volume greater than was reported by the manufacturer.

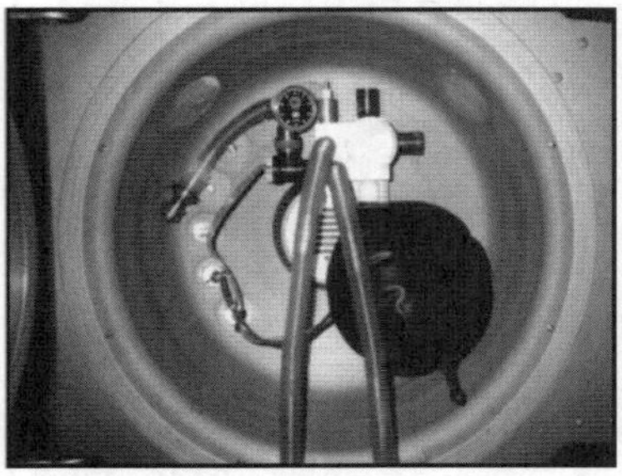

FIGURE 6.

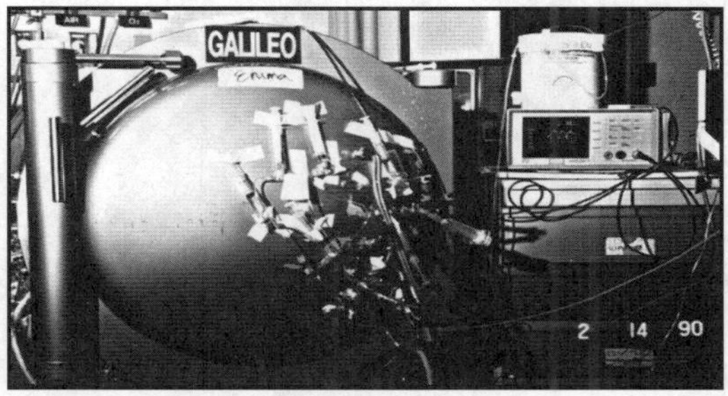

FIGURE 7. Prepared for Compression

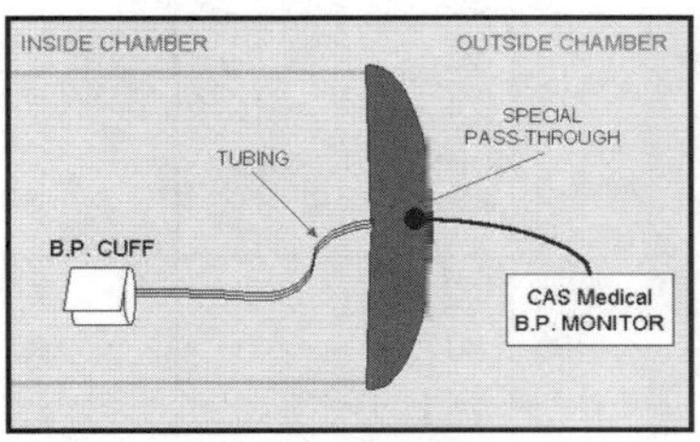

FIGURE 8. Blood Pressure Monitoring Diagram

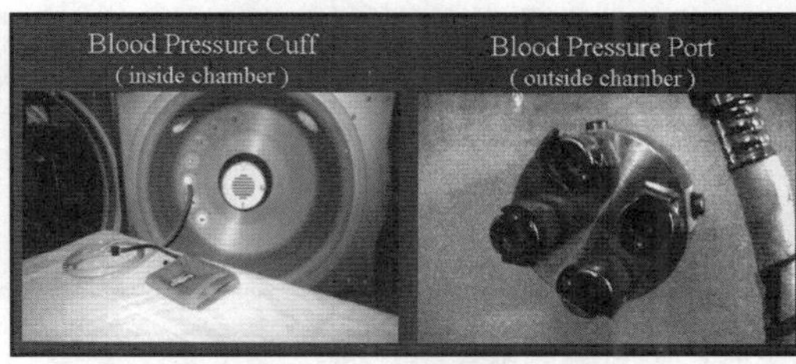

FIGURE 9. Blood Pressure Monitoring

CONCLUSION

Treatment of the critically patient in a monoplace hyperbaric environment requires teamwork. The patients are frequently work-intensive and need dedicated nurses, doctors and technicians who are experienced in both critical care and clinical hyperbaric medicine. Appropriate support services need to be readily available to assist in the care of the patient. Providing monoplace hyperbaric services to these patients should not be undertaken lightly, and needs to be based on a well-thought-out plan of preparedness, staff education, and experience. With this said, it is also very rewarding to play a role in returning a critically ill patient back to their home and life outside a hospital.

APPENDIX

Center for Wound Care
And Hyperbaric Medicine

PATIENT ASSESSMENT
MINI MIND-SET EXAM

	Cognitive Function Exam	Cognitive Tasks	Points
1.	**ORIENTATION** (Maximum score 10) Ask "What is today's date?" Then ask specifically for parts omitted - Ex: "Can you tell me what season it is?" Ask "Can you tell me the name of this hospital?" "What department are we in?" "What town/city are we in?" "What county are we in?" "What state are we in?" (1 point for each correct response for a total of ten points)	Date (ex: July 4th) Month Year Day (Ex: Monday) Season Hospital Department Name Town/City County State	
2.	**REGISTRATION** (Maximum score 3) Ask the subject if you may test his/her memory. Then say "BALL, FLAG, TREE" clearly and slowly - about 1 second for each. After you have said all three words, ask the subject to repeat them. This first repetition determines the score (0 -3), but keep saying them (up to six trials) until the subject can repeat all three words. If he/she does not eventually learn all three, recall cannot be meaningfully tested. How many trials did it take? (1 point for each correct answer)	"BALL" "FLAG" "TREE"	
3.	**ATTENTION AND CALCULATION** (Maximum score of 5) Ask the subject to begin at 100 and count backwards by 7. Stop after 5 subtractions (93, 86, 79, 72, 65). Score one point for each correct answer. **OR** If the subject cannot or will not perform this task, ask him/her to spell "WORLD" backwards (D L R O W). Score 1 point for each letter correctly placed. Ex: DLROW = 5; DLORW = 3 Record how the subject spelled "WORLD" backwards:	"93" "86" "79" "72" "65" **OR** Number of correctly placed letters	
4.	**RECALL** (Maximum score 3) Ask the subject to recall the three words you previously asked him/her to remember (from section 2). Score one point for each word remembered correctly.	"BALL" "FLAG" "TREE"	
5.	**LANGUAGE** (Maximum score 8) ***Naming*** : Show the subject a wrist watch and ask "WHAT IS THIS?" Repeat for a pencil. Score one point for each item named correctly. (2) ***Repetition*** : Ask the subject to repeat "NO IFS, ANDS, OR BUTS" Score one point for correct repetition. (1) ***3-stage command*** : Give the subject a piece of blank paper and say "TAKE THE PAPER IN YOUR RIGHT HAND, FOLD IT IN HALF, AND PUT IT ON THE FLOOR." Score one point for each action performed correctly. (3) ***Reading*** : On a blank piece of paper, print the sentence "CLOSE YOUR EYES" in letters large enough for the subject to see clearly. Ask the subject to read it and do what it says. Score only if he/she actually closes eyes. (1) ***Writing*** : Give the subject a blank piece of paper and ask him/her to write a sentence. It is to be written spontaneously. It must contain a subject and a verb, and make sense. Correct grammar and punctuation are not necessary. (1)	"Watch" "Pen or Pencil" Repeats correctly Takes in right hand Folds in half Puts on floor Closes eyes Writes sentence	

Springhill Memorial Hospital
Mobile, AL
(334) 460-5259

Center for Wound Care
And Hyperbaric Medicine

PATIENT ASSESSMENT
MINI MIND-SET EXAM

	Cognitive Function Exam	Cognitive Tasks	Points
6.	**COPYING** (Maximum score 1) On a clean piece of paper, draw intersecting pentagons, each side about 1 inch. Ask the subject to copy it exactly as it is. All 10 angles must be present and two must intersect to score one point. Tremor and rotation are ignored.	Draws pentagons Example below	
	Rate the subject's level of consciousness: Alert Stupor Drowsy Coma	**TOTAL SCORE** (maximum score 30)	
	Comments:		

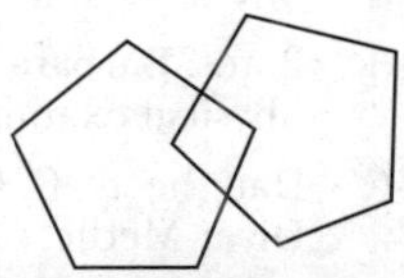

Assessment		Score	Patient's Score
Glasgow Coma Scale			
EYES OPEN			
Spontaneously	eyes open, does not imply awareness	4	
To speech	response to any speech or shout, not necesssarily to command	3	
To pain	response to stimulus applied to limbs	2	
NEVER		1	
BEST VERBAL			
Patient Oriented	aware of self and enviroment; should be oriented x 3	5	
Confusion	attention can be held; conversational responses to questions, but with varying degrees of disorientation and confusion	4	
Inappropriate words	intelligible articulation, but no sustained conversation possible; usually shouting or swearing	3	
Incomprehensible sounds	moaning and groaning without recognizable words	2	
NONE		1	
BEST MOTOR			
Obedience to commands	grasp reflex must be distinguished from response to command	6	
Localization of pain	Pain stimulus causes patient to move limb as to withdraw from stimulus	5	
Flexor withdrawl	withdraws from pain, flexes arms and legs	4	
Abnormal flexion	decorticate; flexion of arms, extension of legs and feet (unless SCI also present)	3	
Extension	decerebrate; extension of arms and legs. Internal rotation of hands and feet	2	
NONE	flaccid; important to R/O SCI	1	
	TOTAL SCORE	3 -15	

Date ________________
Time ________________

____
Signature/Title

Springhill Memorial Hospital
Mobile, AL
(334) 460-5259

REFERENCES

1. Bates, Barbara. Techniques of Examination, The Nervous System, In: A guide to physical examination and history taking, Lippincott 5th ed., pp 514-517.
2. Bates, Barbara. Techniques of Examination, The Nervous System, In: A guide to physical examination and history taking, Lippincott 5th ed., p 51.
3. Means B, Taplett L. Quick Reference to Critical Care Nursing, Aspen Publishers 1986, p 161.
4. Bates, Barbara. Techniques of Examination, The Nervous System, In: A guide to physical examination and history taking, 5th ed., pp 520-530.
5. Bates, Barbara. Techniques of Examination, The Nervous System, In: A guide to physical examination and history taking, Lippincott 5th ed., pp 531-537.
6. Daugherty, C. Gordon. The Neurologic Examination, Field Guide for the Diver-Medic, Coastal Aquatics Publications, pp 131-132.
7. Kindwall E. Gas Embolism. In: Kindwall EP, ed. Hyperbaric Medicine Practice, 1995; 328-341.
8. Weaver LK. Management of critically ill patients in the monoplace hyperbaric chamber. In: Kindwall EP, ed. Hyperbaric Medicine Practice, 1995;174-235.
9. Weaver LK. Appendix V Performance of the Sechrist 500A hyperbaric ventilator in a monoplace hyperbaric chamber. In: Kindwall EP, ed. Hyperbaric Medicine Practice, 1995; 235-245.
10. Reference seven
11. Weaver LK, Howe S, Berlin SL. Normobaric measurement of O_2 tension of blood and saline tonometered under hyperbaric oxygen conditions. J. Hyperbaric Medicine. 190;5(1):29-38.235-245.
12. Holcomb JR, Matos-Navarro AY, Goldmann RW. Critical care in the hyperbaric chamber. In: Problem Wounds. (Davis JC, Hunt TK eds.) New York: Elsevier, 1988; 187-209.
13. Personal communication with Weaver LK 1993.
14. Evans P, Weaver LK. The use of IVAC 530 infusion pumps in the monoplace hyperbaric chamber. Undersea Biomed Res. 1991;18 (supplement):18-19.
15. Ziegler BA, Weaver LK. Intravenous infusion pumps: evaluation for use with the monoplace hyperbaric chamber. Undersea Biomed Res. 1991;18 (supplement):91.
16. Bates, Barbara. Techniques of Examination, The Gastrointestinal System, In: A guide to physical examination and history taking, 5th ed., pp 344-345.
17. Kindwall, Eric. Hyperbaric Medicine Practice, Best Publishing Co., pp 18.
18. Kindwall and Goldman. Hyperbaric Medicine Procedures, Aurora Health Care, pp 68.
19. Kindwall and Goldman. Hyperbaric Medicine Procedures, Aurora Health Care, pp 68.
20. Weaver LK, Howe S. Arterial oxygen tension of patients with abnormal pulmonary function during hyperbaric oxygen therapy. Undersea Biomed Res. 1991;18 (supplement):107-108.
21. Howe S, Hein S, Weaver LK, Larson-Lohr V, Kristo D, Haberstock D. Response of arterial oxygen tension and transcutaneous oxygen to changes in alveolar PO_2. J. Undersea and Hyperbaric Medicine 1995;22 (supplement):76.
22. Weaver LK, Greenway L, Elliott CG. Performance of the sechrist 500A ventilator in a monoplace hyperbaric chamber. In: Kindwall EP, ed. Hyperbaric Medicine Practice, 1995; 235-245.
23. Weaver LK. Air breaks with the Sechrist 500a monoplace hyperbaric ventilator. J. Hyperbaric Medicine 1988;3(3):179-186.
24. Reference nine

CHAPTER VI

EFFECT OF HBO ON GLUCOSE MEASUREMENT: IMPLICATIONS FOR CARE

K. PARKER AND C. FIFE

BACKGROUND

Most observational studies suggest that blood glucose (BG) decreases in diabetics undergoing Hyperbaric Oxygen Therapy (HBOT) (Kakhnovskii, Longoni, Springer, Takahashi, Blackburn, O'Malley, Pontani). This decrease in BG has been a consistent finding in nearly all observational studies, usually on the order of 50 mg/dl. However, it is still not clear whether this drop is causally related to the hyperbaric therapy itself, or merely an effect of the timing of treatment with feeding and medications. Blood glucose does not appear to be significantly affected in non-diabetic patients. How might hyperbaric therapy affect blood glucose in the diabetic patient? Why is this question so hard to answer? The practitioner must first have a basic understanding of glucose metabolism and the role of insulin.

GLUCOSE METABOLISM

The major hormone regulating glucose metabolism is insulin, a hormone synthesized in the beta cells of the pancreas. It stimulates glucose uptake in fat and muscle cells and the conversion in the liver of glucose to glycogen. As blood glucose levels fall in response to insulin, glucagon release from the alpha cells of the pancreas is stimulated. Glucagon stimulates the liver to break down glycogen and amino acids so that glucose is released into the blood. Glucagon also inhibits the uptake of glucose by muscle and fat cells. In non-diabetics the level of blood glucose controls secretion of glucagon and insulin via negative feedback systems. Low blood glucose level stimulates the release of glucagon whereas high blood glucose level stimulates secretion of insulin.

Diabetes mellitus is a group of disorders that all lead to an elevation of glucose in the blood. The two major types of diabetes are insulin-dependent diabetes mellitus (IDDM), and non-insulin-dependent diabetes mellitus (NIDDM). Typically, juvenile onset diabetes is insulin dependent, but some patients with adult onset diabetes also become insulin dependent. In IDDM, there is an absolute deficiency of insulin, and injections are required to prevent death. The cellular metabolism of an untreated patient with IDDM is similar to that of a starving person. Since insulin is not available to aid the entry of glucose into body cells, most cells use fatty acids to produce ATP. Ketones are byproducts of fatty acid catabolism, which causes a form of acidosis called ketoacidosis. The catabolism of stored triglycerides and proteins also causes weight loss.

In non-insulin-dependent diabetes mellitus, the symptoms are generally less severe, and diet, exercise, weight loss, and oral medications may control the high glucose levels in the blood, at least initially. Many patients with NIDDM have a sufficient amount or even a surplus of insulin in the blood. For these patients, the cause of the diabetes is not from a shortage of insulin, but because target cells become less sensitive to it.

For most patients, medication is the key to regulation of the blood glucose levels. In the past, medical therapy for IDDM and NIDDM were quite different. A complete review of diabetes management is beyond the scope of this chapter. However, it is now apparent that, rather than two different diseases, diabetes represents more of a continuum (see Figure 1) which blurs the categories of insulin dependence and non-insulin-dependence. Many physicians are now prescribing oral medications to supplement a patient's insulin regime, and vice versa. Some patients with adult onset diabetes do require insulin. Clearly, this combined therapy complicates the interpretation of studies done to evaluate the effect of HBOT on blood glucose.

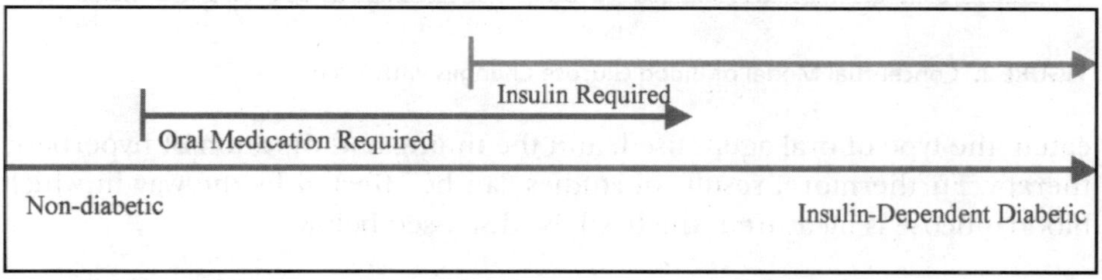

FIGURE 1. Blood Glucose Levels

A further complication in the interpretation of studies is the issue of the timing of medication (whether insulin or oral agents) and hyperbaric oxygen therapy. The goal of diabetic management is a relatively even control of blood sugar throughout the day, and this is usually achieved by using combinations of different types of insulin and/or oral medications. Regular insulin is usually considered to reach its peak activity in the blood about 2 to 4 hours after administration. In contrast, other forms of insulin take longer to peak, but may last longer in the blood stream, thus affecting blood glucose levels for several hours. For example, "NPH" is usually considered to reach its peak activity in 10 to 16 hours. Oral agents also differ in the timing of their peak effect on blood glucose, and in general have even longer lasting effects than the various forms of insulin. For this reason, the timing of the administration of insulin and the administration of HBOT are crucial. A patient undergoing HBOT just as their hypoglycemic agent peaks will obviously be more likely to have a drop in blood glucose than a patient whose medication is past its peak, or has not yet reached its peak (see Figure 2). Add to this the timing of food consumption, which may be altered from the patient's normal schedule as a result of the time required to travel to the chamber and undergo treatment with HBOT. The result is an incredibly complex equation involving several variables including: the amount of insulin, the type of insulin, the amount of food eaten, the time that food is

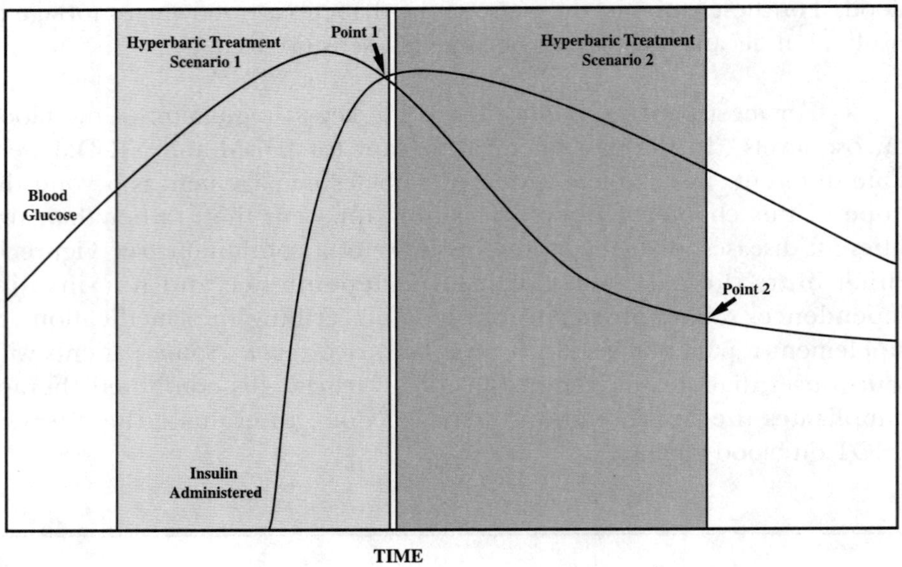

FIGURE 2. Conceptual Model of Blood Glucose Changes with Time.

eaten, the type of oral agent used, and the timing and duration of hyperbaric therapy. Furthermore, results of studies can be affected by the way in which blood glucose is measured which will be discussed below.

MEASURING BLOOD GLUCOSE

In monoplace chambers, blood glucose is usually measured prior to entering the chamber or after exiting. However, in multiplace chambers, it is possible for attendants to measure blood glucose **during HBOT,** either by sending samples out of the chamber to be analyzed at sea level, or by compressing a glucometer inside the chamber to measure blood glucose at depth. The hyperbaric environment may affect the function of glucose monitoring equipment if measurements are done in the hyperbaric chamber. In a study by Shafer, it was noted that the One Touch system was the most accurate overall when exposed to treatment depth of 2.4 ATA. It appears that the high oxygen levels in the chamber affected all the systems available for use at that time, because they all used some form of the glucose oxidase reaction. An important consideration for the researcher would be to note the location of the glucose monitor during testing (in the chamber versus topside). The current One Touch II system does not require the monitor to be placed into the multiplace chamber, but the test strips may be locked in and out for testing during treatment. Unfortunately, many studies involving the effect of HBOT on blood glucose fail to report either the equipment used in testing, or the conditions under which testing occurred.

OBSERVATIONAL AND EXPERIMENTAL DATA

Clinical Studies

Most clinicians agree that there is no significant effect on blood glucose levels in the ***non***-diabetic. The effect of HBOT may also be less on ***non***-insulin dependent diabetes mellitus patients (Zivkovic and Mandic). A study by Springer noted that in a random selection of 25 IDDM patients, an average drop of 51 mg/dl was detected post treatment. Takahashi determined that 5 "severe" diabetic patients monitored continuously during hyperbaric oxygen therapy showed decrease in glucose of 51 mg/dl after 75 minutes of HBOT at 2 ATA with a gradual return to pretreatment levels after decompression. In contrast, four "well-controlled" diabetics and non-diabetics showed a glucose change of less than 50 mg/dl or no change. One further observation was that plasma glucose levels ***decreased*** markedly in diabetic patients while it sometimes ***increased*** in healthy controls.

Longoni observed that insulin requirements were decreased in eleven of fifteen diabetic patients undergoing a series of 15 HBOT at 2.8 ATA, suggesting that blood glucose levels were reduced during the course of HBOT. Insulin requirements returned to normal values when the course of HBOT was completed. Pontani reported a retrospective analysis in which the patients underwent blood glucose screening before, during, and after routine HBOT at 2.4 ATA. ***Non-diabetics*** had a small but significant decrease in blood glucose levels. For the eighteen patients with IDDM, glucose drop on average was 60 mg/dl and was unchanged one hour later.

We retrospectively evaluated pre and post HBOT blood glucose levels of ninety-one consecutive diabetics. We defined "low blood sugar" (LBS) as any blood glucose below 100, regardless of whether the patient was symptomatic. In this analysis, blood glucose dropped below 100 after HBOT in 26.4% of all patients. However, since patients were treated multiple times, this represented only 1.92% of the total HBOT treatments. All patients were asymptomatic. Regression analysis on fifty-two patients with LBS showed that the lower the initial glucose level, the greater the likelihood of a drop in BG after HBOT. Also, insulin-dependent diabetics were more likely to drop. However, the percent drop in blood glucose was medicated by the number of kilo-calories fed prior to HBOT, and the age of the patient (older patients dropped less). Not surprisingly, the risk of patients experiencing LBS increased with the number of treatments they received.

We performed a subsequent prospective analysis of twenty-six diabetic patients who underwent a total of 406 HBOTs at either 2.0 ATA or 2.4 ATA. Fifteen of these patients were insulin-dependent. In a frequency similar to the larger retrospective analysis, 30% of patients experienced a drop in BG below 100 mg/dl, one on at least one occasion following HBOT. However, this represented only 3% of the total treatments. Overall, 77% of total patient treatments (315/406) resulted in some decrease in blood glucose, irrespective of whether the patient was fed beforehand. Again, younger patients were more likely to demonstrate a drop. However, in this small study, ***non***-insulin-dependent diabetics were more likely than insulin-dependent patients to experience a decrease in blood glucose after HBOT. Time of day, treatment depth, and cumulative number of HBOTs were not statistically significant factors. However, BG dropped in 81% of treatments when patients were ***not*** fed beforehand, compared to 63% of treatments where patients **were** fed before HBOT. Post treatment BG ***increased*** in only 19% of treatments when patients were ***not*** fed compared to 37% when they **were** fed. This appears to underscore the importance of feeding on hyperbaric patients with diabetes.

Determinants of Risk

There is currently no validated tool available to assess relative risk of low blood glucose. Clinical data make it difficult to clearly identify risk factors, but the bulk of data suggest the following factors may contribute to a decrease in blood glucose:

1. Young age (which might be related to having juvenile diabetes)
2. IDDM
3. No feeding prior to hyperbaric treatment
4. Blood glucose less than 150 mg/dl initially
5. History of hypoglycemic episode (less than 80 mg/dl) in previous 24 hours

POSSIBLE PHYSIOLOGIC MECHANISMS

None of the above studies attempted rigorous assessment of the timing of diabetic medication, the number of calories consumed, the timing of hyperbaric treatment, or the fluctuations in blood glucose without HBOT during the same part of the day. Therefore, whether HBOT is causally related to these observations is still not clear. Despite the variations in methodology and the limitations of these studies, there does appear to be a population of diabetics whose blood glucose decreases after HBOT. If this were only due to the timing of HBOT with diabetic medications, we would expect to see a similar population of patients with an *increase* in blood glucose after HBOT. Since this is not commonly reported, we will review below the possible physiological mechanisms that might explain how HBOT could result in a decrease in blood glucose. With the exception of a possible change in the half-life of insulin, these mechanisms could affect both insulin-dependent diabetics and non-insulin-dependent diabetics.

Increased Glucose Utilization

Zivkovic suggested that in 152 IDDM patients, insulin needs were reduced by 31% and there was a decrease in blood glucose levels. Although the study was not designed to test this hypothesis, he attributed these finding to increased glucose utilization because of improved tissue oxygenation. This hypothesis would seem to be supported by Martindale's finding that mouse diaphragm muscle cells take up glucose more rapidly at 2.4 ATA than controls.

Alterations in Insulin Receptor Activity

Plasma glucagon levels decrease in diabetics receiving hyperbaric oxygen therapy, perhaps due to alterations in insulin receptor activity. Increased glucose metabolism may also contribute to the drop in blood glucose (Martindale and Dixon). Blood glucose increases in rats just before seizure at 3 or 5 ATA. Torboti postulated that this might be due to activation of the sympathetic adrenomedullary system in oxygen toxicity. Elevated brain glucose has been demonstrated to occur during hyperbaric oxygen therapy (Nolan, Obrenovich).

Change in the Half-life of Insulin

One of the theories postulated, but not yet documented, is the possibility that increased tissue oxygenation could increase the half-life of insulin, perhaps by an effect of oxygen to slow its degradation, thereby altering the peak action. This would explain why patients who report no change in their activity level or eating habits during the course of hyperbaric oxygen therapy do sometimes have to decrease the dose of insulin to prevent hypoglycemia.

Relationship to Pressure

Pressure itself is unlikely to be a significant variable at those depths commonly employed for therapeutic hyperbaric oxygen treatments. Eight non-insulin-dependent diabetics undergoing simulated hyperbaric ***air*** treatments (375 kPa) showed no significant decrease in glucose compared to controls. Furthermore, glucose is not affected in deep-sea divers (Raymond), suggesting that if there is a causal relationship, it be related to the significant increases in tissue oxygen encountered with breathing pure oxygen (as in hyperbaric therapy) versus the respiration of hyperbaric air.

PRACTICAL CONSIDERATIONS

Given the above observations, there are several important nursing considerations to keep in mind when treating the diabetic patient with hyperbaric oxygen therapy. For instance, feeding prior to HBOT may be necessary. To determine this, the timing of the patient's last meal and the approximate kilocalories should be taken into account. It is important to determine the time of day when the patient ate, instead of just asking if the patient ate breakfast or lunch. Also consider the type of food consumed, and how much consumed. Many patients will state that they ate breakfast, but when questioned, that meal consisted of a glass of juice and toast.

Since the type and amount of medication taken also determine the likelihood of a drop in glucose, this should be noted. It is important for the nurse to be familiar with the timing of this peak in relation to the timing of the hyperbaric treatment.

CLINICAL RECOMMENDATIONS FOR TREATING DIABETIC PATIENTS

1. Blood glucose measurement by finger stick using rapid and inexpensive technology should be done prior to hyperbaric treatments on all diabetic patients. A good guideline is that the pre-treatment blood sugar should be greater than 120 mg/dl, and the post-treatment sugar should be greater than 100.
2. Patients with blood glucose of 100 mg/dl or less may benefit from having treatment postponed until the blood glucose rises and should be provided with at least 200 kcal orally.
3. Blood glucose measurement by finger stick should be considered after every hyperbaric treatment, particularly if the blood glucose was less than 150 mg/dl prior to HBOT.
4. No patient should be released with blood glucose less than 100 even if asymptomatic. It is possible that the blood glucose will continue to decrease even after the patient is removed from the oxygen-enriched environment. Patients with post treatment glucose of 100 mg/dl or less should probably be fed prior to leaving the facility.
5. Patients with symptomatic hypoglycemia should not be treated.
6. Glucose gel and intravenous D50 should always be kept available for use.

Finally, the diabetic patient receiving hyperbaric oxygen therapy should be monitored for signs and symptoms of hypoglycemia, and the nurse must be ready to intervene when necessary.

SUMMARY

Even with rigorous screening pre hyperbaric treatment, clinical data suggest that 3% of hyperbaric treatments may result in a blood glucose that falls below 100 mg/dl. Regardless of whether this drop is caused by the effect of elevated oxygen levels in the tissues, or is simply a reflection of the timing of medications and hyperbaric treatment, some sort of glucose monitoring program is warranted. Patients whose blood glucose is less than 150 mg/dl are less likely to experience a drop below 100 mg/dl during hyperbaric oxygen treatment if they are given calories prior to the treatment.

REFERENCES

1. Blackburn E, Williford D, Otto G, Smith L, Parker K, Maus E and Fife C. The effectiveness of a blood glucose screening program for diabetics undergoing hyperbaric oxygen therapy. Undersea & Hyperbaric Med. 2001;28(Suppl): (at printers).

2. Kakhnovskii IM, Efuni SN, Khodas MY, Bolshakova TD and Gitel EP. The mechanism of hypoglycemic effect of hyperbaric oxygenation in diabetes mellitus patients. Klin Med (Mosk) 59(9):83-88; Sept. 1981 HBO Rev 1983 July;4(3):143.

3. Longoni C, Camporesi EM, Buizza M, Carissimi E, Mariani R and Mondini G. Reduction in insulin requirements during hbo therapy. UBR. 1988;15(Suppl): 16-17.

4. Martindale VE and Dixon PA. Fresh dissected mouse diaphragms take up glucose more rapidly during hyperbaric oxygenation. Undersea & Hyperbaric Med. 20 (Suppl):33. Jul 1993.

5. Nolan RJ, Dodd DE and Faiman MD. Cerebral and blood glucose in central oxygen poisoning. Undersea Biomed Res. 1978; 5:87-93.

6. Obrenovich T and Brue F. Effects of different normoxic hyperbaric exposure on glucose, lactate, and glycogen brain concentrations. In: Bachrach AJ, Matzen MM, eds. Underwater physiology VII. Proceedings of the seventh symposium on underwater physiology. Bethesda: Undersea Medical Society 1981:675-684.

7. O'Malley E, Otto G, Berkowicz L, Suttle K, Kulikovsky M, Sparlin S and Fife C. Blood glucose screening in diabetics undergoing hyperbaric oxygen therapy. Undersea & Hyperbaric Med. 1998;25(Suppl):49.

8. Pontani BA, Warriner RA, Tyrrel A, Ricken K, Pliner E, Kennedy M, Barnum S, et al. Hypoglycemia as a complication of hbo therapy: who is at risk and when. Undersea & Hyperbaric Med. 21 (Suppl):33. Jun 1994 (abstract only).

9. Raymond L, Sode J, Johnsonbaugh R, Bower R and Spaur W. Blood glucose in deep-sea divers. Biomedical research and underwater breathing apparatus evaluation dives 10 to 1600 feet, April 1-2, 1974, p5. U.S. Navy Exp Diving Unit, Rep# NEDU-23-74. 1974.

10. Springer R. The importance of glucometer testing of diabetic patients pre and post-dive. UBR. 1991;18(Suppl):20 (abstract only).

11. Takahashi H, Kabayashi S, Sakakibara K, Oshida Y, Sato Y, Iguchi A and Sakamoto N. Effect of hbo on endocrine system and metabolism of diabetic patients. UBR. 1990;17(Suppl):52 (abstract only).

12. Torbati D and Torbati A. Blood glucose as a predictive measure for central nervous system oxygen toxicity in conscious rats. Undersea Biomed Res. 1986;13(2):147-153.

13. Zivkovic M, Mandic B, Denoble P, Kovacevic H, Gosivic S and Ilic A. Influence of hbo on blood glucose level and hba1c in diabetes mellitus type 2. EUBS Proceedings of the XVII Annual Meeting on Diving and Hyperbaric Medicine, Crete, Greece, 1991 Sep 29-Oct 3: 407-410.

CHAPTER I

HYPERBARIC NURSING RESEARCH

C. WRENFORD-BROWN

EARLY HYPERBARIC THERAPY

Hyperbaric therapy has had a checkered career. European chambers in the nineteenth century were used more as spas for the rich and fashionable than as medical treatment modalities for specific disease diagnoses. Subsequently the studies of Paul Bert, Al Behnke, and Ite Boerma et al. established the scientific rationale for the clinical benefits of hyperbaric medicine. Despite the exploitation of Midwest patients by such enthusiasts as Professor Orville J. Cunningham in the 1920s, hyperbaric oxygen is no longer a "cure looking for a disease" but a science-based medical therapy.

ESTABLISHMENT OF UNDERSEA AND HYPERBARIC MEDICAL SOCIETY

It was as recent as 1962 that the Committee on Shock of the Division of Medical Sciences of the National Academy of Science-National Research Council appointed a committee to evaluate the efficacy of hyperbaric therapy.

In 1967, the Undersea and Hyperbaric Medical Society was founded. The Society is an international organization that encourages the intellectual exchange of information on physiology, diving, and clinical hyperbaric medicine. The scientific meetings stimulate the presentation of papers for review, and the results are published in the *Journal of Undersea and Hyperbaric Medicine.*

With pressure from both the reimbursement community and their medical peers, the Society published its first Committee Report on Hyperbaric Oxygen Therapy in 1977. It established appropriate scientific justification for the use of hyperbaric oxygen for the recommended diagnoses.(20) It is this committee that reviews potential diagnoses for additions to the thirteen currently approved indications.

HYPERBARIC NURSING

Hyperbaric nurses entered the arena as the field has become more science-based. Early attendants were divers, medics, medical students, and scientists focused on particular aspects of hyperbarics. The emphasis on physics and physiology, the rigorous physical stipulations, and the autonomy of practice seem to have attracted unique and enterprising individuals. Several of these nurses came with backgrounds in research, and, due to the nature of the patients, critical care experience.

EARLY NURSING ARTICLES

The earliest articles written in the 1960s by North American nurses were essentially descriptive of the nurse's role in a hyperbaric chamber. (37, 45, 48, 69, 70) These articles, often bannered "working under pressure," consider some of the logistical issues involved in blending the technology of hyperbarics with the practice and administration of good medical and nursing procedures. At this time, surgery was often performed in the chamber and nursing was a supportive function. Issues such as staff selection, staff development, informed consent, and laundry are addressed on the same pages as physics and fire prevention. Established programs at the Western Infirmary, Glasgow, Scotland; the Wilhelmina Gasthus in Amsterdam, Holland, and later the Lutheran hospital in Chicago, were used as models.

ESTABLISHMENT OF BAROMEDICAL NURSES ASSOCIATION

In 1973 at the 5th International Hyperbaric Congress in Vancouver, British Columbia, several nurses joined together to present papers and discuss practice. However, it wasn't until 1982, when the Undersea and Hyperbaric Medical Society Associates started arranging regular programs for nurses, respiratory therapists, and technicians, that a formal venue for presentation became established. With the founding of the Baromedical Nurses Association in 1985, the platform for the exchange of information was firmly incorporated. (9)

PATIENT CARE

The care of patients and an holistic approach to their needs has always been a prime nursing function. There have been many articles discussingn nursing practice in the hyperbaric unit, both in this country and abroad, with articles from the United States, Canada, France, Japan, and India. (1, 2, 4, 5, 6, 7, 10, 11, 21, 23, 35, 36, 42, 48, 53, 55, 56, 62, 64, 65, 79, 80) The different diagnoses treated in a hyperbaric chamber have triggered examination of different modalities of pain control (24) and the psychological aspects of confined environment anxiety. (61) The uniqueness of the specific diagnoses demands unique nursing management. The management of a necrotizing fasciitis or gas gangrene patient (59, 60, 66) is very different from that of a diver with decompression sickness or a carbon monoxide victim. (31, 39, 46, 64) The patient does not cease to exist on discharge, and post hyperbaric follow-up gives invaluable information on the effectiveness of care. (71)

COLLABORATIVE RESEARCH

Clinical research has established the indications for hyperbaric therapy. The Undersea and Hyperbaric Medical Society Committee Report on Hyperbaric Oxygen Therapy reviews and revises its extensive and thorough report on the science behind the approved indications. In modern hyperbaric medicine, the relationship between nurse and physician is increasingly collegiate. (74) Nurses have assisted in both the collection and interpretation of data. Retrospective etiological studies looking at differing causes of carbon monoxide poisoning (14, 15, 68) take many patient hours of sifting through records. An interesting review of 17 patients treated for carbon monoxide poisoning after they had been resuscitated from cardiac arrest in the field revealed a depressing zero survivability. (12) In this study as in many, the onerous chore of chart review often falls to the nurse or technicians who may have more time to spend in investigation. The establishment of criteria to treat different diagnoses may involve the mailing of questionnaires to clinicians around the country and phone follow-up to ensure a high response rate. (19, 78) Prospective randomized trials often involve treatments outside routine hours, and the clinical nurse is frequently the one to recruit, consent, and acquire data on potential candidates. Often several persons in the same facility will be enlisted to complete the study.

CLINICAL RESEARCH

Both collaboratively and independently, nurses have participated in the development of valuable clinical data to validate the various diagnoses. Diane Norkool in the mid-1980s reviewed 115 cases of carbon monoxide poisoning. (46) In later years she reviewed with Dr. Neil Hampson various etiologies, such as riding in the back of pickup trucks or the burning of charcoal briquettes in a closed environment. Both of these led to public health initiatives to reduce the incidence of poisoning. (14, 15) Valerie Larson-Lohr assisted Lin Weaver in his studies comparing carbon monoxide treated with and without hyperbaric oxygen. (71) A retrospective 5-year review of anaerobic infections by Australians Cindy Skacel and Martin Boyle revealed two cases occurring after orthopedic plaster of paris casting. (59) The refinement of different hyperbaric treatment protocols begins with the assessment of how different chambers around the country treat such diverse diagnoses. This involves repeated mailings and onerous phone follow-up to achieve a high response rate. It is interesting to examine how different styles of chambers in different locations treat mandibular radionecrosis or carbon monoxide. (13, 78) This, it is hoped, will stimulate comparative outcome studies to evaluate which treatment protocols deliver the best balance of risk/benefit ratio.

TESTING NEW TECHNOLOGY, REFINING THE OLD

Equipment and materials used in the hyperbaric environment are subject to unique conditions and must be evaluated and sometimes adapted to deal with both the high pressure gradients and the complications of high partial pressures of oxygen. With diabetic foot wounds composing a growing part of the patient population in the 1990s, nurses initiated three studies on the effectiveness of glucose reageant accuracy. (40, 47, 57) As cutaneous oxygen measurements became more common to qualify avascular hypoxic wound patients for treatment, studies were conducted to compare different instrumentation and to develop predictive criteria. Although the greater part of research was reported by Paul Sheffield et al. in the Undersea and Hyperbaric Medical Society, nurses contributed to both the actual testing and interpretation of data. (54) Different I.V. pumps have been reviewed for both monoplace and multiplace conditions. The use of ventilators used to treat critically ill children was reported, and the problems of hypotension, bronchospasm, and hemotympanum discussed, and management reviewed. (25) The increase in the use and the reduction in size of cardiac pacemakers and automatic implanted cardiac defibrillators is an ongoing study by Sharil Simmons in Seattle, who is working to establish a resource data base for chambers throughout the country to use when they have patients with implanted devices. (58) Even subjects as routine as medical photography are displayed at the poster sessions to stimulate the exchange of ideas between the members. (77)

As computer chip technology and web-bound information pervades our practice, nurses are designing web pages (29) and will be sharing information on electronic documentation, digital photography, clinical outcomes, and quality control.

As more technology becomes available, nurses will be there beside their colleagues, the Undersea and Hyperbaric Medical Society Associates, assessing, comparing, adapting, and educating.

SAFETY

The potential for injury to both hyperbaric patient and the personnel is unusual in that the consequences can be severe. (38) The first nurse to examine some of the complications of the hyperbaric situation was C. Pittinger in a paper on the problems of anesthesia in 1966. (50) Christy Pirone of Australia has focused her entire career on the establishment of an international database examining reported "incidents" in hyperbaric facilities around the world. (49) Christy, Valerie Larson-Lohr, and Laura Josefsen were all contributors to Tom Workman's book *Hyperbaric Facility Safety*. (76) Nurses have a fundamental responsibility to their patients and peers to provide and be provided a safe environment. (27, 67) Drastic and fatal accidents have occurred because of inadequate attention to safety details.

OFFLABEL

Nurses have not been afraid to step outside the established boundaries of the recognized UHMS indications and to examine other potential diagnoses and uses for hyperbaric therapy. In 1971 G. William reported a newborn resuscitated in a hyperbaric chamber in England. (73) Diana De Jesus-Greenberg looked at hyperbaric treatment of spinal cord injury in 1980 and reviewed the acceptance of the different "medical uses of HBO" in her article in *Critical Care Update* the following year. (8) More recently Michele Reillo reported relief of debilitating fatigue in HIV-infected individuals, although this is not a therapy approved by the Undersea and Hyperbaric Medical Society. (51) Controversial issues such as the treatment of stroke have been reviewed. (3)

ADMINISTRATION

As hyperbaric therapy became more established in this country, nurses became more involved in the planning and administration of the programs. A utilization review study by Wendy Merritt and others examined historical productivity and revenue to establish ongoing tools to monitor and predict efficiency. (33, 34)

Constant review of safety procedures and practice should be part of a responsible hyperbaric program. JCAHO requires that Quality Control is an active ongoing process. These and other issues become "hot buttons" for JCAHO. In 1998 at the Seattle meeting, Laura Josefsen reviewed the JCAHO guidelines for effective nursing leadership. (22)

BNA RESEARCH GRANT

The Baromedical Nurses Association (BNA) awards $500.00 annually to a BNA member to fund hyperbaric nursing research. The Research Committee reviews the applicants and recommends disbursement to the President of the BNA who announces the recipient at the annual meeting of the BNA.

The committee examines the application for grounded theory, relevance to hyperbaric nursing, clarity of purpose and design, sample definition, and ethics. Internal Review Board (IRB) approval is required.

Application may be made by contacting the current Research Committee chairperson by mail or email. The expanded tool that the Research Committee use to evaluate proposals can be found on the BNA webpage.

The scope of the award is broad. The first BNA grant was awarded to establish the research priorities for hyperbaric nurses. In 2001, the grant was awarded for a BNA member's *in vitro* study of Activation of the Complement Protein C5A to predict DCS in SCUBA divers. Interested parties are encouraged to contact the chair of the Research Committee.

NEED FOR MORE RESEARCH

The Baromedical Nurses Association is less than 25 years old. Science-based hyperbaric medicine is completing its first century. There is much more to be done. More clinical outcome trials are needed for support of the diagnoses we treat. Refinement of the treatment protocols is needed to ensure successful outcomes efficiently and economically. Patient care is our prime responsibility, and new techniques to improve and measure satisfaction will need to be investigated and shared among our associates. New equipment must be evaluated and compared to existing technology. Training and education of our hyperbaric peers, our colleagues in allied medical fields, and the general public must addressed. A recent study in New York concluded that better medical education of allied fields is required to develop a better understanding of early hyperbaric oxygen for prophylactic treatment of irradiated patients. The management and administration of hyperbaric programs in today's competitive but heavily regulated medical marketplace is a huge issue to be reviewed against each legislative change.

MONICA HUPALO'S RESEARCH PRIORITIES

In 1997 Monica Hupalo, for her master's thesis at the University of Florida, surveyed the BNA membership to establish priorities for focusing research. (18) The eleven highest ranked priorities were:

1. How can we best inform healthcare professionals about the benefits of HBO_2 for specific disease indications?
2. What strategies work well to promote healthcare team planning (i.e., referring physician, social services, nursing, hyperbaric medicine, physical therapy)?
3. How may we maximize reimbursement within the guidelines of the insuring agencies?

4. Which of the different treatment protocols, including oxygen time, air breaks, and surface intervals are most effective for the different diagnoses?
5. What methods are being used for Continuous Quality Improvement?
6. What benchmarks should be used in critical paths for each approved hyperbaric indication?
7. What is the relationship between educating physicians about current research, and patient outcome?
8. How do you increase the awareness of non-hyperbaric physicians re: the potential outcomes HBO_2 treatments?
9. Does HBO_2 have an effect on the blood glucose level in a diabetic patient?
10. Which of the $tcpO_2$ theories or protocols are most beneficial for patient care in HBO_2?
11. What methods of personnel orientation, ongoing training, and documentation are in use and how effective are they?

As the organization expands and the number of clinical facilities grows to over 400 nationwide in 2000 (63), the need and opportunities for more research arise. As Medicare and other reimbursement organizations become more cost-conscious, the need for controlled studies to examine, refine, and report clinical practice becomes more essential. The tremendous expansion of the Internet has made data sharing simple and immediate. Email has made local, national, and international collaboration between facilities straight-forward and fast. Multi-center outcome research, initiated and coordinated by nurses, seems a logical step in this progression. The next logical step is an autonomous journal to publish papers to share with our peers and to stimulate further research activity.

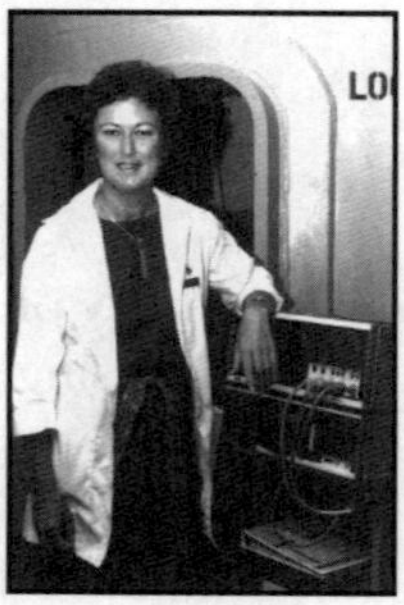

Diane Norkool, RN, MN, CHRN
1942-1996

Virginia Mason Medical Center had just installed a hyperbaric chamber to conduct basic research when Diane took the first hyperbaric course in 1970. As a special project nurse with a critical care background, Diane developed the patient aspect of the hyperbaric facility from the occasional diver into a complete clinical program. (39)

The Virginia Mason Research Center focused on diving physiology. A volunteer subject, as well as investigator, Diane participated in physiological evaluation of deep sea decompression profiles funded by Sub Sea International and the United States Navy from 1972 to 1975.

She wrote her master's thesis at the University of Washington on the effects of intermittent hyperbaric oxygen on small full thickness burns in rats in 1976. (41)

As well as being an avid researcher, Diane developed research-based policies to expand the scope of clinical applications. The nursing staff, working autonomously, developed a clinical program that established Virginia Mason as the leading hyperbaric facility in the Pacific Northwest. She enlisted physicians as the department evolved.

Prolific in her publications, Diane is known especially for papers on carbon monoxide poisoning, radiation cystitis, and critical care in the hyperbaric chamber. (12, 13, 40, 43, 44) Together with Valerie J. Messina, she co-authored a hallmark text on hyperbaric nursing in Dr. Eric Kindwall's *Hyperbaric Medicine Practice.* (25) She wrote several articles on hyperbaric nursing and the physiology of hyperbaric therapy in both medical and nursing journals.

She helped organize the first meeting and presentation of papers by registered nurses at the International Hyperbaric Congress in Vancouver, British Columbia in 1973. In 1981, she encouraged the Undersea and Hyperbaric Medical Society to allow the associate members a more active role which, in 1982, led to the first Associates program being integrated into the annual Undersea and Hyperbaric Medical Society Scientific Meeting. In 1983, she became the vice president of the Undersea and Hyperbaric Medical Society, Pacific Chapter credentials committee. Diane was on the Associates Steering committee and then became a founding member of the Baromedical Nurses Association (BNA), subsequently serving as Director at Large. In that office, she was in the process of rewriting the bylaws of the BNA when she died at the age of 56.

Part of research is the sharing of information, and Diane gave numerous lectures on hyperbaric therapy and diving medicine locally, nationally, and, internationally. The course that she developed in Seattle for orienting new staff was the basis for the annual National Board of Diving and Hyperbaric Medical Technology approved course given there today.

Hyperbaric nurses have the rare opportunity to be involved in a field that is still defining itself. A few, like Diane, are so totally invested and make such an impact by their selflessness and dedication that the practice of those of us who follow is forever changed.

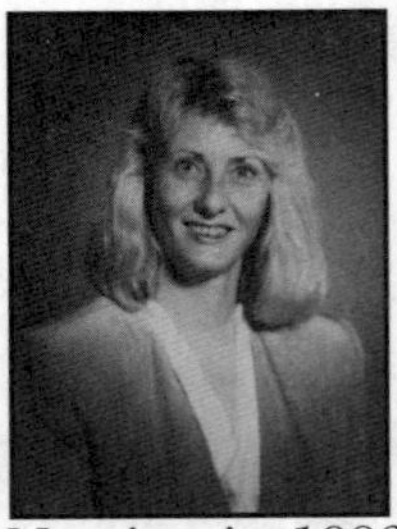

Valerie Larson-Lohr, MSN, APRN, HNC

After graduating from St. Luke's Hospital School of Nursing in Fargo, North Dakota in 1977, Valerie began her life as a nurse in search of excellence. She has advanced her education with a Bachelor of Science in Nursing in 1988, completed the NOAA Dive Medicine Physician Course, and obtained her Master of Science in Nursing in 1993 from the University of Utah. Her Master of Science was a double master in Physiologic Nursing and Informatics. Equipped with the necessary experience, she started her involvement with research in the 1980s. When asked why she first got involved in research, her reply was, "I was asking the question 'why?' and no one gave me a good answer." Her first experience was with Dr. L. Stevens as a clinical research nurse. Their research focused on fibronectin levels and their influence on the trauma patient's immune response, number of complications, and length of stay in the ICU.

Valerie began her work in hyperbaric medicine in 1991 at LDS Hospital in Salt Lake City, Utah working as an advanced practice nurse in wound care and hyperbaric medicine, and served as adjunct professor, School of Nursing, at the University of Utah. Her research experience in Salt Lake City included:

- Family Needs of the Acute Brain Injured and Non-Brain Injured Patients During ICU Admission, principle investigator research project. (72)
- Normobaric Oxygen vs Hyperbaric Oxygen in Patients with Carbon Monoxide Poisoning, co-investigator of clinical trial.
- Long-Term Outcome in Patients with Carbon Monoxide Poisoning, co-investigator of clinical trial. (28)
- Hemodynamic Response of Normal Subjects Exposed to Hyperbaric Air and Oxygen, project manager of clinical trial. (72)
- Long-Term Functional and Cognitive Outcome in ARDS Survivors, co-principal investigator. (16)

She was the 1997 recipient of the Diane Norkool award for consistent excellence in education, research, publication, and clinical operation in the field of wound care and hyperbaric medicine. Her work includes the development of techniques and equipment used to treat critically ill patients in the monoplace hyperbaric chamber and outcome research on the chronic wound patient.

Valerie presently serves as the Director of Clinical Operations for Elsinor Medical Consultants and Director of Warm Springs Hospital's Center for Wound Care. She is an international speaker and recognized expert in the areas of wound care, hyperbaric medicine, and nursing practice. Her future plans for research include outcome studies of the chronic wound patient.

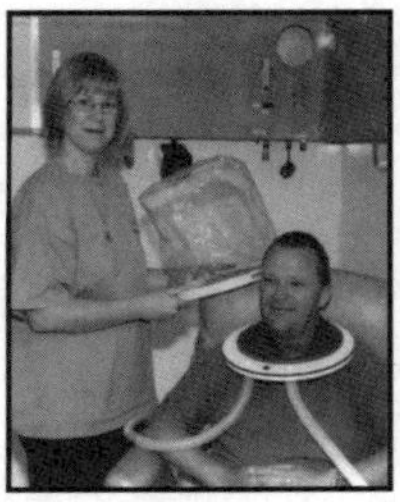

Christy Pirone

In 1982, Christy graduated from Indiana University with a Bachelor of Science in Nursing and started her career in an Adult Critical Care unit at Methodist Hospital in Indianapolis. From the beginning, she was involved with practice committees, education, and quality improvement.

In 1984, she took on the task of the nursing development and operation of her first hyperbaric unit. As she worked to develop the hyperbaric department, her focus remained on education and quality improvement. She saw that nursing did not have an organization to represent them in the specialty of hyperbaric nursing, and she became one of the founding members of the Baromedical Nurses Association.

In 1987, Christy departed for Australia. Always the visionary, she set about developing formal courses in hyperbaric nursing, culminating in the University of Adelaide Graduate Certificate in Hyperbaric Nursing Science. Currently, this is the only Graduate Certificate in Hyperbaric Nursing in the world.

Christy was concerned with the occupational safety of Hyperbaric Nurse Attendants. Little had been done to look at incidents related to inside tenders of multiplace chambers and the factors that contributed to the incidents. In 1992, she launched the Hyperbaric Incident Monitoring Study (HIMS).

HIMS is an anonymous, voluntary reporting system of incidents that could or did affect the safety of hyperbaric staff, patients, and visitors. The intent of the system is to look for factors that have contributed to the incident and correct them, thus preventing another occurrence. All reports are held in strict confidence and are not used in medical/legal issues to assist in assigning blame.

1996 was the international launch of HIMS. By 1997, there were 17 countries participating in the study that had submitted 500 reports. 56% of all reported incidents were related to ear barotraumas. HIMS also documented previously unreported complications such as patient stress reaction after witnessing an oxygen toxic seizure, forceful ejection of a monoplace chamber plug, pulmonary oxygen toxicity in staff, and vision loss in the form of hyperopia.

Factors contributing to the adverse incidents included:

- chance,
- human error,
- no protocols,
- failure to use protocols,
- equipment malfunction, and
- "pressure to proceed."

It is the intent of the database that as more information is collected that strategies to create and develop processes to prevent adverse events will emerge.

The success of HIMS is directly related to the tireless work, perseverance, and commitment of Christy to improving occupational safety of hyperbaric nurse attendants. It was an incredible undertaking which she has made successful. In recognition of her contribution to hyperbaric nursing, in 1999 Christy Pirone was awarded the Diane Norkool Award.

REFERENCES

1. Abbott CC. The use of the hyperbaric chamber as an auxiliary curing aid. AORN Journal. 9(5):80-4, 1969 May.
2. Barois A. [Hyperbaric oxygen therapy]. [French] Revue De L Infirmiere Et De L Assistante Sociale. 16(7):619-27, 1966 Jul-Sep.
3. Borer KM, Borer RC, Strauss MB, Jimenez A, Minkiewitz KM. Hyperbaric Oxygen Therapy For Acute Ischemic Stroke: A Preliminary Clinical Review. Abstract from Baromedical Nurses Association/ Undersea and Hyperbaric Medical Society meeting 1998.
4. Cockerill G, O'Connor R. Hyperbaric Oxygen-a new field for nurses. Nursing Times. 216, 1967 Feb 17.
5. Cogliano J. Diving without water: hyperbaric nursing. Nursing Spectrum (D.C./Baltimore Metro Edition). 8(10):24, 1998 May 18.
6. Daly B. Hyperbaric nursing. Nursing Times. 69(7):203, 1973 Feb 15.
7. De Jesus-Greenberg D. Hyperbaric oxygen therapy. Critical Care Update. 8(2): 8-20, 1981 Feb.
8. De Jesus-Greenberg DA. Acute spinal cord injury and hyperbaric oxygen therapy: a new adjunct in management. Journal of Neurosurgical Nursing. 12(3):155-60, 1980 Sep.
9. Gaul A. Keynote address to first Baromedical Nurses Association meeting. Key Biscayne, FL. April, 1986.
10. Gaul AL. Hart GB. Baromedical nursing combines critical, acute, chronic care. AORN Journal. 21(6):1038-47, 1975 May.
11. Gaul AL. Thompson RE. Hart GB. Hyperbaric oxygen therapy. American Journal of Nursing. 72(5):892-6, 1972 May.
12. Hampson NB, Zmaeff J. Outcome of Patients Experiencing Cardiac Arrest with Carbon Monoxide Poisoning and Treated with Hyperbaric Oxygen. Abstract from Baromedical Nurses Association/ Undersea and Hyperbaric Medical Society meeting 2000.
13. Hampson NB, Dunford RG, Kramer CC, Norkool DM. Selection criteria utilized for hyperbaric oxygen treatment of carbon monoxide poisoning. Journal of Emergency Medicine. 13(2):227-31, 1995 Mar-Apr.
14. Hampson NB, Kramer CC, Dunford RG, Norkool DM. Carbon monoxide poisoning from indoor burning of charcoal briquets. JAMA. 271(1):52-3, 1994 Jan 5.
15. Hampson NB, Norkool DM. Carbon monoxide poisoning in children riding in the back of pickup trucks. JAMA. 267(4):538-40, 1992 Jan 22-29.
16. Hopkins RO, Larson-Lohr V, Weaver LK, Bigler ED. (1998) Neuropsychological Impairments Following Hantavirus Pulmonary Syndrome. Am. J. Crit. Care Med 160: 50-56.
17. Hopkins RO, Weaver LK, Pope D, Orme JF, Bigler ED, Larson-Lohr V. (1999) Neuropsychological Sequelae and Impaired Health Status in Survivors of Severe Acute Respiratory Distress Syndrome. Am. J. Resp and Crit. Care Med. 160:50-56.
18. Hupalo ML. Establishing Research Priorities For The Baromedical Nurses Association. Master's thesis. University of Florida. Abstract from Baromedical Nurses Association/ Undersea and Hyperbaric Medical Society meeting 1998.
19. Hupalo ML. The Utilization Of Hyperbaric Oxygen Therapy As Part Of Routine Burn Care: A Telephone Survey. Abstract from Baromedical Nurses Association/ Undersea and Hyperbaric Medical Society meeting 1998.
20. Hyperbaric Oxygen Therapy Committee. Hyperbaric Oxygen Therapy: 1999 Committee Report. Hampson NB, ed. Kensington, MD: Undersea and Hyperbaric Medical Society; 1999.

21. Illingworth C. Wound sepsis–from carbolic acid to hyperbaric oxygen. Irish Nursing & Hospital World. 32(2):5 passim, 1966 Feb.

22. Josefsen L, Clarke D. Effective Nursing Leadership In The Hyperbaric Unit Per JCAHO Guidelines. Abstract from Baromedical Nurses Association/ Undersea and Hyperbaric Medical Society meeting 1998.

23. Josefsen L, Woodward C, Lewis D, Camporesi EM. The Nursing Role In Hyperbaric Medicine. Abstract from Baromedical Nurses Association/ Undersea and Hyperbaric Medical Society meeting 1997.

24. Josefsen L, Woodward C, Thomas S, Camporesi EM. Hyperbaric Oxygen Therapy/Pain Control: Nursing Responsibilities. Abstract from Baromedical Nurses Association/ Undersea and Hyperbaric Medical Society meeting 1995.

25. Keenan HT, Bratton SL, Norkool DM, Brogan TV, Hampson NB. Delivery of hyperbaric oxygen therapy to critically ill, mechanically ventilated children. Journal of Critical Care. 13(1):7-12, 1998 Mar.

26. Kindwall EP. Hyperbaric Medicine Practice. Best Publishing Company. Flagstaff. 1994.

27. Kraft K, Dear G. Guidelines for the Prevention of Cross Contamination during the Treatment of Patients with VRE and MRSA in a Multi-Place Hyperbaric Setting. Abstract from Baromedical Nurses Association/ Undersea and Hyperbaric Medical Society meeting 2000.

28. Larson-Lohr V, Weaver L, Howe S. Functional Outcome of Hyperbaric Patients at 6 Months After Treatment. Abstract from Baromedical Nurses Association/ Undersea and Hyperbaric Medical Society meeting 1995.

29. Larson-Lohr V. Designing a Web Page for Your Wound Care and Hyperbaric Center. Abstract from Baromedical Nurses Association/ Undersea and Hyperbaric Medical Society meeting 1999.

30. Lawrence G, Bates J, Gaul A. Pathogenesis of Neonatal Necrotizing Enterocolitis. Lancet. 1(8264):137-9, 1982 Jan 16.

31. Lenart S. Decompression sickness and decompression air embolism: treatment with hyperbaric oxygen and nursing management. [Review] [16 refs] Critical Care Nurse. 16(6):40-2, 45-7, 1996 Dec.

32. Mcginn-Merritt W, Bush C, Kim JA, Chung CT, Kellman RM, Camporesi EM. Late Effect Radiation Injuries: A Retrospective Review. Abstract from Baromedical Nurses Association/ Undersea and Hyperbaric Medical Society meeting 2000.

33. Merritt WL, Lewis-Brewster D, Bush C, Hodge J, Adkins J, Camporesi EM. Adoption of a Standard Productivity Tool to Evaluate Hyperbaric Medicine Resource Utilization in a Tertiary Hospital. Abstract from Baromedical Nurses Association/ Undersea and Hyperbaric Medical Society meeting 1998.

34. Merritt WL, Lewis-Brewster D, Bush C, Hodge J, Adkins J, Camporesi EM. Hyperbaric Medicine Resrouce Utilization: A Productivity Tool Coupled with an Associated Financial Tool. Abstract from Baromedical Nurses Association/ Undersea and Hyperbaric Medical Society meeting 1999.

35. Nash M. Hyperbaric medicine. Australian Nurses Journal. 3(8):24-6, 1974 Mar.

36. Nava J, Gamez de Luna P. [Nurse's role in the hyperbaric chamber]. [Spanish] Revista del Colegio Nacional de Enfermeras. 18(1):37-8, 1971 Jan-Feb.

37. Neelon VJ, McIntosh HD. Hyperbaric oxygenation 1. Therapeutic benefits. Cardiovascular Nursing. 7(3):69-72, 1971 May-Jun.

38. Neelon VJ, McIntosh HD. Hyperbaric oxygenation. II. Hazards and implications. Cardiovascular Nursing. 7(4):73-6, 1971 Jul-Aug.

39. Noda T, Sadakiyo S, Muraho I, Sugimoto T, Tahara I. [Hyperbaric oxygenation and nursing care in carbon monoxide poisoning]. [Japanese] Kango Gijutsu - Japanese Journal of Nursing Art. 5:96-104, 1970 May.

40. Norkool DM. Current concepts of hyperbaric oxygenation and its application in critical care. Heart & Lung. 8(4):728-35, 1979 Jul-Aug.

41. Norkool DM. Full thickness burns in rats treated with hyperbaric oxygen. Master's thesis at University of Washington. 1974.

42. Norkool DM. Current concepts of hyperbaric oxygenation and its application in critical care. Heart & Lung. 8(4):728-35, 1979 Jul-Aug.

43. Norkool DM. Fournier's gangrene: assessment and management [letter; comment]. Critical Care Nurse. 16(3):15, 1996 Jun.

44. Norkool DM, Hampson NB, Gibbons RP, Weissman RM. Hyperbaric oxygen therapy for radiation-induced hemorrhagic cystitis. Journal of Urology. 150 (2 Pt 1):332-4, 1993 Aug.

45. Norkool DM. Hyperbaric oxygen therapy: high pressure nursing. Nursing Administration Quarterly. 9(4):57-61, 1985 Summer.

46. Norkool DM, Kirkpatrick JN. Treatment of acute carbon monoxide poisoning with hyperbaric oxygen: a review of 115 cases. Annals of Emergency Medicine. 14(12):1168-71, 1985 Dec.

47. O'Malley E, Otto G, Berkowitz L, Suttle K, Kulikovsky M, Sparlin S, Fife C. Blood Glucose Screening in Diabetics Undergoing Hyperbaric Oxygen Therapy. Abstract from Baromedical Nurses Association/ Undersea and Hyperbaric Medical Society meeting 1998.

48. Oettinger MC. Nursing practice in a hyperbaric unit. ANA Clinical Conferences. 2:9-15, 1965.

49. Pirone C. Occupational Health of Hyperbaric Multiplace Chamber Attendant: A Literature Review. Abstract from Baromedical Nurses Association/Undersea and Hyperbaric Medical Society meeting 1998.

50. Pittinger C. Problems of anesthesia in hyperbaric atmospheres. Journal of the American Association of Nurse Anesthetists. 34(5):321-5, 1966 Oct.

51. Reillo MR. Hyperbaric oxygen therapy for the treatment of debilitating fatigue associated with HIV/AIDS. Journal of the Association of Nurses in AIDS Care. 4(3):33-8, 1993 Jul-Sep.

52. Rogante MM, De Oliveira L. [Nursing care to patients with gas gangrene: treatment in the hyperbaric chamber]. [Portuguese] Revista Enfermagem Em Novas Dimensoes. 4(3):146-50, 1978 May-Jun.

53. Ross MC. Assessing physiological changes from hyperbaric therapy. Dimensions of Critical Care Nursing. 9(1):16-21, 1990 Jan-Feb.

54. Schrader D, Parker K, Otto G, Fife C. The Relationship Between Transcutaneous Oximetry and Laser Skin Perfusion Pressure Utilizing the Vasamedics Laser Doppler 2000. Abstract from Baromedical Nurses Association/ Undersea and Hyperbaric Medical Society meeting 1997.

55. Schweisheimer W. [Hyperbaric oxygenation methods]. [German] Agnes Karll-Schwester - der Krankenpfleger. 25(6):241, 1971 Jun.

56. Serrano Ferrer Y, Valiente Gonzalez MA, Ramirez Lopez F, Valdivia Chinea A, Morales Cudello S. [Work of nurses in hyperbaric oxygenation]. [Spanish] Revista Cubana de Enfermeria. 9(1):39-44, 1993 Jan-Jun.

57. Shafer MR. 1991 Federal Nursing Service Award recipient. The effect of increased atmospheric pressure on glucose reagent strip accuracy. Military Medicine. 157(4):162-5, 1992 Apr.

58. Simmons S. Review of Permanent Pacemakers in Hyperbaric Chambers. Abstract from Baromedical Nurses Association/ Undersea and Hyperbaric Medical Society meeting 1998.

59. Skacel C, Boyle M. A five year review of anaerobic, necrotizing soft tissue infections: a nursing perspective. Australian Critical Care. 5(4):15-7, 18-20, 1992 Dec.

60. Soaper L, Hastee L. Necrotizing Soft Tissue Infections with Hyperbaric Medicine. Abstract from Baromedical Nurses Association/ Undersea and Hyperbaric Medical Society meeting 1998.

61. Sullivan N, Zarikos A. Psychological aspects in the confined environment: managing the patient, the diver, the diver-patient. Abstract from Baromedical Nurses Association/ Undersea and Hyperbaric Medical Society meeting 1999.

62. Sunakura M, Matsuzawa T. [Hyperbaric oxygen radiotherapy and its nursing care]. [Japanese] Kango Gijutsu - Japanese Journal of Nursing Art. 5:88-95, 1970 May.

63. Undersea and Hyperbaric Medical Society 2000 membership directory ed. Kensington, MD: Undersea and Hyperbaric Medical Society; 2000.

64. Usher K. Carbon monoxide poisoning: nursing priorities and treatment. Journal of Psychosocial Nursing & Mental Health Services. 32(7):41-3, 1994 Jul.

65. Vadalkar S. Hyperbaric oxygenation. Nursing Journal of India. 57(11):321 passim, 1966 Nov.

66. Valesi M, Belletti M, Traballi L, Rainier C, Vezzani G. Mortality Rate in Soft Tissue Infections: A Seven Year Review. Abstract from Baromedical Nurses Association/ Undersea and Hyperbaric Medical Society meeting 1997.

67. Valesi M, Belletti M, Traballi L, Rainieri C, Nuletti T, Nasi O, Vezzani G. Microbiological Monitoring of the Air in Hyperbaric Chamber. Abstract from Baromedical Nurses Association/ Undersea and Hyperbaric Medical Society meeting 2000.

68. Valesi M, Belletti M, Traballi L, Rainieri C, Vezzani G, Pizzola A. Carbon Monoxide (Co) Poisoning in Children: An Eight Year Revue. Abstract from Baromedical Nurses Association/ Undersea and Hyperbaric Medical Society meeting 1998.

69. Venger MJ. Hyperbaric oxygenation: nursing responsibility in planning for a new clinical service. Nursing Clinics of North America. 1(1):131-42, 1966 Mar.

70. Venger MJ, Jacobson JH. A Nursing Challenge. American Journal of Nursing. 1964 Oct.

71. Weaver LK, Hopkins RO, Larson-Lohr V. (1996) Neuropsychological and Functional Recovery from Severe Carbon Monoxide Poisoning without Hyperbaric Oxygen Therapy. Annals of Emergency Medicine, 27:(2) 736-740.

72. Weaver L, Larson-Lohr V. (1994) Hypoxemia During Hyperbaric Oxygen Therapy: A Case Report. Chest 105:(4) 1270-1271.

73. Williams GF. Resuscitation of the newborn by hyperbaric oxygen. Nursing Mirror & Midwives Journal. 133(6):30-1, 1971 Aug 6.

74. Wills-Long SL, Long CH. Laybourne M. Hyperbaric oxygen therapy–nursing opportunity. [Review] [4 refs] Dimensions of Critical Care Nursing. 8(3):176-82, 1989 May-Jun.

75. Woodward C, Josefson L, Lewis D, Hodge J, Chiles P, Camporesi EM. Flap Preservation Both Ears. Abstract from Baromedical Nurses Association/ Undersea and Hyperbaric Medical Society meeting 1997.

76. Workman W. Hyperbaric Facility Safety. Best Publishing Company. Flagstaff. 1999.

77. Wreford-Brown C. Review of 35mm Photography of Chronic Wounds, Technique and Technology, a Cookbook Approach. Abstract from Baromedical Nurses Association/ Undersea and Hyperbaric Medical Society meeting 1997.

78. Wreford-Brown CE, Hampson NB. Hyperbaric Oxygen Treatment Protocols for Mandibular Osteordionecrosis. Abstract from Baromedical Nurses Association/ Undersea and Hyperbaric Medical Society meeting 2000.

79. Zilm G. [Hyperbaric oxygenation therapy: high pressure nursing]. [French] Infirmiere Canadienne. 11(3):24-7, 1969 Mar.

80. Zilm G. Hyperbaric oxygen units-high pressure nursing. Canadian Nurse. 65(2):37-40, 1969 Feb.

CHAPTER I

PATIENT EDUCATION

H. NORVELL, V. LARSON-LOHR, S. FABUS, AND L. JOSEFSEN

INTRODUCTION

Education of the patient and his/her family improves patient health outcomes. It does this by helping to promote a healthy behavior and involving the patient in care and care decisions. The Joint Commission on Accreditation of Healthcare Organizations (JCAHO) includes education as one of its standards for hospital accreditation. Clear, goal-directed processes of patient and family education are defined to clarify what a hospital should do to meet this standard. In the hyperbaric environment, patient education also includes safe practice and the patient's responsibility in guaranteeing that safety. JCAHO's goals that substantiate education of the patient in the hyperbaric environment encompass, but are not restricted to:

- Formulating patient education program goals
- Allocating resources for patient education
- Determining and prioritizing specific patient educational needs
- Providing education to meet the identified patient needs

Activities involved in addressing the above goals include, but not restricted to:

- Promoting interactive communication between patients and providers
- Improving the patient's understanding of his/her health status, options for treatment, and anticipated risks and benefits of treatment
- Enhancing patient participation in continuing care

Psychosocial, spiritual, and cultural values also affect patients' response to care and their willingness to participate actively in care and education. When the impact of these values is recognized, a hyperbaric facility can encourage patients' involvement in their care and educational process. The facility should make sure its education plan encourages an ongoing interaction between patients and staff. A plan that views education as an interaction in which both parties are learners is valuable.

Patient education helps to maximize the benefit of hyperbaric therapy's integration into the total healthcare delivery system and helps to improve cost effectiveness and patient care. To be effective, education must be coordinated among all disciplines involved in the patient's care. Patient education has demonstrated its potential to increase consumer satisfaction, improve quality of life, and ensure continuity of care, by reducing the incidence of complications with illness, promoting adherence to treatment plans, and decreasing patient anxiety. It is accepted as an essential component in the safe practice of hyperbaric oxygen therapy. Objectives of patient care in the hyperbaric environment involve safety, effective treatment outcomes, patient adherence to the treatment plan, treatment comfort, and clear comprehension. Training of healthcare providers in the hyperbaric environment helps to achieve these objectives. Success of these objectives is increased by effective patient and family education to familiarize the patient and/or significant others to the treatment, its effects, benefits, risk factors, and safety considerations relating to his/her treatment.

The basic principles of education are in accordance with patient rights. All patients have rights of access to care, respect, confidentiality, and dignity. They also have the right to be involved in all aspects of their care-planning including decision-making. Healthcare providers must carry out the processes that attend to these rights in a manner that is acceptable to the individual patient and that meets patients' needs.

Patient education involves the entire staff of a hyperbaric facility, including the physicians, nurses, technicians, respiratory therapists, and part-time patient care staff. The staff should help the patient understand and accept the reasons he or she needs hyperbaric oxygen therapy. The physician must be able to communicate with his patient in a way that fosters the patient's learning.

Patients who misunderstand their diagnosis and treatment plans exhibit poor compliance. JCAHO requires that instruction be given on a level understandable to the patient. Healthcare providers often give too much information on too high a level for many patients to understand. Speaking in simpler language, repeating instructions, and demonstrating key points while avoiding too many directives enhance a patient's understanding. Combining easy-to-read written patient education materials with oral instructions has been shown to greatly enhance patient understanding. Patient education materials should be short and simple, contain culturally sensitive graphics, and encourage desired behavior. Compliance with therapy also improves by including family members in the patient education process. The purpose of patient education is to provide the patient with the knowledge needed for self-care.

Patient/family education is ideally started prior to initiating hyperbaric oxygen treatment, and is continued and reinforced throughout the entire treatment course. The documentation of patient safety education and patient understanding for each treatment is important as a tool for standardization and evaluation of patient safety. Teaching may be facilitated with the use of audiovisual aids such as videos, handouts, pamphlets, and computerized instructions. Other effective methods include one-on-one teaching or group teaching. A guided format can be utilized to assure that all pertinent information is reviewed on a consistent basis. Effective patient education is a necessary component of patient satisfaction and has proven instrumental in decreasing hospital stays while improving clinical outcomes.

KEY ISSUES FOR THE EDUCATION PROCESS

When evaluating the teaching process, key points to remember are:

- Introduce all caregivers to the patient.
- Ask the patient what he/she knows about hyperbaric oxygen therapy.
- Assess the patient's readiness to learn, incorporate age-specific issues.
- Assess the physical and emotional needs of the patient.
- Assure that anxiety levels are controlled, and determine that any discomfort/pain is relieved such that the patient can tolerate the treatment.
- Adapt the teaching process to the individual patient and family.

PATIENT EXPECTATIONS

Patients should know what is expected of them. Ask patients if they have any questions regarding their treatments. Have patients discuss their expectations of the treatment and plan of care. Compliance with the treatment plan is needed for optimal outcomes.

PATIENT PREPARATION

The patient should be able to verbalize the purpose and indication for treatment.

Risks and Benefits

Risks involved with hyperbaric oxygen therapy should be discussed prior to consent of the patient and any family members present. The discussion between the hyperbaric physician and the patient, related to the itemized risks, hazards, and benefits, is the key component. This education should include the potential for and preventative measures of the risk factors due to increased concentrations of oxygen under pressure and the pressurization itself. These risk factors include fire, barotrauma, and oxygen toxicity of the central nervous system, and pulmonary and ophthalmic function. Emphasize the importance of breathing normally during pressure changes. Instruction in ear equalization techniques is also an important educational element to assure patient comfort and success in the initial treatment.

DEPARTMENT EDUCATION

Patients should (where applicable and appropriate) be given a tour of the hyperbaric unit. Answer any questions they might have concerning the treatments. Most patients have never heard of hyperbaric oxygen therapy. An explanation of the treatment scheduling and duration should be discussed with the patient and family. Be sure that patients know what time they are expected to arrive for treatments. Explain that patient emergencies can alter the schedule.

CHAMBER ORIENTATION

Educate patients on what they should expect to feel, hear, and experience during a treatment. The patient should be educated about the rationalization of emptying the bladder before a treatment. Explain that a treatment should feel no different from traveling in an airplane or at high elevations, except for possible ear discomfort.

Explain the following:

Temperature Changes
As stated in Charles' Law of physics, when pressure is increased and the container remains constant, the temperature will increase. Instruction to the patient about temperature changes during compression and decompression should be discussed.

Noises
Noises in the monoplace chamber will include the background noise of the oxygen entering the chamber topressurize and maintain the treatment pressure. Any noises made in the chamber area or while manipulating the chamber, such as closing the door or returning the mike after talking to the patient will be amplified because of the enclosed space. The staff should inform the patient that the noise is normal and explain the source if known. If you do not know the source of the noise, investigate it to assure that nothing is improper with the chamber operation.

In a multiplace chamber, the same is true about noise amplification. Other noises that can be of concern to the patient are opening and closing pressure valves to maintain constant pressure. Assure the patient that they are normal noises and explain how the chamber pressure is maintained by opening and closing the valves.

Middle Ear Equalization

The patient should be able to demonstrate an effective technique for "clearing ears" (swallowing, chewing, yawning, tilting head back, modified valsalva/toynbee maneuver), and be made aware of the possible need to take a decongestant and/or a nasal spray. Return demonstration is a good tool to assess patient understanding and ability to perform the task during compression. Patient history should also include questions of ear surgery. Instruct the patient to notify the attendant of any sinus or tooth pain during pressurization. Upper respiratory infections and chronic sinusitis make it difficult for the patient to clear the ears and sinuses. These patients can often be compressed if ,decongestants are used, or may require myringotomy or PE tubes performed bilaterally.

Claustrophobia/Confinement Anxiety

Patient preparation includes psychological adaptation to the hyperbaric chamber. Patients should be able to verbalize self-control for exiting the chamber as needed, identify/refine their own relaxation techniques, demonstrate the technique for calling the nurse or technician, and be able to discuss when/how to request a sedative for relaxation, if needed. Many people feel anxious in a confined space. Several measures can be taken to decrease anxiety. These measures may include anti-anxiety medications, talking to the patient with a soft voice, establishing eye contact with the healthcare provider, reassuring the patient that he/she is safe, and teaching the patient relaxation methods (such as visualization, distraction, listening to music, relaxation videos). It is important to satisfy the patient that he/she is in full control at all times and that the treatment can be terminated at any time he/she feels too anxious to continue. It is rare that a patient cannot continue therapy due to confinement anxiety. Patients with true claustrophobia, however, may be unable to go into the hyperbaric chamber at all. Emphasize to patients that they will be under continuous observation during the entire hyperbaric treatment.

For optimum comfort and safety, the patient should be instructed to notify the healthcare provider of any flu- or cold-like symptoms that include fever, cough, sore throat, runny nose, fever blisters, sores, nausea, vomiting, diarrhea, or ache-all-over feelings. Animal studies have shown respiratory viral infections to be more debilitating when the animal is exposed to hyperbaric oxygen, perhaps because of synergistic oxygen irritation of the lung. For this reason, it is suggested that patients who develop colds and whoare receiving hyperbaric oxygen therapy for a chronic disease, which does not require urgent therapy, take a break in therapy until they are over the acute symptoms.

FIRE HAZARDS

Because of the rapid increase in combustibility of materials as ambient PO_2 rises, specific safety measures must be implemented to minimize the risk of fire in hyperbaric chambers. For the monoplace chamber, a review of items and substances not allowed in the chamber should be explained to the patient along with the rationale. A sign displaying the fire hazard items should also be visible to the patients and staff on a daily basis.

APPROPRIATE CONSENT FOR TREATMENT

Informed consent is a basic right of the patient or guardian. To be educated of his/her diagnoses, treatments, and prognoses necessary, enables him/her to take part in treatment decisions that reflect his/her wishes. It is also the right of the patient to be informed of any human experimentation or other research/educational projects affecting his/her care or treatment and to refuse participation in such experimentation or research.

INFORMED CONSENT

Informing patients of the expected outcomes and of the risks and the side effects that may occur related to their therapy is an important component in both the emotional and physical tolerance of their care. Options related to other forms of treatment available, or the expectations of outcome if no therapy at all is provided, need to be discussed with the patient as well. Informed consent implies that a dynamic and interactive relationship occurs between the patient and the hyperbaric physician. This interaction is the basis from which the patient is able to make an informed decision relative to his/her care. For this to occur, the information provided to the patient needs to be in format context and language that the patient can clearly understand. In situations of impaired decision-making ability or mental state, a surrogate decision-maker should be identified, usually a spouse or other family member.

This process is not simply obtaining a signature on a "release" or "consent form" and cannot occur between anyone but the physician and patient or surrogate. All of the nursing and technical interactions involved in instructional preparedness for chamber therapy are supportive to this process, but in no way supplant it. Further, if patients develop questions related to outcomes or risk, it is the responsibility of the physician to redirect explanations.

SAFETY POLICIES AND PROCEDURES

Safety policies and procedures are an essential component of personnel training in a hyperbaric facility. Healthcare personnel have the responsibility to check each patient prior to each treatment. Awareness of these policies and procedures by the patient and the family provides an added safety factor.

Patient/family education should include the following issues and return demonstration knowledge of fire-related safety protocols:

- Patients are to wear only 100% cotton gown/clothing provided by the hyperbaric unit
- No personal garments or unnecessary items are accepted
- Toiletries (alcohol, oil, or petroleum-based products) are removed
- All jewelry is removed (rings may be taped)
- A grounding strap is affixed
- Items that contain batteries are not allowed (including but not limited to watches, hearing aids, TENS units, external pacemakers, external pumps, etc.)
- No hard contact lenses

MEDICATIONS

Patients must inform their hyperbaric physician of all their current medications. Medications that are absolute contraindications in hyperbaric oxygen therapy are:

- Mafenide Acetate (Sulfamylon)
- Disfulfiram (Antabuse)
- Doxorubicin (Adriamycin)
- Cis-Platinum

A third chemotherapeutic agent, bleomycin sulphate, is intimately associated with oxygen-induced pulmonary toxicity. Patients who have received oxygen therapy at 1.0 ATA several days or weeks following bleomycin have exhibited pulmonary toxicity and fibrosis which may progress to irreversible respiratory failure.

Narcotics

In general, narcotics can decrease respiratory drive that can lead to an increase in PcO_2. Oxygen will also decrease respiratory effort, further increasing PcO_2. Elevated PcO_2 can dilate cerebral blood vessels, causing increased diffusion of oxygen into the brain. This can lead to an oxygen toxic seizure.

In a choice of I.V. versus I.M. injection, the preferred route of administration of narcotics and sedatives is I.V. During and immediately after hyperbaric oxygen therapy, generalized vasoconstriction is present. The effect of vasoconstriction on medication given by an I.M. route is a decrease in drug absorbency that may lead to subsequent injections for relief of pain/anxiety. This could potentially lead to over-sedation of the patient.

STEROIDS

Use of high-dose steroids can increase the risk of seizure activity from oxygen toxicity.

ANTICONVULSANTS

The use of anticonvulsants, in connection with hyperbaric oxygen therapy, may be either prophylactic or for the treatment of seizures which do not stop when oxygen inhalation is terminated.

SEDATION

Sedation can be used to increase the seizure threshold in those patients at greater risk of oxygen toxic seizure, and is also used to assist in control of claustrophobia or confinement anxiety. Xanax, Ativan, or Valium may be prescribed and should be taken by the patient 30-60 minutes prior to treatment. During this time and for several hours after the hyperbaric oxygen treatment, the patient should not drive a car or operate any type of equipment or machinery.

OXYGEN TOXICITY

Each tissue is uniquely sensitive to oxygen. Some toxic manifestations occur with exposure to hyperoxia at ambient pressures, whereas others are limited to hyperbaric oxygen environments. Only pulmonary, CNS, and ophthalmologic effects have been shown to be clinically significant.

Patients should be aware of the signs of pulmonary oxygen toxicity. These include tightness in the chest; dry, hacking cough; difficulty inhaling a full breath; and difficulty breathing-increased rate or depth of respirations. The use of air breaks should be discussed with the patient when indicated. Instruction in the correct use of an air break device (mask, hood, trach collar, face tent) should be effectively covered.

PNEUMOTHORAX

A person suffering a spontaneous pneumothorax, especially in the monoplace chamber, is in a very serious predicament. In the multiplace chamber, the pneumothorax may be reduced in the usual way by inserting a chest tube. In the monoplace chamber, this is not possible and the patient must not be decompressed until all preparations have been made to immediately insert a chest tube to relieve the pneumothorax at surface. The proper department procedure for emergency decompression needs to be followed. Previous thoracic surgery may have produced air-trapping lesions which could cause problems during decompression; therefore, these patients need to be accepted for treatment on a case-by-case basis. Slow decompressions must be used to avoid the possibility of air-trapping and the patients should preferably be breathing oxygen during decompression in these cases. Patients with any kind of pulmonary lesions on x-ray, even if asymptomatic, should be decompressed slowly. Rapid pressure changes in these patients might produce serious consequences.

Patients should be aware of premonitory signs and symptoms of CNS oxygen toxicity. These include anxiety, behavioral changes, sweating, nausea, twitching of the lips and face, visual field and auditory changes, vertigo, syncope, and tonic-clonic seizures, which also may occur without prodrome.

Seizure-prone patients should receive prophylactic anti-convulsant therapy prior to hyperbaric oxygen treatments. Depending on the patient's need for hyperbaric oxygen therapy, the physician can decide to continue hyperbaric oxygen treatments at a lower atmospheric pressure and prescribe anti-convulsant medication during the course of hyperbaric oxygen.

When hyperbaric oxygen exposures above 2.0 ATA are required, such as in the treatment of necrotizing infections, air embolism, or decompression sickness, the risk of oxygen-induced seizures may be decreased by allowing the patient to breathe air intermittently during the treatment. These "air breaks" may be included in the treatment of any patient who is at high risk for seizures, such as patients with underlying seizure disorders or high fever.

Preventive measures should be taken and include:

- Close observation and monitoring for early s/s of oxygen toxicity such as unexplained tachycardia, anxiety, speech or visual disturbance, etc.
- Air breaks – the physician may choose to use a 10-minute air break instead of a 5-minute break

SMOKING

Smoking cessation for the duration of the hyperbaric oxygen treatment series needs to be emphasized because of its effect on tissue oxygenation. The patient should be instructed in what resources/mechanisms assist with cessation.

SERUM GLUCOSE LEVELS FOR ALL DIABETIC PATIENTS

Serum glucose levels need to be checked on all diabetic patients prior to each hyperbaric oxygen treatment to prevent possible CNS toxicity (seizure activity) due to hypo/hyperglycemia.

- The patient's blood glucose should be monitored before and after each hyperbaric treatment.
- Insulin doses may need to be altered during the hyperbaric oxygen course of therapy.
- During the hyperbaric oxygen treatment, the staff may have the patient take orange juice into the chamber in case he/she starts to feel hypoglycemic.
- Patient departure from the hyperbaric center may have to be delayed if sugar is too low after treatment. The staff should not release the patient from the center if they feel there is a risk of a hypoglycemic event.

INSULIN

Medicine does not fully understand the effects of hyperbaric oxygen on insulin secretion and metabolism. It has been observed during the course of hyperbaric oxygen therapy that blood glucose levels consistently fall and insulin dosing may need to be adjusted.

Plasma glucagon levels have also shown a decrease during the hyperbaric oxygen course.

CONTRAINDICATIONS FOR TREATMENT

ABSOLUTE

- An untreated pneumothorax, unless it can be surgically relieved before decompression is carried out
- The concomitant administration of doxorubicin (Adriamycin TM) or cisplatin (Platinol) as chemotherapeutic agents for cancer

Pregnancy was thought to be a contraindication because high oxygen partial pressure is associated with closure of the patent ductus arteriosus, and as the unborn fetus is by definition a "premature" infant, retrolental firoplasia was a theoretical danger. However, work carried out in the Soviet Union in which mothers with congenital heart disease who could not carry babies to term were treated intermittently throughout their pregnancy with hyperbaric oxygen, has shown that there appeared to be no complications associated with the use of the chamber. Additional anecdotal reports continue to support this view.

RELATIVE CONTRAINDICATIONS

Conditions in which caution must be observed but which are not absolute contraindications to hyperbaric oxygen therapy are:

- Upper respiratory infections
- Chronic sinusitis
- Seizure disorders
- Emphysema with CO_2 retention
- Uncontrolled high fever
- History of spontaneous pneumothorax
- History of thoracic surgery
- History of reconstructive ear surgery
- Pulmonary lesions on routine x-ray or CT scan
- Viral infections
- Congenital spherocytosis
- Sickle cell anemia
- History of optic neuritis

In some persons with COPD and CO_2 retention, there is a possibility that with the addition of more-than-normal quantities of oxygen the patient may stop breathing spontaneously due to a loss of the hypoxic drive. In patients with severe pulmonary disease who are suffering from CO_2 retention, a hyperbaric treatment may be carried out if the patient is intubated and on a ventilator. Not all patients with abnormal pCO_2 will experience this problem, and a 100% O_2 challenge may be useful.

Uncontrolled high fever can predispose a patient to oxygen seizures, but in such cases aspirin or acetaminophen and a hypothermia blanket can minimize this possibility. Also, anticonvulsant medication can be given prophylactically.

In congenital spherocytosis, the red cells are extremely fragile and hyperbaric oxygen may be followed by considerable hemolysis. Patients with spherocytosis have been successfully treated and simply monitoring the patient for signs of hemolysis is probably adequate. If it is an absolute requirement to treat such a patient (i.e., gas gangrene), one should not be deterred but should be prepared to manage the complication. Hereditary spherocytosis is therefore termed a relative contraindication to therapy. If the patient is carefully followed for evidence of hemolysis and adequate nutritional supplementation is provided, the patient can be successfully treated.

Multiple authors have noted that sickle cell patients are notorious for manifesting oxygen toxicity in the form of seizure activity. Sickle cell patients themselves are more seizure-prone and appear to be much more likely to seize in hyperbaric environments than the average patient. The question of whether or not sickle cell is aided or exacerbated by pressurization has been argued for some time. In the setting of the patient who requires hyperbaric management who also has sickle cell disease, seizure prophylaxis should be considered. It should also be noted that sickle cell patients, because of their chronic hemolysis and turnover of hemoglobin, will frequently have elevated carboxyhemoglobin levels in the absence of a source of external carbon monoxide poisoning.

Blindness has been associated with hyperbaric treatment in some patients with a history of optic neuritis, even if not active at the time of treatment. However, these have been extremely rare and the only reports are anecdotal. If a person gives a history of optic neuritis, exercise caution. We do know of one case of a woman being treated for MS who went completely blind during a course of hyperbaric treatments and remained so. One should immediately halt any further hyperbaric treatment at the slightest suggestion of any visual changes related to the retina. A consult should be obtained at such a time. Some units defensively insist on an ophthalmologist's evaluation on all patients prior to submitting to multiple treatments.

Ear surgery, with the placement of a wire or plastic strut in the ear after stapedectomy, may be a contraindication as changes in pressure could disrupt the implant. In such cases, a consult should be obtained from an ear, nose, and throat surgeon who can prophylactically place a polyethylene tube through the eardrum to avoid problems.

WOUND CARE

Ongoing wound management includes patient education on wound care, including patient awareness of contraindications of materials not allowed on the wound during hyperbaric treatments and the verbalization and recognition of infection control during dressing changes.

NUTRITIONAL ASSESSMENT

As part of the patient education evaluation for a wound care and/or hyperbaric center, a nutritional assessment may be performed. This assessment is done to evaluate the patient's nutritional assessment as it pertains to wound healing. Generally, a nutritional assessment includes taking a sample of blood and collecting a 24-hour urine sample to evaluate nitrogen balance. To promote optimal wound treatment, the patient needs to be in a positive nitrogen balance that would suggest adequate protein for wound repair.

General Nutrition Information

Protein:

- Low protein will prolong the inflammatory response and delay healing.
- Edema can develop secondary to hypoalbuminemia, which can adversely affect the diffusion of oxygen and cause hypoxia to the non-healing wounded tissue.
- Protein is associated with collagen synthesis, and inadequate protein can interfere with collagen synthesis and prolong the healing process.

Adequate Caloric Intake:

- Inadequate caloric intake can adversely affect wound healing by promoting catabolism (breakdown of protein for energy instead of carbohydrates).
- Weight loss with associated subcutaneous fat loss that can potentially cause further wounding of tissue.
- Glucose is the primary fuel for cellular metabolism of leukocytes, fibroblasts, and macrophages; if not available, the body catabolizes protein. This will also occur in diabetics if there is not enough insulin present to allow glucose to be utilized by the cells.

Vitamins & Minerals:

Recommend a balanced daily vitamin intake during patient treatment.

Vitamin A

- Required for adequate inflammatory response
- Plays a role in collagen synthesis
- Counteracts the catabolic effect of glucocorticosteroids on wound healing
- Important in maintaining normal defense mechanisms and limiting complications associated with infected wounds
- Essential for epithelial integrity

Vitamin C

- Role in collagen synthesis and fibroblast mitosis
- Increases activation of leukocytes and macrophages to injured site
- Affects tensile strength and generation of extracellular matrix

Zinc

- Needed for collagen synthesis
- Cofactor in over 100 enzyme reactions
- Deficiency in zinc will reduce rates of epithelialization and decrease wound strength

Vitamin E

- Should be taken on a daily basis during the course of hyperbaric oxygen therapy, shown to be effective in animal research to decrease the risk of oxygen toxic seizures

REFERENCES

1. Joint Commission 1999 Hospital Accreditation Standards pp. 113-120.
2. Bastable, SB. "Overview of Education in Health Care." Nurse as Educator: Principles of Teaching and Learning. p. 7, 1997.
3. Gaynor, S. Patyk, M. Putting the pieces in place: the patient education puzzle. J Nurs Care Qual, 12(3): 64-8, 1998 Feb.
4. Mayeaux EJ Jr., Murphy PW, Arnold C, Davis TC, Jackson RH, Sentell T. Improving patient education for patients with low literacy skills. Am Fam Physician, 53(1): 205-11, 1996.
5. Hussey LC. "Strategies for effective patient education material design." J Cardiovasc Nurs. 11(2):37-46 1997 Jan.
6. Fitzgerald K. "Instructional Methods: Selection, Use, and Evaluation." Nurse as Educator: Principles of Teaching and Learning. pp. 261-285, 1997.
7. Kindwall EP. "Contraindications and Side Effects to Hyperbaric Oxygen Treatment." In: Hyperbaric Medicine Practice (Kindwall EP, ed) Best Publishing Company, Flagstaff, AZ, 1994.
8. Norkool DM. "Care of the Patient Receiving Hyperbaric Oxygen Therapy." Manual of Patient Care Standards. Reiner, Ann, Editor. Aspen Publishers, Inc., Gaithersberg, MD, 1988.
9. Pinchcofsky-Devin G. "Nutritional Assessment and Intervention." In Chronic Wound Care (Krasner D, Kane D, eds) Health Management Publication, Wayne PA.
10. Shilotry PG. Phagocytosis and leukocyte enzymes in ascorbic acid deficient guinea pigs. Journal of Nutrition 1977;107:1507.
11. Ehrlich HP, Hunt TK. Effect of cortisone and Vitamin A on wound healing. Annals of Surgery 1968;167:324.
12. Kindwall EP. "The Use of Drugs Under Pressure." In: Hyperbaric Medicine Practice (Kindwall EP, ed) Best Publishing Company, Flagstaff, AZ, 1994.
13. Messina VJ, Norkool DM. "Hyperbaric Nursing." In: Hyperbaric Medicine Practice (Kindwall EP, ed) Best Publishing Company, Flagstaff, AZ, 1994.
14. Bastable SB. Nurse as Educator. (Bastable SB, ed) Jones and Bartlett Publishers, Sudbury, Massachusetts, 1997.
15. Hyperbaric Oxygen Therapy: A Committee Report (Camporesi EM, ed) Undersea and Hyperbaric Medical Society. Kensington, Maryland, 1996.
16. Fife CE, Piantadosi CA. "Oxygen Toxicity." Problems in Respiratory Care, Clinical Applications of Hyperbaric Oxygen. Vol 4, No 2, 1991.
17. Moon RE, Camporesi EM. "Operational Use and Patient Monitoring in a Multiplace Hyperbaric Chamber." Problems in Respiratory Care. p. 182-183, June, 1991.
19. Weaver LK. "Hyperbaric Oxygen-Monoplace Chamber Use." Problems in Respiratory Care. p. 192, June, 1991.
20. Camporesi EM. "Therapeutic Use of Hyperbaric Oxygen." Respiratory Physiology. Ch 9, pp. 2-3.

NOTES

CHAPTER I

REGULATORY AGENCIES THAT IMPACT THE PRACTICE OF NURSING IN THE FIELD OF HYPERBARICS

W.T. WORKMAN

INTRODUCTION

Over the past 30 years, the clinical hyperbaric medicine community has witnessed a rather dramatic increase in indirect regulatory awareness; direct regulatory involvement; and the number of professional organizations or agencies with varying levels of special interest in the field. This has been driven in large part to the growth of the specialty. In the early 1970s there were fewer than 30 clinical hyperbaric facilities in the United States. In 1998, according to the Department of Health and Human Services, there were over 500. (1) Today, there are no less than 15 organizations that have either direct or indirect input to the operation of a clinical hyperbaric medicine facility. Some these organizations have overlapping areas of influence, while others act totally independently. There are those that the average clinical hyperbaric facility will not come into contact with as well as those whose input impacts the daily operation of every facility. Though not all organizations will directly influence the practice of hyperbaric nursing, they all influence, in their own way, the safe operation of a clinical hyperbaric medicine facility.

DEFINITIONS

To establish a common understanding of the hierarchy of regulatory terms that one may come into contact with, the following definitions are provided (see Figure 1, Hierarchy of Governing Directives):

- **Law** – a rule that must be obeyed or some form of punishment will result. The enforcement of laws is usually by a governmental agency.
- **Code** – a compliance document that contains only mandatory provisions using the word "shall" to indicate a requirement. Codes are generally written in a form that is suitable for adoption into law by a governmental agency.
- **Standard** – a compliance document that contains mandatory provisions using the word "shall" to indicate a requirement. Non-mandatory provisions using words such as "should" and "is recommended" are provided in an appendix.
- **Recommended practice** – a document that is similar in content to either a code or standard, but uses only non-mandatory language in the text to indicate recommendations.
- **Guideline** – a document that contains information that is advisory or informative in nature and contains only non-mandatory provisions.

Although not part of the hierarchy of regulatory terms, there is another useful definition:

Authority Having Jurisdiction (AHJ) – The organization, office, or individual responsible for approving equipment, an installation, or procedure. (2)

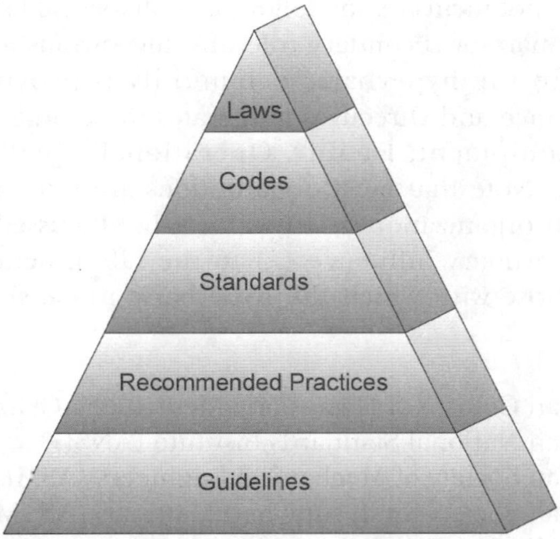

FIGURE 1. Hierarchy of Governing Directives

GOVERNING DIRECTIVES

The field of hyperbaric medicine is somewhat unique in that not only are there bureaucratic requirements applied to various aspects of the specialty, but notable industry involvement produces consensus standards as well. There are few medical specialties with established consensus standards to guide all or a portion of their discipline. Hyperbaric medicine is fortunate in that it has two such consensus documents: the American Society of Mechanical Engineers' *Safety Standard for Pressure Vessels for Human Occupancy* (ASME/PVHO) and the National Fire Protection Association's NFPA 99, *Standard for Health Care Facilities.* These two standards will be discussed in greater detail later in this chapter. Hyperbaric medicine is not unique in the number of different organizations or agencies that have something to say or do with the safety and/or quality of care provided in a clinical hyperbaric medicine setting. What has been of particular concern to this author is that there does not seem to be a single organization or agency with ultimate authority or the empowerment to ascertain the field's ability to meet the collection of laws, codes, standards, recommended practices, and guidelines levied upon it. This deficiency is changing as the Undersea and Hyperbaric Medical Society (UHMS) is in the process of developing a voluntary clinical hyperbaric facility accreditation program that will assess a given facility's compliance with existing laws, codes, standards, etc. An expanded discussion of facility accreditation will be provided later in this chapter. Meanwhile, an overview of agencies and organizations that have something to say about patient safety and quality of care for the hyperbaric patient is first required. Since the hyperbaric nurse is often the common bond between the patient and the hyperbaric facility, the nurse must have a general working knowledge of how these organizations influence daily activities within the hyperbaric department.

Although not inclusive, the following alphabetical list of organizations with either a primary or secondary role offering various levels of guidance and direction to the hyperbaric community is provided. Table 1 – Governing Guidance and Directives, integrates these organizations into the categories of Equipment, Facility, Operational, Quality of Care, and Reimbursement. Note that most organizations are referenced in multiple categories. Each organization listed will not be discussed in this chapter, only those with primary influence (*) to the safe practice of hyperbaric medicine and those with which the hyperbaric nurse should be directly acquainted.

- American College of Hyperbaric Medicine (ACHM)*
- American National Standards Institute (ANSI)
- American Society of Mechanical Engineers (ASME)*
- American Society for Testing and Materials (ASTM)
- Baromedical Nurses Association (BNA)*
- Centers for Medicare and Medicaid Services (CMS – formerly the Health Care Finance Administration)*
- Compressed Gas Association (CGA)
- Food and Drug Administration (FDA)*
- International Fire Marshal's Association (IFMA)
- Joint Commission on Accreditation of Healthcare Organizations (JCAHO)
- National Board of Boiler and Pressure Vessel Inspectors (NBBI)
- National Board of Diving and Hyperbaric Medical Technology (NBDHMT)*
- National Fire Protection Association (NFPA)*
- Occupational Safety and Health Administration (OSHA)*
- Undersea and Hyperbaric Medical Society (UHMS)*
- Uniform Boiler and Pressure Vessel Laws Society (UBPVLS)

Table 1
Governing Guidance and Directives

Organization	Equipment	Facility	Operational	Quality of Care	Reimbursement
NBBI	X				
UBPVLS	X				
ASME*	X				
ANSI	X	X			
ASTM	X	X			
IFMA	X	X			
CGA	X	X	X		
NFPA*	X	X	X		
OSHA*	X	X	X		
JCAHO*	X	X	X	X	
NBDHMT*			X	X	
BNA*			X	X	
ACHM*			X	X	X
FDA*	X			X	X
CMS*		X	X	X	X
UHMS*	X	X	X	X	X

American Society of Mechanical Engineers

The development of safety standards for the design, fabrication, testing, and stamping of boiler and pressure vessels dates back to 1911 when the ASME first established the Boiler Code Committee. The years between 1901 and 1905 were tragic for industry in that there were over 13,000 deaths reported from over 1,700 boiler and pressure vessel explosions. (3) Reflective of the level of technological sophistication at the time, most did not appreciate the types of hazards involved in the use of these pressurized devices and felt that such catastrophic accidents were "acts of God" and could not be prevented. It was not until two major explosions in Massachusetts, one in 1905 and the other in 1906, which were fatal to 59 people, injured more than 180, and resulted in extensive loss of property, that the state legislature passed the first legislation to regulate the construction, installation, and inspection of boilers in 1907. The Boiler Code was approved as the first safety standard in 1915. It is now known as the ASME Boiler and Pressure Vessel Code. (4)

One of the first major changes to the Boiler Code occurred in 1925 when Section VIII, Unfired Pressure Vessels was added. This was further modified in 1968 when Section VIII was changed to Pressure Vessels, Division 1 and supplemented by Division 2, Alternative Rules for Pressure Vessels. Until the early 1960s most hyperbaric chambers were designed, fabricated, and tested by ASME Section VIII rules. However, as commercial diving activities increased during the early years of offshore oil exploration, it became readily apparent that the existing rules for the design and fabrication of hyperbaric chambers were not sufficient. Issues such as quick-opening hatches, lighter metals, lower allowable temperatures for metal selection, and acrylic viewports were not addressed in Section VIII rules. Therefore, the Technical Committee on Pressure Vessels for Human Occupancy (PVHO) was established in 1971 to tailor these requirements to PVHOs. The committee published its first consensus standard in 1977.

Operating under the guidelines set forth by the American National Standards Institute, the ASME/PVHO committee is one of two consensus committees that impact the field of hyperbaric medicine. Committee members represent a broad cross section of the industry ranging from designers, fabricators, suppliers, commercial and military diving, and regulatory and medical personnel. This arrangement is preferred so that no one special interest industry group can dominate or unduly influence the resulting standards that are developed at the committee level. The following subcommittees complete most of the PVHO committee's actions: General Requirements, Design, Piping, Diving, Quality Assurance, Viewports, Post Construction, and Medical Systems. Each of these committee's recommendations are submitted to the Main Committee for letter ballot action. The Main Committee subsequently reports to the Board of Pressure Technology for final resolution. The PVHO safety standard is currently revised on a three-year review cycle but plans are underway to adopt a two-year revision cycle.

The scope of PVHO is very specific in that it provides the rules for the new construction of a pressure vessel for human occupancy (5). More specifically, it covers the design, fabrication, inspection, testing, and stamping of PVHOs, and establishes the criteria for welding, piping, acrylic viewports, and general design considerations for PVHOs intended for medical use. Its application is very precise. The standard is applied to any pressure vessel designed to contain humans while under internal or external pressure, regardless of the pressure magnitude. Even though there is an exemption in Section VIII of the Boiler and Pressure Vessel Code for pressure vessels designed for operation at 15 psi or less, this exemption does not apply to PVHOs. Therefore, even low-pressure hyperbaric chambers designed for operational pressures of 3 psi are to be designed, fabricated, tested, and stamped in accordance with the rules found in ASME/PVHO-1. Unfortunately, most PVHOs in this low-pressure category are not currently in compliance with the standard.

As of this publication date, the ASME Boiler and Pressure Vessel Code is adopted in 48 states, 13 Canadian provinces and territories, and 58 countries. ASME/PVHO has been adopted in 11 states, 3 cities, and 5 Canadian provinces or territories. (3) They are:

States

- Arkansas
- California
- Delaware
- Georgia
- Hawaii
- Minnesota
- North Carolina
- Oregon
- Tennessee
- Washington
- Wisconsin

Cities

- Denver
- Seattle
- District of Columbia

Canadian Provinces and Territories

- Alberta
- British Columbia
- New Brunswick
- Nova Scotia
- Ontario

National Fire Protection Association

The second set of consensus committee standards that directly impact the safe practice of hyperbaric medicine are those developed by the NFPA's Technical Committee on Hyperbaric and Hypobaric Facilities. The requirements found in NFPA 99, *Standard for Health Care Facilities,* Chapter 19 – Hyperbaric Facilities (2) are the cornerstone of a comprehensive hyperbaric safety program and represent time-honored practices that should be followed on a daily basis. It is vital for the hyperbaric nurse to have a working knowledge of these requirements to assure the highest possible safety standard for the department.

The first recorded hyperbaric system fire was in 1923. (6) However, it was not until 42 years later that fire risks in the hyperbaric environment caught the industry's attention. In 1965, a fire occurred in a chamber at the United States Navy Experimental Diving Unit and was fatal to two divers. This tragedy prompted a significant research effort into a variety of issues related to hyperbaric fire risk including the classical effort to evaluate burning rates of materials at different gas mixtures and pressures. The knowledge gained from these efforts is as valid today as it was over 30 years ago.

There were two subsequent events that prompted the community to join together to establish minimum fire safety standards for hyperbaric operations. The first happened on January 27, 1967, when a fire occurred in the Apollo 1 Command Module, which was fatal to Astronauts Roger Chafee, Virgil "Gus" Grissom, and Edward White. Their capsule was pressurized with 100% oxygen at 20 psia. The second tragedy happened four days later (January 31, 1967) in a United States Air Force hypobaric chamber with an environment of 100% oxygen at 0.2 ATA. Airman Bartley and Airman Harmon died as a result of a fire caused from a short in the electrical cord of a portable lamp. These two events led directly to the NFPA's creation of fire safety standards for hyperbaric facilities.

The first NFPA standard for hyperbaric fire safety was adopted in 1968 as a tentative standard (NFPA 56DT) and became a full standard in 1970 with the introduction of NFPA 56D. Due to the projected growth of clinical hyperbaric medicine, NFPA 56D was incorporated into NFPA 99, *Standard for Health Care Facilities* in 1984 where it currently resides. Though the hyperbaric facility safety standard is due to be relocated in the standard in the 2002 edition, it can currently be found in Chapter 19 - Hyperbaric Facilities. The NFPA standard is revised every three years.

This safety standard is unique in that it addresses requirements for hyperbaric equipment, the facility in which the equipment is located, the operation of the equipment, and general management of the hyperbaric department. It is the most comprehensive hyperbaric safety standard known to exist. Further, it has proven its usefulness because there has been no reported fatality due to fire in any North American hyperbaric facility that follows its requirements and recommendations since its initial release in 1968.

Areas of Emphasis. It is not the intent of this text to replicate the contents of Chapter 19 - Hyperbaric Facilities. Every hyperbaric facility should obtain a copy of the current standard for ready reference and application. However, for those readers unfamiliar with its contents, the general issues that are addressed in the standard are listed below:

- Purpose, scope, and application of the standard
- Classification of chambers
- Nature of hazards
- Construction and equipment
  - Housing for hyperbaric chambers
  - Fabrication of hyperbaric chambers
  - Illumination
  - Chamber ventilation
  - Fire protection in Class A chambers
  - Fire protection in Class B and C chambers

- Electrical systems
- Communications and monitoring
- Other equipment

• Administration and maintenance
- Recognition of hazards
- Responsibility
- Rules and regulations
- General requirements
- Personnel
- Equipment
- Handling of gases
- Maintenance logs
- Electrical safeguards
- Furniture
- Conductive accessories
- Fire protection equipment
- Housekeeping

The general purpose of NFPA 99, Chapter 19 is to establish the minimum safeguards for the protection of patients, hyperbaric medical personnel, equipment, and surrounding facilities from the dangers of fire. It also provides guidance for rescue personnel who may not be familiar with the intricacies of hyperbaric chamber operation and their unique requirements.

The scope applies to hyperbaric chambers and related support systems used for medical and experimental purposes at pressures from 0 psig to 100 psig. It covers recognition of, and protection from, hazards associated with electrical, explosion, and implosion as well as fire. It applies to both single and multiple patient occupancy chambers and to animal chambers whose size precludes human occupancy. It is only applied to new construction, new equipment added to new facilities, and new equipment added to existing facilities. It does not require the alteration or replacement of existing construction or equipment.

Chambers are generally classified according to occupancy. A Class A chamber is considered a multiple occupancy chamber, a Class B chamber is a single occupancy chamber, and a Class C chamber is animal occupancy only. Animal chambers that are equipped for human access are considered as Class A chambers by the standard.

The greatest distinction between building requirements for Class A chambers and Class B chambers is in the firewall requirement. A Class A chamber requires 2-hour, fire-resistant rated construction and a B-label, 1-hour fire-door rated construction. These requirements are not currently imposed on a Class B chamber installation. Other room requirements for both classes of chambers are, exclusive use of the room for hyperbaric operations, floor support for the weight of the chamber, and room sprinkler protection.

As previously mentioned, all chambers used for clinical application are to be designed, fabricated, and installed in accordance with ASME/ PVHO, *Safety Standard for Pressure Vessels for Human Occupancy.* Additionally, specific guidance is provided on flooring material, antistatic flooring properties, bilge installation, interior painting, viewports, access ports, electrical enclosures, illumination, environmental control, humidification, and minimum chamber ventilation rates. The need for an individual breathing apparatus for each occupant of a Class A chamber is also cited in case the chamber environment becomes fouled for any reason. This apparatus must be immediately available and provide breathing gas independent from the chamber environment. Alternative breathing air sources for outside personnel of Class A chambers will also be available. To help minimize the chance of contaminated chamber air, sources of air for the chamber atmosphere must be toxin-free and flammability-free. Compressor intakes are to be located in places to avoid air contamination from exhaust from vehicles, internal combustion engines, building exhaust outlets, etc.

Patient Handling. NFPA 99, Chapter 19 does not prescribe a detailed procedure for patient handling. The majority of safeguards listed are aimed at minimizing the amount of hazardous materials that a patient can introduce into the chamber environment. One direct way of exercising control is to have patients change from their street clothes into special clothing provided by the hyperbaric facility. Silk, wool, or synthetic materials may not be worn in either Class A or Class B chambers unless the fabric meets the flame resistance requirements as stated in NFPA 701, Standard Methods for Fire Tests for Flame-Resistant Textiles and Films. (7) Therefore, personal clothing should never be allowed into the chamber. Only garments fabricated of 100 percent cotton, special anti-static blends of cotton and polyester, or fire resistant garments made of materials such as Durette Gold, etc., should be used in any class of chamber. In addition to the requirement for textiles, the design of the garment shall be such that it is of the overall or jumpsuit type, completely covering as much of the skin as possible. Street shoes shall never be worn into the chamber because of the risk of sparking and introduction of hazardous hydrocarbons and solvents into the chamber from residue collected on the soles and heels of the shoes.

The use of flammable hair sprays, hair oils, and skin oils (cosmetics) are forbidden for all chamber occupants, patient and medical observer alike. Synthetic undergarments are also discouraged. Due to the length of treatment, patients are often allowed to bring into a Class A multiplace chamber a book or magazine to read during the course of treatment. Newspapers are never allowed due to the type of paper and inks used for printing. No reading material of any type is ever allowed to be used in a Class B chamber.

Operational Procedures. Although detailed operational procedures are not covered in the NFPA standard, general guidelines for administration and maintenance are. It is not enough to define how a hyperbaric system is to be designed, fabricated, and installed. In order to create the safest environment possible for hyperbaric systems, careful attention must also be placed on how the facility is routinely operated and maintained. There are many good operational models available that provide representative pre and post treatment checklists and outline solid maintenance programs that operators can follow. Many of these operational guides were developed by the U.S. military and have been successfully used for many years. They are routinely adopted for general use.

One of the strongest cornerstones of any hyperbaric safety program is hazard recognition. Hazards can only be mitigated when all personnel involved, from the hospital administrator down to the most junior technician, clearly understand the nature of hazards that are possible in any hyperbaric facility. A partial description of these hazards is found in Appendix C-19 of the standard.

Even though the hazards and operational procedures are similar between one facility type and another, it is highly recommended that all personnel (administrative, technical, and professional) jointly develop a series of operational procedures to follow for both routine and emergency situations. It is not enough just to develop the procedures; they must also be practiced. Although proficiency can be achieved for routine procedures, emergency procedures must be practiced on a recurring basis to imprint the necessary steps that must be taken to deal appropriately with any emergency situation. In the case of fire, representative checklists are also included in Appendix C-19. Fire drills should be practiced frequently. These drills should also involve activation of the deluge fire suppression system in Class A chambers at least annually.

Personnel Issues: Training, Staffing, Etc. The one area that is less well-defined is that of staffing and training. The NFPA standard is very clear that the ultimate responsibility for hyperbaric facility safety is placed on the governing board of the medical facility. It is incumbent on that body to insist that adequate rules and regulations are in place and that all personnel follow them. The standard also stipulates that a Safety Director be designated and made responsible for all hyperbaric equipment. The Safety Director has the authority to restrict hazardous materials, supplies, or equipment from the interior of the chamber. (Refer to "How to Manage Your Hyperbaric Facility Safety Program" for additional information on the duties and responsibilities of the Safety Director.) There are no minimum staffing or training requirements mandated by the current standard.

The Food and Drug Administration

The Medical Device Amendments of 1976 (Public Law 91-295) established a comprehensive system for the regulation of medical devices intended for human use.(8) Specifically, they mandated that the FDA classify all medical devices into three categories: Class I, General Controls; Class II, Performance Standards; and Class III, Pre-market approval. Devices in commercial distribution prior to May 28, 1976 are not required to comply with this law and are "grandfathered" as preamendment devices. However, devices developed after this date are required to establish either validated performance or substantial equivalency to devices already in commercial distribution.

The FDA Anesthesiology Panel categorizes hyperbaric chambers as Class II medical devices. As such, before being placed into commercial sales, the manufacturer must submit a 510(k) Pre-Market Notification request. This application can be based on an entirely new design or by establishing substantial equivalency. The majority of clinical hyperbaric chamber manufacturers are in compliance with this requirement; however, there are some that are not. Efforts are underway to ensure compliance by all manufacturers. As of June 30, 2001, of the 34 hyperbaric chambers and accessories that have been cleared for marketing since 1976, half have been cleared since 1996. Postmarket compliance activity (warning letters, etc.) has increased accordingly.

In addition to being defined as a Class II medical device, clinical hyperbaric chambers are also considered "Prescription Devices" by the FDA. A "Prescription Device" is one in which a physician must be involved in its procurement and must issue a prescription for the use of high-pressure oxygen.

The manufacture, packaging, storage and installation of hyperbaric chambers are to be in compliance with the Quality Systems Regulations (QSRs) as described by the FDA. Failure to comply with any of the requirements of the QSR directives renders the device adulterated. Such a device, as well as the person responsible for the failure to comply, is subject to regulatory action. Any written or oral complaint under the FDA's mandatory Medical Device Reporting program or its voluntary MedWatch program concerning a hyperbaric chamber relative to its quality, reliability, safety, effectiveness, or performance shall be reviewed, evaluated, and documented. This includes taking action on a hyperbaric chamber manufacturer for promotion and advertisement of their chamber for medical conditions that are not recognized as approved indications by the Undersea and Hyperbaric Medical Society (UHMS). Failure to comply with these requirements may result in the hyperbaric chamber being withdrawn from commercial distribution.

In addition to the above, the FDA also establishes criteria for evaluating the use of hyperbaric oxygen for indications not yet recognized by the UHMS. FDA clearance for such research is generally accomplished through submission of an Investigational New Drug (IND) application. Due to the unique interaction of hyperbaric systems and the classification of oxygen as a drug, these applications are jointly reviewed by the Center for Drug Evaluation and Research (CDER) and the Center for Devices and Radiological Health (CDRH). In such an instance, CDRH would maintain marketing authority with the CDER consultation on the efficacy of the use of hyperbaric oxygen for the treatment of a particular condition.

Although the above process is available for organizations to utilize, thus allowing the role of hyperbaric oxygen to be properly validated, there is much attention being placed on the "off-label" use of HBO. In such cases, some organizations aggressively promote the use of HBO in such conditions without providing HBO therapy under an approved IND application. The FDA has been very clear that they do not regulate the practice of medicine; however, they have also made it very clear that they do regulate the promotion and advertising of the devices themselves.

The "dos and don'ts" promotion and advertising for hyperbaric medicine are not well understood. Under current FDA policies, a company (a hyperbaric chamber manufacturer, for example) may be held liable if its printed material or website refers to or provides a link to a third-party site that specifically promotes off-label uses of HBO. The FDA considers a company responsible for the material it produces or provides on its website to which it promotes a direct reference or link. However, it is acceptable to refer or link to a site such as the National Library of Medicine (NLM), but one should not provide a reference or link from a product page to a specific article on the NLM website that discusses an off-label use for hyperbaric oxygen. This policy also extends to practitioner and facility promotional material and websites that discuss off-label uses.

Companies and facilities can also be held responsible for the content of testimonial statements or case studies and should not include patients who have undergone hyperbaric therapy for an off-label indication in all types of promotional material including websites.

Another aspect not well understood is a hyperbaric facility's reporting responsibilities should death or serious injury occur to a patient while undergoing HBO therapy. In accordance with 21 CFR Part 803, the requirements for Medical Device Reporting apply to both hyperbaric chamber manufacturers and user facilities. (9) First, one must understand what qualifies as a reportable event. The FDA generally expects for information that reasonably suggests that a hyperbaric chamber has or may have caused or contributed to the death or serious injury to a patient to be reported.

The agency also expects for malfunctions that could contribute to death or serious injury, should they recur, to be reported. In this case, caused or contributed means that a death or serious injury was or may have been attributed to a hyperbaric chamber, or that it was or may have been a factor in a death or serious injury, including events occurring as a result of failure, malfunction, improper or inadequate design, manufacture, labeling, or user error. Further, serious injury means injury or illness that is life threatening, results in permanent impairment of a body function or permanent damage to a body structure, or necessitates medical or surgical intervention to preclude permanent impairment of a body function or permanent damage to a body structure.

Centers for Medicare and Medicaid Services (formerly the Health Care Finance Administration)

On June 14, 2001, the Health Care Finance Administration, better known as HCFA, changed its name to the Centers for Medicare and Medicaid Services (CMS). Under the new organizational scheme, HCFA has been restructured into three different centers. A Center for Beneficiary Choices will distribute information to beneficiaries on Medicare managed programs, while traditional Medicare fee-for-services will be managed out of the Center for Medicare Management. State-based programs such as Medicaid and the State Children's Health Insurance Program will be managed in the newly created Center for Medicaid and State Operations.

Historically, the guidance issued from CMS has been limited to specifying covered disease conditions for which the use of HBO is indicated and subsequently recommended for reimbursement. CMS has generally relied on the recommendations provided in the UHMS Hyperbaric Oxygen Therapy Committee Report. Its Coverage Instruction Manual (CIM) Section 35-10 contains the conditions for which the use of hyperbaric oxygen therapy is reimbursed. Identification of a hyperbaric procedure is based on the American Medical Association's CPT code 99183 for physician supervision or a facility revenue center code 413. Reimbursement for facility costs is typically part of the diagnosis related group (DRG) payment if the treatment was provided as part of hospitalization or cost-based if treatment was provided as an outpatient service. Dramatic changes are underway for reimbursement and it is not wise to further speculate on its uncertain future.

The Joint Commission on Accreditation of Healthcare Organizations

The Joint Commission, better known as JCAHO, was founded in 1951 as an independent, non-profit organization to establish standards for and to accredit healthcare organizations. For the past 50 years, JCAHO has developed professional standards and evaluated healthcare organizations against these benchmarks. Specifically, they provide accreditation services for general, psychiatric, children's, and rehabilitation hospitals; healthcare networks; home care organizations; assisted living residencies; behavioral healthcare organizations; ambulatory care providers; and clinical laboratories.

JCAHO standards are too broad to cover in this chapter. Even so, most hyperbaric nurses, especially those who work in a hospital-based facility are at least familiar with their requirements. Therefore, only one special emphasis area has been selected to describe because it has a direct link to overall hyperbaric facility safety and thus complements the information presented on developing and managing a comprehensive hyperbaric facility safety program. This area is patient safety. In many instances, it is the hyperbaric nurse who provides continuity for patient safety and bridges elements of the facility, the patient, and practitioner to ensure that quality of care is maintained in the safest environment possible.

Effective on July 1, 2001, JCAHO increased its emphasis on patient safety and efforts at patient risk reduction. To do so, it created a multi-factorial, coordinated approach to a facility's leadership and its accountability to facilitate a comprehensive organizational safety program that includes all activities of the organization that have a role to play in the maintenance and improvement of patient safety. Representative elements of this integration are performance improvement, environmental safety, and risk management.

To effectively reduce errors in the healthcare environment, JCAHO feels that in order to cultivate an environment where real and potential risks to patient safety can be identified and managed, the organization must be able to recognize and acknowledge the risks, introduce actions to reduce the risks, establish reporting systems with means of follow-up, focus on process improvement, and facilitate organizational learning. Though newly established specific probe areas are extensive, a review of those added in 2001 under the "Leadership" section provides a good overview of the issues involved. Namely, the leadership of a healthcare organization is to ensure that the patient safety program includes the following (10):

- Designation of one or more qualified individuals or an interdisciplinary group to manage the organization-wide patient safety program.
- Definition of the scope of the program activities, that is, the types of occurrences to be addressed, typically ranging from "no harm," frequently occurring "slips" to sentinel events with serious adverse outcomes.
- Description of mechanisms to ensure that all components of the healthcare organization are integrated into and participate in the organization-wide program.

- Procedures for immediate response to medical/healthcare errors, including care of the affected patient(s), containment of risk to others, and preservation of factual information for subsequent analysis.
- Clear systems for internal and external reporting of information relating to medical/healthcare errors.
- Defined mechanisms for responding to the various types of occurrences, i.e., root cause, analysis in response to a sentinel event, or for conducting proactive risk reduction activities.
- Defined mechanisms for support of staff that have been involved in a sentinel event.
- At least annually, a report to the governing body on the occurrence of medical/healthcare errors and actions taken to improve patient safety, both proactively and in response to actual occurrences.

Nowhere are the objectives of this initiative more important than in a hyperbaric facility. The analysis of fire-related accidents in hyperbaric chambers by Sheffield and Desautels (6) reveals that the majority of hyperbaric fires since the early 1980s have been related to operational oversight and contraband allowed in the chamber. It is logical to think that an aggressive safety program may have prevented many of these tragedies. Additionally, recent mishap data collected through the Hyperbaric Incident Monitoring Study (HIMS) supports the notion that many incidents and "near-misses" that have been documented may have been avoided if such a program had been in place and diligently applied. (11)

JCAHO offers a number of publications and periodicals that should become part of the hyperbaric nurse's library. These references are important source documents for improving the quality of nursing in general and more specifically of hyperbaric nursing. Representative examples of these are:

- *Nursing Practice and Outcomes Measurement* (ISBN: 0-86688-499-8)
- *Nursing: Hospital Examples of Compliance for Patient-Focused Standards* (ISBN: 0-86688-616-8)
- *Environment of Care News*
- *Joint Commission Perspectives*
- *Joint Commission Perspectives on Patient Safety*
- *Joint Commission Benchmark*
- *Joint Commission Journal on Quality Improvement*

The Occupational Safety and Health Administration

The Occupational Safety and Health Administration (OSHA) is the agency of the U.S. Department of Labor that promotes safe and healthful working conditions. Their chief responsibility is to develop and enforce job safety and health regulations. Even though OSHA provides directives for commercial diving (STD 1-23.3-29 CFR 1910.401-1910.441, Subpart T – Commercial Diving) (12) they have no direct program or regulation that deals specifically with hyperbaric facilities.

Though they have no specific directives targeted at hyperbaric facilities, they have established numerous directives that deal with specific health and safety issues associated with healthcare facilities. Some of their directives include bloodborne pathogens and biological hazards, potential chemical and drug exposures, waste anesthetic gas exposures, ergonomic hazards from lifting and conducting repetitive tasks, laser hazards, hazards associated with laboratories, and radioactive material and x-ray hazards. A detailed list of these directives can be found at http://www.osha-slc.gov/SLTC/healthcarefacilities/index.html.

The Undersea and Hyperbaric Medical Society

The Undersea and Hyperbaric Medical Society is an international medical society whose purpose is to:

- Provide a forum for professional scientific communication among individuals and groups involved in basic and applied studies concerned with life sciences and human factors aspects of the undersea environment and hyperbaric medicine
- Promote cooperation between the life sciences and other disciplines with undersea activity and hyperbaric medicine
- Develop and promote educational activities and other programs which improve the scientific knowledge of matters related to undersea and hyperbaric environments and the accepted indications of hyperbaric oxygen therapy for the membership, as well as physicians and allied health professionals, divers, diver technicians, and the public at large

An important role played by the UHMS is to evaluate the use of hyperbaric oxygen in specific diseases or conditions and to list those that are supported by prevailing scientific evidence. The Hyperbaric Oxygen Therapy Committee meets annually to consider research and clinical data to render recommendations as to the clinical efficacy and safety of HBO in a particular disease or condition. The committee also reviews the cost-effectiveness of HBO and establishes guidelines (utilization review) for each listed indication. The Centers for Medicare and Medicaid Services (formerly the Health Care Finance Administration), the FDA, and many third-party payers have adopted the recommendations of this report as a basis for indications of use and reimbursement.

Another important function of the Society is to enhance hyperbaric facility safety. Over the years, the Hyperbaric Safety Committee has been very active in establishing a leading role in promoting hyperbaric facility safety. Practical guidelines on both monoplace and multiplace hyperbaric facility operations have been published and widely distributed. These common-sense documents contain valuable information for the hyperbaric nurse and should be required for every hyperbaric facility.

Recognizing the need for a comprehensive set of "Standards of Practice" for use throughout the U.S. hyperbaric medicine community, the UHMS recently established the Operations Committee and tasked it to develop consensus criteria on minimum training, staffing, skills verification for each specialty level, and for overall facility safety. First published in 2000, the Operations Committee Report contains extensive guidance for critical, core elements for a clinical hyperbaric medicine facility. (13) Though the guidelines are too lengthy to produce in this chapter, the following sections provide an in-depth overview of its contents:

Recommended Training Guidelines

- Physician personnel
  - Clinical hyperbaric medicine physician
  - Physician continuing medical education requirements
- Nurse personnel
  - Clinical hyperbaric registered nurse (entry-level)
  - Nursing director/manager
  - Clinical nurse specialist
- Allied healthcare personnel
  - Allied healthcare provider (entry-level)
  - Safety director
  - Technical director
  - Program manager

Job Descriptions and Responsibilities

- Medical job descriptions
  - Hyperbaric physician
  - Medical director
- Nursing job descriptions
  - Hyperbaric nurse
  - Hyperbaric nurse manager/director
- Technical job descriptions
  - Technical personnel
  - Safety director
  - Technical director
  - Program manager

Staffing Guidelines

- Physician staffing
- Nurse staffing
- Technical staffing

Safety Program Guidelines
Physician Credentials Privilege List (sample)
Quality Assurance Check List

- Quality of care
- Quality assessment and improvement
- Infection control
- Rights and responsibilities of patients
- Teaching, research, and publication activities
- Clinical administration

Adoption of these standards will, for the first time, provide a national set of guidelines for the appropriate and safe application of hyperbaric medicine.

The American College of Hyperbaric Medicine

Unlike the UHMS with its broadly based membership, the American College of Hyperbaric Medicine (ACHM) is specifically for hyperbaric physicians. The College promotes and develops liaisons with individuals and groups with similar interests in the field of hyperbaric medicine. A primary goal of the College is to enhance the exchange of scientific and therapeutic information related to the specialty of hyperbaric medicine in a manner that will encourage national and international goodwill and social and cultural exchanges.

The Baromedical Nurses Association

Established in 1985, the mission of the Baromedical Nurses Association (BNA) is to provide nurses with a professional organization to define, develop, maintain, and promote the status and standards of the practice of hyperbaric nursing. Today, the BNA has member representation in the United States, Europe, Asia, Africa, South and Central America, and the South Pacific.

In ten short years, the BNA has progressed in importance and recognition to justify creation of the Baromedical Nurses Association Certification Board (BNACB) in 1995. This board provides a means for nurses to obtain certification specifically in hyperbaric nursing instead of the previously established Certification in Hyperbaric Technology (CHT) offered by the National Board of Diving and Hyperbaric Technology (NBDHMT). The NBDHMT manages the certification process on behalf of the BNACB.

For a nurse to qualify as a certified hyperbaric registered nurse (CHRN), the following criteria must be met:

- RN who graduated from an accredited school and who is current in the state in which they practice hyperbaric nursing
- Current certification in basic life support
- Completion of a 40-hour-NBDHMT- or UHMS-approved primary course in hyperbaric medicine
- Minimum of one year hyperbaric nursing experience with a minimum of 400 hours
- Letter of recommendation from employer including validation of hyperbaric experience
- Successful completion of the hyperbaric nursing certification examination

In contrast to the single certification level for CHT, the BNACB has established three levels of certification to recognize varying levels of experience. The three levels are certified hyperbaric nurse, advanced certified hyperbaric nurse, and hyperbaric nurse clinician. To qualify for the entry-level certification, the criteria are listed above. However, to meet the qualifications of the advanced certified hyperbaric nurse, the nurse must have the following:

- Three years experience working a minimum of 20 hours per week in the practice of hyperbaric nursing
- Written documentation of at least two of the following:
  - Contributions to the administrative activities of the hyperbaric unit
  - Teaching in the field of hyperbaric nursing or hyperbaric medicine
  - Providing primary responsibility for planning hyperbaric care

In order to satisfy the requirements to become a hyperbaric nurse clinician, the nurse must meet the following criteria:

- Master's degree in nursing- or health-related field from an accredited program
- Minimum of five years experience in the field of hyperbaric nursing with a minimum of 20 hours per week devoted specifically to hyperbaric nursing
- Written documentation of three of the following:
  - Responsibility for administrative activities of the hyperbaric unit
  - Speaker at regional/national hyperbaric conferences
  - Publication history in journals, manuals, or videos for regional and/or national distribution
  - Active participation in the professional activities of the BNA, UHMS, or Associates of the UHMS as an officer or committee member
  - Principle investigator or co-investigator in a hyperbaric research project

To retain certification as a CHRN, a nurse must obtain 20 CEUs during each registration period. At least ten hours must be directly related to undersea, hyperbaric, or aerospace medicine. Continuing education credits can be one of two types: Category A or B. At least ten hours must be Category A credits which are directly related to functions as a CHRN and to undersea, hyperbaric, or aerospace medicine. The remaining credits can be from Category B which includes subjects that are related to one's base specialty. In addition to the validation of CEUs, a CHRN must also have employer verification of at least 200 hours per year in hyperbaric nursing.

To further establish the BNA as an organization devoted to improving the quality of care in hyperbaric medicine, they have established guidelines for "Standards of Care for the Hyperbaric Patient Receiving Hyperbaric Oxygen Therapy." (14) These guidelines provide recommended nursing interventions and their related desired outcomes for 14 different diagnoses and problems. These are:

1. Anxiety related to knowledge deficit of hyperbaric oxygen therapy and treatment procedures
2. Potential for injury related to transferring patient in/out of chamber, explosion of equipment, fire, and/or medical support equipment
3. Potential for barotrauma to ears, sinuses, teeth, and lungs or cerebral gas embolism related to changes in atmospheric pressure inside hyperbaric oxygen chamber
4. Potential for oxygen toxicity related to delivery of 100% oxygen at an increased atmospheric pressure
5. Potential for inadequate therapeutic gas delivery related to delivery system and patient's needs/limitations
6. Anxiety and fear related to feelings of confinement anxiety associated with hyperbaric oxygen chamber
7. Pain related to associated medical problems
8. Discomfort related to temperature and humidity changes inside hyperbaric chamber
9. Potential for ineffective individual coping related to stresses of illness and/or poor psychosocial support systems
10. Potential for dysrhythmia related to disease pathology
11. Potential for fluid volume deficit related to dehydration and fluid shifts
12. Altered cerebral tissue perfusion related to:
    - Carbon monoxide poisoning
    - Decompression sickness
    - Acute necrotizing infection
    - Gas embolism
    - Other

13. Potential for alteration in comfort, fluid, and electrolyte balance related to nausea and vomiting
14. Altered health maintenance related to knowledge deficit for:
    - Management of chronic wound
    - Restrictions following decompression illness
    - Symptoms to report after carbon monoxide poisoning

All hyperbaric nurses are encouraged to contact the BNA to request a complete copy of these guidelines. Also, individual hyperbaric units are further encouraged to adapt them to specific facility application.

The Operations Committee Report of the UHMS has set the standard that either a CHT or CHRN will be present in the hyperbaric department whenever a hyperbaric chamber is operation. As of March 17, 2001, there were 170 nurses certified in hyperbaric nursing.

The National Board of Diving and Hyperbaric Medical Technology

With its origins rooted in the National Association of Diving Medical Technicians, the National Board of Diving and Hyperbaric Medical Technology (NBDHMT) was formed in 1991. Soon after formation, the Board introduced its certification program in hyperbaric technology (CHT) and established minimum approval criteria for introductory training for those wishing to enter the field. As originally conceived, certification is considered validation of "added qualifications." NBDHMT certification has proven to hold widespread appeal to a cross section of specialists and healthcare providers ranging from chamber technicians, diving medical technicians, paramedics, and respiratory therapists to researchers and even physicians. As of April 26, 2001, there were 1,060 CHTs throughout the world.

The following requirements must be met to become NBDHMT certified as a CHT:

- Be at least 18 years old
- Have a high school diploma or equivalent
- Complete an NBDHMT-approved Hyperbaric Medicine Introductory Course
- Complete a clinical internship with at least 480 hours of emphasis in undersea, hyperbaric, or aerospace technology or medicine
- Provide a letter of recommendation from present employer, administrator, or medical director
- Successfully complete the clinical hyperbaric technologist's certification examination.

Clinical Hyperbaric Facility Accreditation

As previously stated, there were fewer than 30 hyperbaric facilities operational in this country in the late 1970s. Most were military, commercial, or highly specialized research facilities. There are now over 500 in operation. We have seen the primary role of hyperbaric facilities transition from the treatment of diving-related disorders to providing an important primary and adjunct treatment modality for multiple medical conditions. Refined research efforts will no doubt validate continued efficacy, and perhaps even support new indications. The location of facilities is expanding from hospital-based to nonaffiliated outpatient settings, some with appropriate medical supervision, others without. In the past decade, certification in hyperbaric technology and hyperbaric nursing has become a staffing requirement in many programs. After years of dedicated efforts by many members of the UHMS, the American Board of Preventive Medicine recently approved certification for physicians in Undersea and Hyperbaric Medicine. Minimum recommended staffing and training standards did not exist two years ago. Now, thanks to the efforts of the UHMS Operations Committee, they are an important part of a more comprehensive set of guidelines and recommended practices. The Operations Committee Report sets the foundational standards of practice for hyperbaric medicine. Progress is being made but the field must not stop here.

Each of these milestones reflects a continuing maturation and professional recognition of clinical hyperbaric medicine in the United States. As in any growth process, success has not come easy. There are still many challenges that must be faced. The UHMS is the primary professional organization that represents a broad constituency base for clinical hyperbaric medicine and should be proactive in dealing with these problematic issues. It must position itself to grow with, and reflect the needs of, the community it serves while providing the leadership this specialty needs. There are many in the field who feel that the next evolutionary level should be one that provides a measured means of quality assurance: a formal clinical hyperbaric facility accreditation program. Programs that evaluate the adequacy of the facility and equipment, the appropriateness of the staff and their training, quality of care, and patient safety have proven useful to professional organizations in ensuring that quality is maintained within their specialty. The UHMS has accepted this challenge and, at the time of this publication, is moving quickly to establish a professional, comprehensive clinical hyperbaric facility accreditation program.

The Society believes that such a program is the most efficient method to ensure that:

- Clinical hyperbaric facilities are staffed with the proper specialists who are well-trained
- Clinical hyperbaric facilities are using quality equipment that has been properly installed and maintained, and is being operated with the highest level of safety possible
- Clinical hyperbaric facilities are providing high quality of patient care

- Clinical hyperbaric facilities are maintaining the appropriate documentation of informed consent, patient treatment procedures, physician involvement, etc.

There are many advantages that can result from accreditation. Advantages impact the regulatory environment, individual hyperbaric facilities and programs, and the specialty of hyperbaric medicine. Of immediate importance is the community response to the current regulatory climate. In October 2000, the Office of the Inspector General (OIG) of the Department of Health and Human Services released a report on "Hyperbaric Oxygen Therapy: Its Usefulness and Appropriateness." (1) Among its findings, the OIG reported that a lack of testing and treatment monitoring raised a variety of quality of care concerns, and that CMS (HCFA) guidance to the field of hyperbaric medicine was limited. Specific OIG recommendations were for CMS (HCFA) to initiate a national coverage decision policy for HBO, improve policy guidance (i.e., practice guidelines and physician attendance policy), improve oversight by requiring contractors to initiate edits and consistent medical review procedures, and explore the creation of a national registry of facilities and/or physicians. Without doubt, this report lays the foundation for increased government involvement and intervention. By creating a national clinical hyperbaric facility accreditation program, the UHMS is responding proactively to the OIG findings and recommendations and is sending a signal to the various regulatory agencies that the organized hyperbaric medical community is concerned with our current situation and is responding to the recognized need to assure quality of care across the continuum of clinical hyperbaric facilities. It also minimizes the possibility that governmental agencies such as CMS would develop further regulatory criteria with which the community must comply.

Equally important are the advantages that an individual clinical hyperbaric facility may recognize. Though not all inclusive, some of the more immediate are:

- Improved quality of care
- Increased efficiency at the facility level
- More effective risk management programs
- Lower liability insurance premiums
- Staff motivation and *esprit de corps*
- Maximized public relations and marketing efforts
- Ability to recruit and retain quality staff
- Develop alliances with other provider groups
- Establish credibility of legitimate nonaffiliated outpatient facilities among their professional referral base

Achieving the regulatory and facility level advantages provides the foundation for significant advancements in the acceptance and credibility of hyperbaric medicine as a growing, recognized medical specialty, thus enhancing professional organizations such as the UHMS, ACHM, BNA, NBDHMT, etc., who are at the forefront of the field. Further, a successful accreditation program will bring hyperbaric medicine in line with other specialties such as the American College of Radiation Oncology that sponsor specialty-specific accreditation programs and will establish nationally recognized Standards of Practice for clinical hyperbaric medicine.

In summary, everyone wins from the development of a comprehensive accreditation program. The regulatory community has a non-government mechanism for ensuring that the issues identified in the OIG report are minimized, thus reducing the need for further intervention. Individual clinical hyperbaric facilities can be recognized for creating and managing a top-quality clinical hyperbaric medicine program. The field of hyperbaric medicine benefits from enhanced credibility among its professional peers. However, the most important winner is the patient. Thousands of patients throughout the nation can be confident of the quality of care they are receiving from an accredited hyperbaric medicine program.

CONCLUSION

With at least 15 different organizations and agencies that influence the safety of hyperbaric operations and the quality of care administered in hyperbaric facilities, it is no wonder that confusion often exists with what is actually required. In the midst of this confusion, it is important for the hyperbaric nurse to be very familiar with the requirements of the Centers for Medicare and Medicaid Services, the National Fire Protection Association, and the Joint Commission as they daily impact the safety, quality of care, and reimbursement climate of the hyperbaric facility. Since the hyperbaric nurse is often designated as the unit's Safety Director, nurses should be keenly aware of the responsibilities that accrue to that position and should avail themselves to as many training opportunities as possible to assume this role in a responsible manner.

A growing reflection of the maturation of hyperbaric nursing is specialty certification. All hyperbaric nurses are strongly encouraged to pursue certification by the Baromedical Nurses Association Certification Board. Equally important is for the hyperbaric nurse to support facility-specific accreditation. A third-party accreditation program is a viable mechanism to ensure that quality of care provided to the hyperbaric patient is not compromised across the ever-changing continuum of hyperbaric facilities.

REFERENCES

1. Hyperbaric Oxygen Therapy: Its Usefulness and Appropriateness, Office of Inspector General, Department of Health and Human Services, October 2000.
2. Standard for Health Care Facilities, NFPA 99, 1999 Edition, National Fire Protection Association, Quincy, MA, 1999.
3. Swanson, Raymond P., Governing Directives, in Hyperbaric Facility Safety: A Practical Guide, W.T. Workman, Ed., Best Publishing Company, Flagstaff, AZ, 1999.
4. ANSI/ASME Boiler and Pressure Vessel Code, 1990 Edition, American Society of Mechanical Engineers, New York, NY, 1990.
5. ANSI/ASME Safety Standard for Pressure Vessels for Human Occupancy, PVHO-1-1997, American Society of Mechanical Engineers, New York, NY, 1997.
6. Sheffield, Paul J. and D.A. Desautels. Hyperbaric and hypobaric chamber fires: a 73-year analysis. Undersea Hyper Med 1997; 24(3): 153-164.
7. Methods for Fire Tests for Flame-Resistant Textiles and Films, NFPA 701, 1996 Edition, National Fire Protection Association, Quincy, MA, 1996.
8. Federal Food, Drug, and Cosmetic Act, Section 201.[321](h), DHHS Publication FDA 93-1051.
9. 21 CFR Part 803, revised as of April 1, 1998.
10. Official website of the Joint Commission on Accreditation of Healthcare Organizations, www.jcaho.org, July 10, 2001.
11. Hyperbaric Incident Monitoring Study (HIMS), Royal Adelaide Hospital, Adelaide, Australia.
12. STD 1-23.3-29 CFR 1910.401-1919.441, Subpart T – Commercial Diving, Occupational Safety and Health Administration, U.S. Department of Labor, Washington, D.C.
13. Operations Committee Report, Undersea and Hyperbaric Medical Society, Kensington, MD, 1999.
14. Standards of Care for the Hyperbaric Patient Receiving Hyperbaric Oxygen Therapy, Baromedical Nurses Association.

CHAPTER II

HOW TO MANAGE YOUR HYPERBARIC FACILITY SAFETY PROGRAM

W.T. WORKMAN

Author's Note: In many clinical hyperbaric facilities, it is common for the hyperbaric nurse to be responsible for the development and management of the unit's hyperbaric safety program. Due to the importance of a well-conceived and properly managed program, this chapter has been reproduced in its entirety from ***Hyperbaric Facility Safety: A Practical Guide****. The reader will note that there has been no effort to eliminate repetition or redundancy from the material in this chapter and the information contained in "Regulatory Agencies that Impact the Practice of Nursing in the Field of Hyperbarics." Retaining this information is felt to be important in maintaining the continuity of the chapter and serves as reinforcement to the role of these regulatory agencies and the guidance for which they are responsible.*

A key component of any successful operational or clinical hyperbaric medicine program is a strong safety program with a well-defined plan. Such a program is multifaceted, incorporating a variety of complementing program elements: carefully controlled operational procedures, attention to detail, practice, preventive maintenance, vigilance, training, equipment knowledge, etc. It is not sufficient to simply have a well-crafted program; staff members must fully understand their responsibilities in maintaining the highest level of safety. Maintaining a safe environment for patients and staff is not automatic; it results, in part, from a focused mind-set. Creation of this mind-set generally begins by learning the fundamentals that any hyperbaric safety program should embrace.

MULTIFACETED PROGRAM

As mentioned above, a properly developed safety program is multifaceted. Although there can be a variety of program elements depending on the specific setting and need, there are several common aspects that are elementary in program design and execution. These basic elements are:

- **Operational procedures** – managers should develop a comprehensive set of operational procedures that cover the complete spectrum of issues based upon the type of equipment employed by a given facility. Not only should these procedures cover all items of medical equipment to include the chamber or chamber system, they should address patient care activities as well. Written operating instructions form the foundation of any proper safety program.

- **Attention to detail** – procedures should address every aspect, no matter how mundane, of operating and maintaining a given type of chamber system, medical device, or patient treatment process. The level of detail should be sufficient to ensure that no critical process or procedure has been omitted. Being thorough is a time-consuming process and one that some can easily justify not completing; however, thoroughness is absolutely necessary.

- **Vigilance** – an organization may have the most comprehensive safety plan possible; but, if the staff is not constantly aware of their surroundings and the consequence of their actions or the actions of others, it means little. As noted in the chapter on "How Accidents Happen" in *Hyperbaric Facility Safety: A Practical Guide,* mishaps are rarely the result of a single event but usually result from a chain of events that lead to an accident. Maintaining constant awareness of one's situation may help break a link in this chain.

- **Preventive maintenance** – keeping all equipment in peak working order depends directly on a comprehensive preventive maintenance program. In general, hyperbaric equipment is well designed and highly reliable, requiring relatively little maintenance (except perhaps for large multiplace hyperbaric complexes). As a result, in times of fiscal restraint, preventive maintenance often is relegated to a lower priority. Such management decisions usually prove to be very costly. Senior management must fully support routine maintenance expenditures since it is generally cheaper to keep equipment in good working order than to face the higher cost of repairing a component after a major failure.

- **Proper training** – the importance of this element cannot be overly stressed. Safety awareness begins in the classroom and is applied in the facility. Mishap data clearly points to the dominance of operator errors in recent hyperbaric accidents. Proper initial instruction and timely continuing education can help mitigate these tragic findings in the future. Minimum training standards must be developed, adopted, and enforced throughout the international hyperbaric community. Training outcomes should be focused on providing all staff members with sufficient information for them to know when to question a particular action or situation. It is neither practical nor desired to educate every staff member to be an expert on every aspect of hyperbaric operations. However, if a person notes that something does not seem right, and stops and investigates the situation, then a major training objective has been met. This person may have broken the chain of events leading to an accident. The ones that should cause concern are those staff members whose knowledge level is not high enough to recognize that something is not right and continue to allow the situation to exist, perhaps ending in a tragic mishap.

- **Practice, practice, practice** – the proper response to an emergency situation should be calculated and immediate. Although it is not practical for each staff member to memorize every emergency procedure, it is important for them to routinely practice planned reactions to a range of emergency situations.

Each should be familiar enough with all department or equipment emergency procedures to allow them, with the aide of emergency checklists, to deal with any quick response situation. Being aware of others' responsibilities is crucial in that anyone may find oneself in a position of having to respond to an incident when the staff member normally responsible for that particular function is not immediately available. Practicing as a group helps the staff to better appreciate the responsibilities of others and fosters development of the hyperbaric team. As difficult as it is, time should be set aside on a recurring basis for focused unit safety training. Although monthly staff safety training is recommended, the minimal interval should be no more than quarterly.

- **Safety mind-set** – attention to the above elements helps cultivate a safety mindset for the entire hyperbaric facility staff. This obvious attitude then becomes very evident to the patient, helping to instill confidence and easing any fear they may have. Safety must be an overriding philosophy that guides the attitudes and actions of the entire staff.

PRECEDING SAFETY ELEMENTS (EQUIPMENT)

Thanks to the extremely hard work done over the years by many people representing a variety of engineering and safety disciplines, there are codes and standards working behind the scenes to ensure the safety of the equipment installed in hyperbaric facilities. These various groups exert their influence before the doors of the hyperbaric facility are open for business.

The first group coming into contact with the basic equipment for a hyperbaric facility is the American Society of Mechanical Engineers (ASME) and the standards developed by the Pressure Vessel for Human Occupancy (PVHO) Committee. It is not the intent of this chapter to go into detail on the specific role of that committee; that issue has been reserved for elsewhere in this text. In summary, the ASME/PVHO establishes the design and fabrication rules for hyperbaric chambers. Although not recognized throughout the world as the internationally accepted standard, it is considered by many as the premier guidance governing this issue. The reader is referred to other portions of this text for a detailed description of other pressure vessel design and fabrication standards used throughout the world. Additionally, a comprehensive discussion of the regulatory status of ASME/PVHO is provided in the introduction to the chapter on governing directives. Unfortunately, compliance with ASME/PVHO is not yet mandatory in all 50 American states. Of primary importance, however, is that a pressure vessel intended for human occupancy be designed and fabricated in accordance with some sort of recognized safety standard.

A second group having tremendous influence on the safe design of a hyperbaric system is the National Fire Protection Association and their fire safety standard for hyperbaric facilities. Also covered in detail earlier in this text, it establishes minimum performance criteria for ancillary hyperbaric support equipment and systems such as the fire suppression system, intercommunications system, air quality monitoring, electrical requirements, etc. Though ASME/PVHO is not yet mandatory in all 50 American states, NFPA 99 is. It requires that any hyperbaric chamber installed in a healthcare facility be in compliance with ASME/PVHO.

A third group which, in this author's opinion, is underestimated and certainly not well understood for the role it plays, is the Food and Drug Administration. The FDA classifies hyperbaric chambers as Class II medical devices and requires that manufacturers comply with 510(k) Pre-market Notification Requirements before a specific chamber design can be legally placed into commercial sales. A well-written chapter on FDA requirements is presented earlier in this text and no attempt will be made to improve on that discussion. Unfortunately, not all U.S. hyperbaric chamber manufacturers are in compliance with these requirements. Any healthcare organization considering purchase of a hyperbaric chamber or hyperbaric system should require the manufacturer to produce evidence of pre-market clearance. Such documentation verifies that the manufacturer surpassed a rigorous third party review of design and fabrication adequacy and that the system complied with recognized industry standards. If a hyperbaric system under consideration for purchase does not have a cleared 510(k), or is not "grandfathered" (few are), it is suggested that other equipment alternatives be considered. Similar requirements, such as CE Marking in Europe, are being established in other world regions that will ultimately raise the level of quality of hyperbaric systems. Improved quality leads directly to improved safety.

Guidelines developed by the American Society for Testing and Materials (ASTM) are used extensively to direct designers of oxygen equipment and oxygen system components to proper material selection, design, and maintenance. These guidelines help ensure that consideration is given to these elements to minimize the risk of fire due to improper materials, inadequate design, or sub-optimal maintenance. More information on ASTM interests is found in the chapters titled "The Role of Oxygen in Hyperbaric Chamber Fire Safety and Hyperbaric Fire Risk Assessments and Forensics," *Hyperbaric Facility Safety: A Practical Guide.* The Compressed Gas Association (CGA) sets guides for the installation of primary and secondary gas delivery systems and gas purity. Compliance with these standards gives the new operator assurance that the necessary steps have been taken to ensure delivery of high quality gas supplies to either the patient or the chamber.

Additionally, the Undersea and Hyperbaric Medical Society (UHMS) produced companion safety guidelines for both monoplace and multiplace hyperbaric chamber systems. Originally intended to provide a potential purchaser with a better understanding of the issues that needed to be understood when contemplating installation of a hyperbaric system, they have now become valuable source documents for users and engineers alike. Referring to these documents in the early stages of facility planning has proven to be a valuable effort by many.

Though hyperbaric medicine is poised for rapid expansion into developing areas of the world, comprehensive safety standards like those mentioned above are not in place in most of these countries to help establish and support the growth of the specialty. Aggressive efforts are underway to promote adoption of comprehensive safety standards throughout the world.

PRECEDING SAFETY ELEMENTS (FACILITIES)

Not only are there codes and standards that govern the design and fabrication of hyperbaric chambers and their affiliated component systems, there are also standards in the United States and a few other countries that establish minimum facility requirements that must be met before the hyperbaric chamber can be installed. These requirements are summarized in the chapter on governing directives. However, at present, the building requirements as set forth in NFPA 99, Chapter 19 are only for those facilities in operation in designated healthcare facilities. Efforts are currently underway to apply the requirements in NFPA 99, Chapter 19 to business-classed occupancies as well. The UHMS monoplace and multiplace safety guidelines previously mentioned also address general facility issues that should be considered. In reality, the type of building into which a hyperbaric chamber is installed is immaterial – there are basic facility standards that should be met to ensure continued safe operation regardless of arbitrary classification.

PRECEDING SAFETY ELEMENTS (STAFF TRAINING)

The previous elements that frame equipment and facility requirements generally work quite well, and for the most part are conducted behind the operational scene. Most hyperbaric staff personnel are not even aware of many of the details of the above requirements. However, it all comes together with the initial training the staff receives before beginning hyperbaric chamber operations. Although these aspects of a viable hyperbaric safety program are all important in their own right, training is, in this author's opinion, the most critical element.

As in any discipline, training is central to successful outcomes. The operator must acquire the knowledge to understand the *what, why, when, where,* and *how.* Raising the knowledge level of each hyperbaric operator high enough to know when to ask a question when something does not seem right has already been stressed. Experience also contributes to this higher-order awareness. I encourage the reader's support in adopting the philosophy to obtain a thorough hyperbaric knowledge and to expand it through experience. More basic, however, is the need to have a minimum skill and knowledge level in place before hyperbaric operations even begin. Training after the fact, although better than no training at all, leaves an organization open to all sorts of potential legal pitfalls should an accident occur involving a person who has not been properly trained.

More directly, training is one of the links in the accident chain of events over which the management of any hyperbaric facility has direct control. At present, there are no mandatory requirements in the United States for minimum training standards for all hyperbaric staff. Though there are efforts underway to establish these minimums, there is much work that needs to be done. This is a universal need recognized by the international hyperbaric medicine community and movement in this direction among our peers encourages the author.

CORE PROGRAM ELEMENTS

The basic elements of any comprehensive hyperbaric facility safety program should include at least the following:

- Defined responsibilities
- Documented safety procedures based on the type and size of the facility
- Documented in-service training
- Documented maintenance
- Documented measurement and validation

Responsibilities

Borrowing from the preceding discussion on training, one of the first individual responsibilities is to ensure that each person directly involved in hyperbaric operations is knowledgeable of all potential hazard sources. If there is ever doubt about a particular situation or procedure, then stop and ask for clarification. Do not continue blindly down what may be the beginning of the accident chain of events. Once again, each individual has direct control over his or her level of hyperbaric knowledge and understanding.

Broadly speaking, each organization should develop a program that includes four major checkpoints. Unfortunately, this is generally not the case. The development, execution, and management of the safety program is usually left entirely up to the hyperbaric facility. It is important to do all that is practically possible to indoctrinate everyone from the most senior hospital executive to the most junior technician on the hyperbaric program. The more they understand about what hyperbaric medicine is, what its limitations are, and what the requirements are to provide high quality care safely, the better they can serve as an advocate for the program. The four checks are:

- The governing body (Hospital Board of Directors, etc.) should set a firm hyperbaric safety policy
- The hyperbaric facility management should develop comprehensive safety procedures
- The technical staff of the hyperbaric facility should implement the procedures
- Accrediting agencies (such as the Joint Commission for Accrediting Healthcare Organizations, or JCAHO, in the United States and similar organizations in other countries) should survey for compliance

As mentioned above, the Governing Body should establish a firm hyperbaric safety policy. Within a given institution, the ultimate responsibility resides with this senior management group. They must work closely with the Safety Director (SD) to ensure that these policies are developed and rigidly adhered to. Adherence implies there is an ongoing dialog between the Governing Body and the hyperbaric facility. This should be encouraged. Developing a close working relationship between the Governing Body and the SD is extremely important in that it helps establish the credibility of the SD with senior institutional management. Again, the more institutional management understands your program, the better they can serve as your spokesman.

Continuing down the hierarchy, the Administrator of the host institution plays an important role as well. Specifically, the institution's administration should adopt and correlate regulations and standard operating procedures to ensure that both the physical qualities and operating maintenance methods pertaining to the hyperbaric facility meet the standards required of other departments of the institution. In particular, administration must have an appreciation of the unique compliance issues cited by various codes and standards pertaining to hyperbaric facilities. The more administration understands of the requirements, they better they can offer support and funding for major department expenditures such as periodic maintenance, etc.

As this hierarchy becomes more functional, the hyperbaric medical staff is not exempt from responsibility. The department medical director should work closely with the Safety Director to develop department-specific regulations and procedures. Other medical personnel should also make themselves available to the SD to assist in this effort. Finally, the Medical Director should adopt and ensure that all staff adhere to the procedures developed.

Perhaps the most visible position of a comprehensive hyperbaric safety program is that of the designated Safety Director. This is the only position directed by NFPA 99, Chapter 19. Every facility, regardless of size or the type or number of chambers employed, shall have a Safety Director. This individual has a tremendous responsibility to ensure safe order and discipline among the staff and patients. Specific responsibilities of the SD are covered later in this chapter.

Documented Safety Procedures

There are a variety of issues that should be documented in your safety program. It is not the intent of this text to provide a specific list for your use. Instead, you are encouraged to think through each process, procedure, concern, activity, etc., and to conduct a step-by-step analysis of each. From that detailed assessment, construct a set of guidelines for each action that is appropriate for your facility. There will be many procedures that you will have in common with all other hyperbaric facilities, but there will also be those that are unique to your department.

There are a few general and specific areas identified in NFPA 99, Chapter 19 that are recommended for inclusion in your documentation.

General facility safety

- Conduct of personnel – this area should address such issues as staff performance and evaluation, conduct around patients, etc.

- Apparel and footwear – based on documented mishap data, this is also an area of great concern. It was mentioned earlier that training is one aspect over which any hyperbaric department has direct control; this is another. The Sheffield and Desautel analysis of recent mishaps indicates a high percentage of accidents where contraband or unauthorized items and synthetic materials were allowed into the chamber interior. Research is very clear on the benefits of fire resistant or fire retardant materials in minimizing the fuel available to help propagate a fire. Garments made of 100% cotton are widely used because of their ability to reduce the buildup of static electricity. Unfortunately, many hyperbaric facilities throughout the world allow patients to enter the chamber in regular street clothes, shoes, etc. **This practice is highly discouraged.**

Garments made from anything other than natural fibers are a potential source of increased fuel. Many argue that it takes too much time to have the patient change from their regular clothing into prescribed garments provided by the facility and that the staff is too limited to assist those patients unable to change clothes on their own. ***It is this author's opinion that you CANNOT AFFORD NOT TO!*** As long as the process of assisting patients in the change of clothing is planned, any well-managed program can afford the few extra minutes and effort to perform this vital function.

- Contraband can also more easily be managed by having the patient wear only garments provided by the facility. Personal clothing may have numerous pockets where items such as cigarette lighters, matches, fuel or chemical warmers, etc., may go unnoticed. If the patient is given a garment to wear that has had the pockets sewn closed, or better yet, no pockets at all, then the likelihood that contraband could be brought into the chamber is greatly minimized. Once again, this is an action that you can control!

- Posting of procedures – although it is not recommended to post all emergency procedures throughout the facility for the patients and others to see, there are key procedures that should be posted in public view. Procedures such as building evacuation routes, etc., fall into this category. For multiplace hyperbaric chambers with auxiliary control stations, the chamber operator should post emergency procedures at each control station in a quick-reading flip chart folder for ready access. Any chamber operator, whether monoplace or multiplace, should have immediate access to a complete series of emergency procedures for use in any emergency situation.

- Staff familiarity with procedures – the operative words here are **practice, practice, practice!** Though each person has his or her specific responsibility within the unit, each should be aware enough of the duties of others to be able to respond to any emergency that might happen when they may be the only one around. Frequent practicing, playing the role of other staff members, etc., will help develop an esprit de corps and a sense of being a member of the hyperbaric team that will be advantageous in the event of an accident. During mishaps, things may happen very quickly, possibly leaving little time to contemplate your next action. Practice helps minimize this hesitation and facilitates one's confidence in dealing with the adverse situation regardless of how drastic.

In many organizations, it is difficult to set aside sufficient time to conduct in-service safety training. If an organization, from the very beginning, weaves recurring in-service safety training into the fabric of its organizational structure, it then becomes second nature and part of the routine. For those organizations that seldom or never devote the time necessary to hone staff safety skills, there is, in this author's opinion, higher risk for a mishap.

Specific facility safety

- There should be specific procedures developed, based on the unique characteristics of your hyperbaric chamber or system, that cover situations such as fire in the chamber, patient egress, contaminated air, equipment component failure, fire in the building, etc. Failure to develop these specific response actions will add to the confusion that generally accompanies a mishap situation and will certainly increase one's response time necessary to interrupt the accident chain of events. As noted earlier, these procedures should also be posted at auxiliary control stations for multiplace hyperbaric chamber systems.

- In addition to developing a comprehensive response posture to mechanical or operational emergency situations, a companion list should also be developed to address physiological emergencies such as ear/sinus pain, confinement anxiety, oxygen toxicity, etc. The reader is referred to the chapter on emergency procedures for a more detailed discussion on developing these crucial operational safety aides.

DOCUMENTED IN-SERVICE TRAINING

The familiar theme of practice, practice, and more practice cannot be stressed too strongly. Having said that, it is realized that it may be easier said than done. Time must be routinely set aside; otherwise, in-service training will often take the backseat to other important activities. Ideally, an organization should devote time to monthly safety training. However, if this is not feasible, it is recommended to establish the frequency best suited to your needs, but no less than quarterly. The important thing is that training be done routinely. Safety must be given priority in the ongoing business of a hyperbaric facility.

Examples of training topics are as varied as the mind is creative. Several suggestions are offered to stimulate thinking:

- Fire drills – not only should your fire suppression system (FSS) be exercised periodically (for multiplace chambers so equipped), the local fire department should be frequently involved.

All too often, the FSS is ignored, sitting idle for months and then being expected to perform flawlessly when needed. They must be routinely activated to maintain peak efficiency. There have been several mishaps in which a faulty FSS has been implicated in the accident chain of events. Activating the FSS every six months (preferably) or annually (at minimum) will help instill operator confidence in the system and better assure proper function when needed.

Some organizations are reluctant to invite local fire department personnel into their facility. This attitude is foolish. The patient egress requirements for a hyperbaric environment are different from those of a regular healthcare facility setting. This is especially true in multiplace hyperbaric chamber facilities, where both patients and chamber operators may be required to stay with the chamber longer than usual in order to decompress the chamber safely. Fire department personnel need to understand these unique requirements and be given the opportunity to practice them. Otherwise, they will be unable to provide the quality support necessary during any mishap situation. The needs are different; they need to be able to practice their response to that difference.

- Mock patient emergencies – the staff must be capable of responding to the complete spectrum of patient emergencies such as confinement anxiety, ear/sinus pain, oxygen toxicity reactions, etc. Practice helps the staff develop those reflexive actions necessary to deal with a patient emergency in a timely fashion.

- Simulated equipment failure – although hyperbaric equipment is generally reliable, they are mechanical devices and are subject to failure. A good example for multiplace chamber operations is to practice the steps necessary to deal with a failed viewport. A good example for monoplace chamber operations is the operator's response to loss of pressure control. There are numerous other equipment failures for any type of chamber that can be simulated for practice.

- Contaminated air – usually, the quality of the air produced for hyperbaric chamber operations depends on the quality of the air ingested for compression and proper function of the compressor. Fortunately for the human, one of the most sophisticated alarms for air contamination is the nose. Hydrocarbon-based contaminates can be easily detected. Of concern, of course, is carbon monoxide, which is odorless. Regardless, dealing with contaminated air should be routinely practiced.

- Updates on codes and standards – fortunately for the in-service trainer, change in this area is very slow, making it easy for the trainer to stay current. Changes do occur, however, and hyperbaric personnel are encouraged to be aware of them. The advantage here is that emphasizing these issues in your training program helps broaden your staff's knowledge base for factors that influence the everyday world of hyperbaric medicine.

Vital to an effective ongoing hyperbaric training program are those sessions for which continuing education credits are offered. This is especially crucial for technical personnel. Generally, there is no problem with professional medical staff personnel in satisfying continuing medical educational credits. Unfortunately, technical staff do not often have the administrative support to routinely participate in these ongoing educational activities. They can rarely afford to attend these functions at their own expense, and as a result, they usually do not attend. This situation needs to change. As an alternative, larger clinical hyperbaric medicine programs are encouraged to apply to organizations such as the National Board of Diving and Hyperbaric Medical Technology for continuing education credits for their on-going in-service training program. This approach will help ensure that staff members have the opportunity to maintain currency for minimal cost and less time away from the facility. Further, it is highly recommended that technical personnel attend courses such as the ASTM course *Fire Hazards in Oxygen Delivery Systems,* or International ATMO's *Advanced Course in Hyperbaric Safety.* There are others. If a good working relationship has been established with the institution's administrative management, it is easier for the director of hyperbaric medicine to advocate on the technician's behalf to help justify funding the educational need.

Continuing to grow in importance is certification in hyperbaric technology. A detailed discussion of this program is provided elsewhere in this text and will not be replicated here. Suffice it to say this is a valuable tool to recognize staff competence and should be a priority for every hyperbaric facility. Developing a comprehensive in-service training program assists those technicians not yet certified to achieve the background preparation necessary to successfully complete the certification exam.

Finally, there is an old military saying: "If you did not write it down, you did not do it!" That speaks for itself. It is very important for you to document what you do. This is the one thing surveyors have to review to determine department activity in this area. Additionally, one tends to be more organized in program development and execution when documentation is required.

Documented Maintenance

Preventive and responsive maintenance of any component of a hyperbaric chamber or system is required. Considering the total number of hyperbaric facilities in the United States, few are fortunate enough to maintain sufficient technical expertise on staff to handle the majority of maintenance needs in-house. Generally, third-party contractors or the chamber manufacturer is relied upon. Regardless of your particular situation, all aspects of maintenance ranging from daily inspections to major component overhauls should be documented in detail. Failure to maintain detailed maintenance records often makes future repairs more costly since historical system actions cannot be validated.

Documented Measurement and Validation

In setting up any program for which outcomes are important, the processes developed to achieve those outcomes must be measurable. If they are not, there is no mechanism for feedback to determine if the process is actually needed, if it is achieving the desired result, or if it is as efficient as it can be. It is relatively easy to measure outcomes in an industrial setting where a product is produced. You can measure machining tolerances, component rejection rates, etc. It is more difficult to measure management outcomes, yet this is still attainable. If an organization has no tool by which it can assess performance, regardless of the measurement area, then it is omitting an important tool that management can use to ascertain the success of a given program. This is equally true with the need to assess outcomes of a hyperbaric safety program. Compliance organizations such as JCAHO traditionally review such inter-departmental documentation to assist with their survey of a particular department or patient service. Good documentation cannot be stressed too strongly.

Safety Director

As previously mentioned, one of the key positions of every hyperbaric facility is that of the Safety Director. Every hyperbaric facility, regardless of type, should have a designated Safety Director. Due to the extensive nature of responsibilities of the Safety Director, no attempt will be made to provide a detailed discussion of each. Instead, these responsibilities are provided in list form.

Knowledge and Experience:

- Completion of a recognized course in hyperbaric medicine (Undersea and Hyperbaric Medical Society, American College of Hyperbaric Medicine, National Board of Diving and Hyperbaric Medical Technology, etc., or similar nation-specific requirement)
- Training or experience in hyperbaric chamber maintenance and operations (primarily for multiplace hyperbaric facilities)
- Working knowledge of safety codes and decompression requirements
- Certification in Hyperbaric Technology (**highly desired**)

General Responsibilities:

- In charge of all hyperbaric equipment in the absence of a Technical Director. (Note: there is no requirement in NFPA 99 for a designated Technical Director as there is for the Safety Director. Generally, monoplace hyperbaric facilities do not have a Technical Director whereas multiplace hyperbaric facilities do. This is due, in part, to the increased complexity of multiplace systems.)
- Responsible for the safe/effective operation and maintenance of the hyperbaric chamber and related support systems and ancillary components
- Works closely with facility management and hyperbaric physician(s)
- Recommends and implements safety procedures as appropriate
- Serves on institutional Safety Committee (recommended)
- Has authority to restrict or remove potentially hazardous items or supplies from inside the chamber
- Provides training and leadership
- Maintains all safety-related codes and standards as required by various licensing and regulatory agencies

Specific Responsibilities:

- Ensures compliance with NFPA 99, Chapter 19, Hyperbaric Facilities (or other country equivalents as appropriate) and unit safety policies and procedures
- Reviews safety incidents, collects information on equipment/patient safety, reports relevant incidents, and provides periodic in-service training on accident prevention
- Works closely with the medical, nurse, and technical directors to develop and annually review and revise documents pertaining to policies, procedures, operations, and maintenance
- Fosters positive relationships between department personnel and local regulators such as the local fire marshal, director of emergency services, pressure vessel inspector, etc.
- Works with the Technical Director to coordinate/approve all upgrades, modifications, and repairs to the hyperbaric chamber or hyperbaric system
- Interacts with hospital maintenance personnel and outside contractors to ensure all maintenance is performed in accordance with applicable codes and standards
- Ensures that all system modifications are tested prior to manned chamber operations
- Evaluates equipment and supplies before they are used inside the chamber
- Maintains a safe environment for the staff and patients alike
- Monitors to ensure that appropriate decompression procedures are used for all persons with hyperbaric exposure to inert gases

- Informs personnel of any special work conditions such as infection control, hazard control, etc.
- Serves as technical trainer for full-time and part-time staff
- Provides in-service training on aspects of hyperbaric physiology, equipment operations, safety, decompression requirements, and treatment protocols
- Validates in-chamber safety training of new staff before their initial entry into the hyperbaric chamber (multiplace)
- Generates and supervises safety drills which are tailored to the special needs of the facility
- Conducts annual review of safety-related events in order to identify trends and monitor improvements
- Sets up procedures to assist the medial director in reviewing, documenting, and reporting safety-related events to the staff to facilitate learning

SUMMARY

A well-structured safety plan consists of a variety of components, each with its relative importance. Not to diminish the other elements, proper training serves as the foundation for continued safety.

In order to maintain a safe operational hyperbaric environment, everyone must realize it is a team effort. Though a particular aspect of daily operation may not be a specific person's responsibility, each must appreciate the role of another. Each person must do his or her part by developing a safety mindset to strengthen the chain of mishap avoidance.

The Safety Director is a key figure in any hyperbaric medicine department's safety program and has wide-ranging responsibilities to ensure that the functions of hyperbaric safety are properly planned, executed, documented, and validated.

REFERENCES

1. ANSI/ASME PVHO-1-1997, Safety Standard for Pressure Vessels for Human Occupancy, American Society of Mechanical Engineers, New York, 1997.
2. GCA Pamphlet G-7.1-1989, Commodity Specification for Air, Compressed Gas Association, Inc., Arlington, Virginia, 1989.
3. Guidelines for Clinical Multiplace Hyperbaric Facilities. UHMS, Kensington, MD, 1994.
4. Health Care Facilities Handbook, 5th Edition, Burton R. Klein, Ed., National Fire Protection Association, Quincy, Massachusetts, 1996.
5. Hyperbaric Facility Safety: A Practical Guide, W.T. Workman, Ed., Best Publishing Company, Flagstaff, AZ, 1999.
6. Monoplace Hyperbaric Chamber Safety Guidelines. UHMS, Kensington, MD, 1997.
7. Sheffield PJ, Desautels, DA. Hyperbaric and hypobaric chamber fires: a 73-year analysis. Undersea Hyper Med 1997; 24(3): 153-164.
8. Standard for Health Care Facilities, NFPA 99, 1996 Edition, National Fire Protection Association, Quincy, Massachusetts, pp. 108-119.

NOTES

CHAPTER I

TRANSCUTANEOUS OXYGEN MEASUREMENTS

M. NICASIO, V. LARSON-LOHR, AND P.N. KIMBRELL

INTRODUCTION

Several key developments have led to our ability to perform measurements of tissue oxygenation. Clark[1] using an electrode model developed by Davies and Brink[2] modified the electrode, placing both the anode and cathode together in an electrolyte fluid behind a membrane. Huch et al.[3] further modified the Clark electrode by adding a heating element and a thermistor. Baumberger et al.[4] demonstrated the ability to diffuse oxygen through the skin into a heated (45 degrees) buffered solution.

Today, transcutaneous oxygen measurements (TCOM) are used in the wound center environment to evaluate degree of tissue hypoxia in patients with non-healing wounds, to aid in selection of those patients who require further vascular evaluation, to evaluate response to normobaric and hyperbaric oxygen, and to determine amputation levels.

HOW DOES THE MODIFIED CLARK ELECTRODE WORK?

The modified Clark electrode contains a heating element and a thermistor that is preset and able to maintain a temperature of 42 to 45 degrees centigrade. Maximum arterialization of capillaries occurs at 45 degrees. Due to the fragile nature of the patient's skin, 44 degrees centigrade is commonly used to prevent blistering. The electrode is applied to the skin through a fixation ring. Contact fluid is placed in the fixation ring and the Clark electrode is secured to the fixation ring. The skin is heated, dilating the capillaries, shifting the oxyhemoglobin curve to the right and allowing oxygen to diffuse through the skin and into the contact fluid. The heat will dissolve the dead lipid layer of the epidermis, improving the diffusion of gas through the skin. The oxygen that has diffused through the skin and is dissolved in the contact fluid is then reduced to a measurable current. That current is equivalent to the oxygen given off by the skin, thus measuring PO_2 in a contact liquid which will be in equilibrium with the underlying dermal tissue 10 to 15 minutes after the skin application.

EQUIPMENT

In the United States, there are three models of TCOM machines that are commonly used: the Radiometer (Copenhagen, Denmark) (Figure 1), the PeriMed (Stockholm, Sweden) (Figure 2), and the Novametrix (Wallingford, CT) (Figure 3). In 1991, the Radiometer used a Clark electrode, and modified the equipment so it could safely be used in oxygen-pressured chambers (monoplace hyperbaric chambers). The PeriMed monitor uses the same Clark electrode as Radiometer and can also be used in the pressurized oxygen environment. The Novametrix electrode cannot be used in a pressurized oxygen environment.

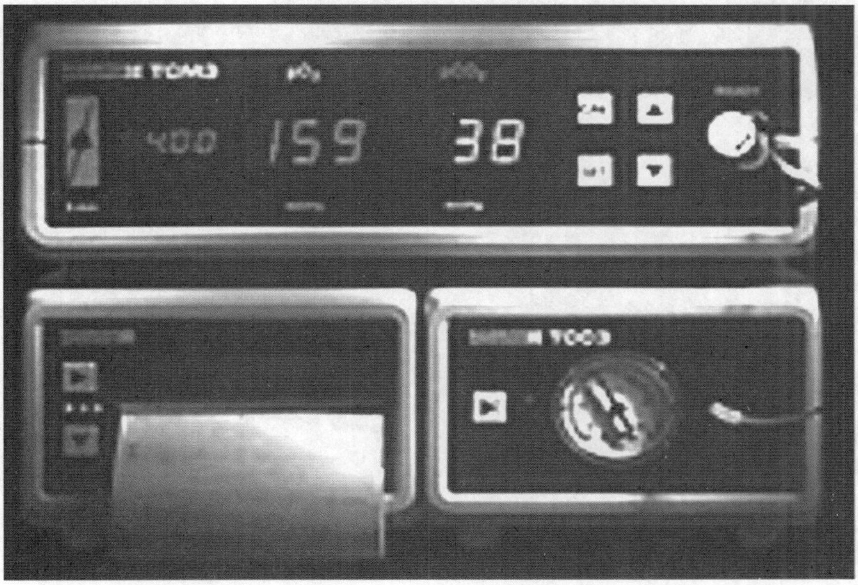

FIGURE 1 Radiometer

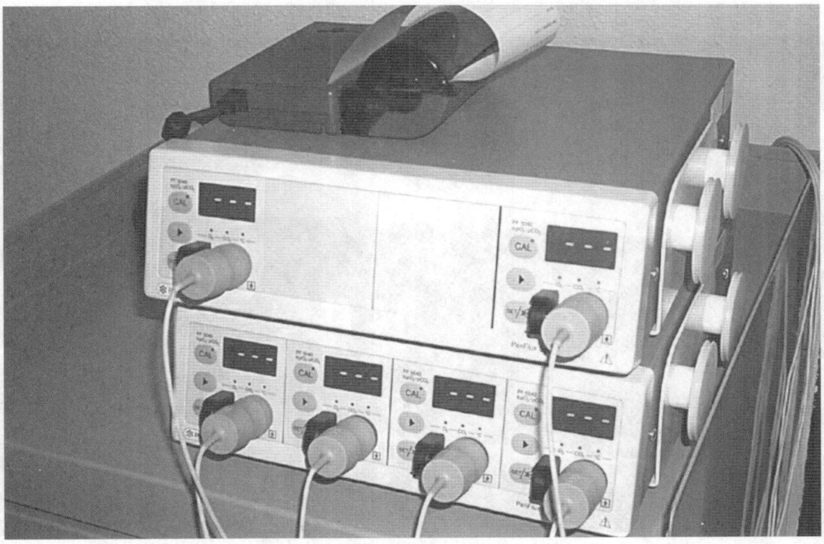

FIGURE 2 PeriMed

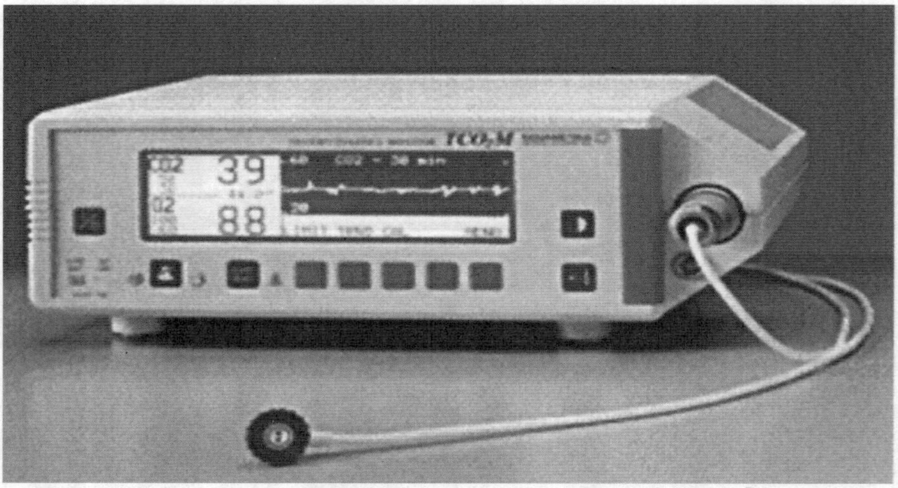

FIGURE 3 Novameter

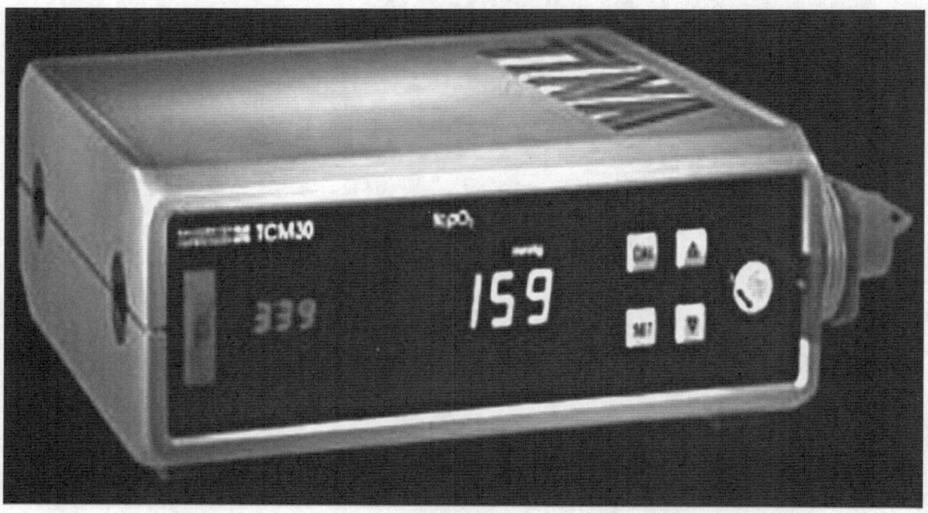

FIGURE 4 TCM 30

Radiometer

Radiometer currently manufactures two machines, the TINA 3 and the TCM 30. The TINA 3 consists of a monitor unit and an electrode. The electrode can be oxygen-only or dual gas (carbon dioxide and oxygen). When the monitors initially came on the market a 2-point calibration was required. Due to improvements in design, a single-point calibration is now done. If the electrode will be used in hyperbaric oxygen environment or a PO_2 in excess of 1,000mmHg is anticipated, the electrode will need to be half-calibrated to extend the range. The TCM 30 (Figure 4) is an oxygen-only machine. This machine is able to measure values greater than 1,000 so does not need be half calibrated.

PeriMed/PeriFlux

The second monitor is the PeriFlux System 5000. The PeriFlux system 5000 consists of a main unit that can be equipped with one, two, three, or four function units. The base unit will accommodate the TCOM modules or laser doppler with thermistor. This main unit contains a diode laser emitting laser light that is transmitted to the PF5110 LDPM unit(s). The 5002 Basic Unit can also be equipped with the same functional units except the PF5010 LDPM Unit. The function unit types are the PF5010 LDPM unit for one laser doppler probe and the 5020 Heating Unit used for one or two heat probes/sensors as well as for heat provocation test temperature stabilization or temperature measurement. The PF5040 $tcpO_2$ unit is for one $tcpO_2$ electrode or one combination $tcpO_2/tcpCO_2$ electrode. The PeriMed printer is the DPU3445 Thermal Printer.

Novametrix

The Novametrix System 800 transcutaneous oxygen monitor can link up two separate three-electrode sensor units, allowing up to six measurements to be made simultaneously. The monitor has an attached recorder as well as a display of the transcutaneous oxygen measurements. This monitor can be used only in a multiplace chamber and not in a monoplace chamber.

PRACTICAL APPLICATION

Preparing the Equipment

Turn the unit on. Calibrate the electrode and set parameters using the manufacturer's guidelines. Connect the electrode plug to the electrode connector on the unit. Insert the membraned electrode into the electrode holder and turn clockwise. Push the CAL button on the unit to initiate the calibration. The calibration indicator light will flash and the *C light will be illuminated until set temperature is reached. When pre-set temperature is reached, the value is displayed. After two–four minutes, the calibration indicator light on the unit will be continuously illuminated to indicate that the system is calibrated. Most machines now recommend only a one-point calibration. One-point calibration is to air, barometric pressure, and humidity. Temperature can also be adjusted. To have maximum arterialization of capillaries without causing thermal damage to the patient, a temperature of 44 degrees centigrade is recommended. It is important to use a consistent temperature between patients and between tests. Studies done at 44 degrees centigrade will have reading 2% less than a test done at 45 degrees centigrade.

Preparing the Client

Provide a position of comfort while maintaining the patient supine with legs horizontal. Limit activities by patient, keep warm and calm, control pain, and decrease patient anxiety. It is recommended to limit visitors or distractions as they may interfere with test results. Ensure that the staff is calm and quiet. Encourage the patient not to smoke two hours prior to exam or values can be 10% less than a non-smoking value. Limit caffeine intake prior to exam. Instruct the patient on what to expect during the exam, that it is painless, requires minimal movement during the testing, and will take approximately one hour.

Site Selection

Site selection is best done by a combination of physician selection and protocol selection. This takes into account anatomical structures, wound location, and condition of surrounding tissue. Bony prominences, large superficial vessels and pulse sites, callous areas, areas with significant edema, soles of feet, and palms should be avoided as they can falsely lower or elevate the reading. The best electrode contact will be on flat or slightly convex areas. The number of electrodes to be used is largely determined by what is available. The authors of this chapter recommend a minimum of six electrodes to obtain an adequate study and efficient use of human resources.

Skin Preparation

First, remove body hair from the site. A dry razor is usually sufficient. Second, clean the skin with a mild soap or alcohol prep pads to degrease the skin. The third step is removal of dry scaling skin. Repeated applications of clean paper tape until the tape remains clear will effectively denude the skin of this relative barrier. Removal of dry scaling skin will optimize both electrode contact and oxygen diffusion. Use extreme care when preparing the fragile or paper-thin skin so as not to cause further open wounds. Do not use a harsh tape such as adhesive or packing tape.

Electrode Application

Carefully apply the fixation ring to the measuring site as follows: remove the protection film from the adhesive disk; press the center of the fixation ring onto the measuring site with a finger; run a finger or cotton tip applicator around the rim circumference; press firmly to prevent air bubbles that can cause leaks. To ensure the seal, cover ring or tape may be used over fixation ring. Do not apply tape over electrode head, as this will alter readings. Fill the hole in the fixation ring with three to five drops of the contact fluid. To place the electrode on the fixation ring, align the arrow on the electrode with one of the big marks on the fixation ring and turn the electrode 1/4 clockwise to fasten it in the fixation ring. Wait for a stable reading. The typical physiological stabilization time of a patient is ten to fifteen minutes for the $tcpO_2$ reading.

Recording Results

Results should be recorded on a form that allows the physician to clearly see the anatomical position of the electrode, flow of readings from stabilization, elevation, and oxygen challenge (see Figure 5). The technician or the nurse should record any problems that occurred during the test, condition of the sites, and status of the patient. The nurse or technician should not record an interpretation. Only the physician or other provider who is credentialed to interpret should do so. A simultaneous flow recording should be printed and attached to the back of the recording form.

Pictures

A digital photograph of the placement of electrodes will provide a visual reference if a comparative study needs to be performed. It will also provide a record of the test for reimbursement purposes.

Reference Site

A reference site is used to identify any problems with the cardiopulmonary system affecting oxygenation. Traditionally, a reference site has been a chest lead placed at the mid-clavicular, third intracostal space position. This can also be easily evaluated using a pulse oximetry. By using pulse oximetry you will free up an electrode to be used in mapping of the extremity. The physician may choose to do a contralateral reference. This is placing an electrode on the unaffected extremity. In doing a contralateral reference, information can be obtained that will identify a tissue oxygenation problem before a wound develops. A reference site may also be used to calculate a regional perfusion index (RPI), which is a limb-to-chest ratio. The RPI first came into use with the vascular specialists who were used to view numbers as a ratio or index such as the ankle-brachial index (ABI). There remains debate as to the best method by which to review the data, though the use of RPI is decreasing.

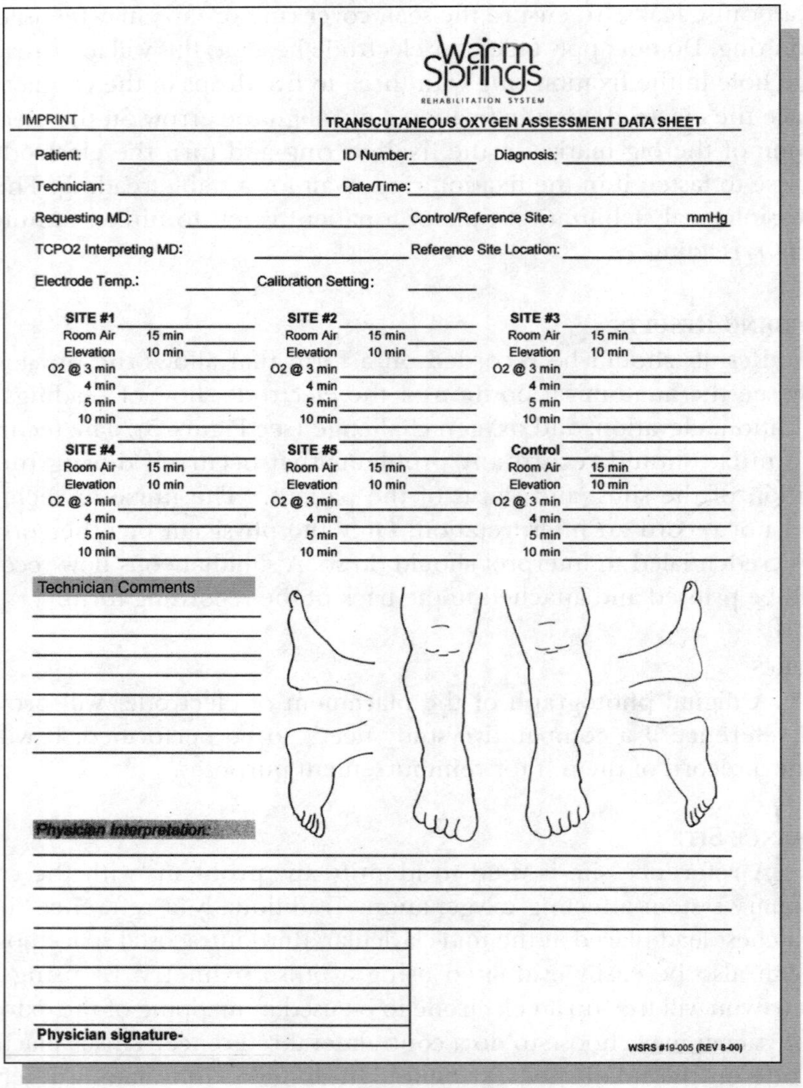

Warm Springs
REHABILITATION SYSTEM

IMPRINT

TRANSCUTANEOUS OXYGEN ASSESSMENT DATA SHEET

Patient: ______ ID Number: ______ Diagnosis: ______

Technician: ______ Date/Time: ______

Requesting MD: ______ Control/Reference Site: ______ mmHg

TCPO2 Interpreting MD: ______ Reference Site Location: ______

Electrode Temp.: ______ Calibration Setting: ______

SITE #1		SITE #2		SITE #3	
Room Air	15 min	Room Air	15 min	Room Air	15 min
Elevation	10 min	Elevation	10 min	Elevation	10 min
O2 @ 3 min		O2 @ 3 min		O2 @ 3 min	
4 min		4 min		4 min	
5 min		5 min		5 min	
10 min		10 min		10 min	

SITE #4		SITE #5		Control	
Room Air	15 min	Room Air	15 min	Room Air	15 min
Elevation	10 min	Elevation	10 min	Elevation	10 min
O2 @ 3 min		O2 @ 3 min		O2 @ 3 min	
4 min		4 min		4 min	
5 min		5 min		5 min	
10 min		10 min		10 min	

Technician Comments

Physician Interpretation:

Physician signature-

WSRS #19-005 (REV 8-00)

FIGURE 5

EQUILIBRATION AND PROVOCATION

Adequate time needs to be allowed for equilibration at the baseline and with each provocation. In individuals with normal circulation, ten to fifteen minutes are required for oxygen to diffuse through the capillaries and into the contact fluid.[5] In patients with compromised circulation, up to twenty minutes may be required. It is best to observe the digital reading to determine when it has stabilized.

There are three provocations to be used that can provide added specificity to the exam. The first is elevation. The involved extremity is elevated 45 degrees, taking care to support the extremity. Initially a drop in tissue oxygen is seen. If there is no disease, the level of tissue oxygen should recover. A 10% change in the tissue oxygen reading from the supine position is indicative of medium- to large-sized arterial occlusive disease.

The second provocation is 100% oxygen at surface. The oxygen is delivered by a non-rebreather or aviator's mask. The fit of the mask should be as snug as possible. The oxygen provocation is used to assess the potential for response to adjunctive hyperbaric oxygen. Guidelines for obtained response values on 100% oxygen at surface are as follows:

>300 mmHg	excellent response
>200 mmHg	good response
100-200 mmHg	adequate response, non-limb threatening ischemia
51-99 mmHg	significant ischemia
0-50 mmHg	demonstrates high-grade ischemia/hypoxia

The third provocation is a trial of HBO at 2.0 to 2.5 ATA. Both the value obtained and the rate of rise is observed. There is initial data suggesting that a more rapid rate of rise of tissue oxygen can be related to improved response to HBO. Minimum response values of 100-450 mmHg have been reported in literature as a positive response to healing.[6,15]

REMEMBRANING

The membrane on the electrode will need to be replaced on a regular basis. Manufacturers' recommendations vary between seven to fourteen days. Factors that affect the frequency of remembraning are: the number of studies per week, care of the membrane between studies, if the membrane comes in contact with patient drainage, or if there is difficulty calibrating the electrode. If the membrane is allowed to dry out between studies, oxygen will not effectively diffuse across the membrane. The electrode heads should be stored in the protective caps provided. The caps are filled with contact fluid to keep the membranes moist. If the membrane comes in contact with a wound or wound drainage, it should be changed to prevent cross contamination of patients. If there is no contact with wound drainage, there is no need to change the membranes between patients.

WHAT DO THE NUMBERS MEAN?

Over the last twenty years, a tremendous volume of literature has addressed TCOMs and improved our knowledge and ability to interpret the values we have obtained. A selection of the research is presented in this section.

Sheffield[7] in 1982 confirmed the tissue hypoxia in wounded areas with TCOMs. A rise is tissue oxygenation under HBO was also documented using TCOM measurements.

In 1983, Dowd et al.[8] compared 161 volunteers without known peripheral vascular disease to 62 patients with ischemic skin due to peripheral vascular disease. The hypothesis was that the transcutaneous oxygen pressure would reflect the fall in cutaneous blood flow and perfusion allowing for an accurate assessment of skin viability. Findings of the study demonstrated that $TCPO_2$ was related to the degree of ischemia and was a many times more accurate guide to skin viability than clinical assessment. This was also one of the first studies to define a $TCPO_2$ level of greater than or equal to 40 mmHg as necessary for healing in patients with peripheral vascular disease.

Wyss et al.[9] compared diabetic patients with peripheral vascular disease to non-diabetic patients with the same disease. They reported that those patients whose foot or leg $TCPO_2$ was below 20 mmHg were more likely to have ulcers, rest pain, or require an amputation as compared to those limbs with $TCPO_2$ greater than 20 mmHg.

In 1990, Grouden et al.[10] examined $TCPO_2$ ability to accurately reflect tissue perfusion. Ankle-brachial indexes (ABI) and absolute ankle and toe pressures were compared to foot and calf $TCPO_2$'s in 51 patients who were referred for vascular testing. In ABIs of 0.50 and greater, this study showed good correlation. Conclusions of this study indicate that $TCPO_2$'s are useful in the assessment of ischemia, but further work was needed to define their role in patients with intermittent claudication.

Pecoraro et al.[11] prospectively studied the course of healing of full-thickness lower extremity ulcers in 46 diabetic patients. They determined that periwound perfusion is a critical physiologic determinant of diabetic ulcer healing, with a 39-fold increased risk of early healing failure when the periwound $TCPO_2$ was less than 20 mmHg.

Bacharach et al.[12] looked at $TCPO_2$ and whether it could be used to predict amputation site healing in lower extremities with arterial occlusive disease. Ninety extremities were evaluated. The results of the study demonstrated that $TCPO_2$ equal to or greater than 40 mmHg was associated with primary or delayed healing in 98% of extremities, while $TCPO_2$ less than 20 mmHg was universally associated with failure. In patients with $TCPO_2$ between 20-40 mmHg, it was found that measurements obtained during elevation improved predictability.

Ballard et al.[13] did a prospective evaluation of transcutaneous oxygen measurements in the management of the diabetic foot. The focus of the study was to determine whether $TCPO_2$ could accurately predict severity of foot ischemia and if it could be used to select appropriate treatment. Fifty-five patients with sixty-six limbs were prospectively mapped. Those patients with $TCPO_2$ greater than 30 were managed with wound care, debridement, or minor foot amputation. In the patients with $TCPO_2$ less than 30 evaluations for vascular reconstruction were done. The conclusion of the study was that $TCPO_2$ can prospectively determine severity of foot ischemia and aid in selecting appropriate treatment and decrease total cost of care.

Watel, Mathieu, and Neviere[14] questioned whether they could use $TCPO_2$ to determine if a group of patients would benefit from hyperbaric oxygen therapy. Twenty patients with arterial or mixed wounds that had failed to heal after medical treatments were selected. Results showed no difference in $TCPO_2$ between the group that healed with HBO and those that did not when the $TCPO_2$ measured was on room air or breathing 100% oxygen at surface. In patients where the $TCPO_2$ was measured at 2.5 atmospheres absolute (ATA), and found to be greater than 100 mmHg, it was demonstrated that healing was consistently successful.

Smith et al.[15] also looked at the ability of $TCPO_2$ measurements to predict the healing of leg wounds with hyperbaric oxygen therapy. Periwound measurements were obtained before treatment and after ten hyperbaric treatments on twenty-six patients. Patients who had a 5% reduction in wound score were identified as responders. Nine patients were responders. In the wounds examined, periwound measurements correlated directly with improvement in wound score per treatment (p=0.03), and elevated periwound TCOM at 2.4 ATA and reduced periwound TCOM at surface were associated with a more rapid response to HBO treatments.

CONCLUSION

Work over the last twenty years has demonstrated the effectiveness of TCOMs in the evaluation and management of the chronic or non-healing wound. It must be remembered that it is a tool to be used in the hands of an experienced clinician. TCOMs represent only one piece of data, and should be used together with all information gained during the initial evaluation of the patient to generate a plan of care.

REFERENCES

1. Clark CL, Wolf R, Granger D, et al. Continuous recording of blood oxygen tensions by polarography. *J Appl Physiol* 6:189-193 1953.
2. Davies PW, Brink F. Microelectrodes for measuring local oxygen tension in animal tissues. Rev SCI Instru. 13:524-533 1942.
3. Huch R, Lubbers DW, Huch A. Quantitative continuous measurements of partial oxygen pressure on the skin of adults and newborn babies. Pflugers Arch 337:185-198 1972.
4. Baumberger JP, Goodfriend RB.
5. Sheffield PJ. Measuring tissue oxygen tension: a review. *Undersea & Hyperbaric Medicine* 1998 25(3):179-188.
6. Strauss MJ, Breedlove JW, Hart GB. Use of transcutaneous oxygen measurements to predict healing in foot wounds. *Undersea & Hyperbaric Medicine,* 24(suppl):15, 1997.
7. Sheffield PJ. Tissue oxygen measurements. In Problem Wounds: The Role of Oxygen. JC Davis and TK Hunt, (Eds) New York: Elsevier. 1988; 17-51.
8. Dowd GSE, Liknge K, Bentley G. Measurement of transcutaneous oxygen pressure in normal and ischemic skin. *J Bone & Joint Surg* 1: January 1983.
9. Wyss CR, Matsen FA, Simmons CW, Burgess EM. Transcutaneous oxygen tension measurements on limbs of diabetic and non-diabetic patients with peripheral vascular disease. *Surgery* 95(3):339-345, 1984.
10. Grouden MC, Fitzpatrick P, Stanley ST, Colgan MP Burke PE, et al. Do transcutaneous oxygen tension pressure measurements accurately reflect tissue perfusion? *J of Vascular Technology* 14(5):221-23, 1990.
11. Pecoraro RE, Ahroni JH, Boyko EJ, Stensel VL. Chronology and determinants of tissue repair in diabetic lower-extremity ulcers. *Diabetes* 40:1305-13, 1991.
12. Bacharach JM, Rooke TW, Osmundson PJ, Gloviczki P. Predictive value of trancutaneous oxygen pressure and amputation success by use of supine and elevation measurements. *J Vasc Surg* 15:558-563, 1992.
13. Ballard JK, Eke CC, Bunt TJ, Killeen JD. A prospective evaluation of transcutaneous oxygen measurements in the management of diabetic foot problems. *Journal of Vascular Surgery* 22, 4:485-492, 1995.
14. Watel FE, Mathieu DM, Neviere RR. Transcutaneous Oxygen Pressure Measurements. *J Hyperbaric Medicine* 1990, 221-223.
15. Smith BM, Desvigne LD, Slade JB, Dooley JW, Warren DC. Trancutaneous oxygen measurements predict healing of leg wounds with hyperbaric therapy.

CHAPTER II

LASER DOPPLER FLOWMETRY (LDF)

A.L. ZIEMBA

WHAT IS LASER?

Laser is an acronym that stands for Light Amplification by Stimulated Emission of Radiation. A laser has unique properties. The light it produces is monochromatic and contains only one specific light wave. The light produced can be low power used for measurements or it can be high power light allowing laser devices to even cut metals. Currently, laser devices are used in medicine for cutting and sealing in various surgical procedures as well as in many analysis instruments.

WHAT IS LASER DOPPLER FLOWMETRY?

Laser Doppler Flowmetry (LDF) is a technology that uses a small beam of laser light to obtain information from beneath the skin surface where it penetrates to a depth of 1-2 mm. Because LDF measures the movements of particles in living tissue, all particles including blood cells that move and reflect light are recorded. Therefore, LDF measures the total microvascular blood perfusion in local tissue including capillaries, arterioles, venules, and shunts in a volume of approximately 1 mm^3.

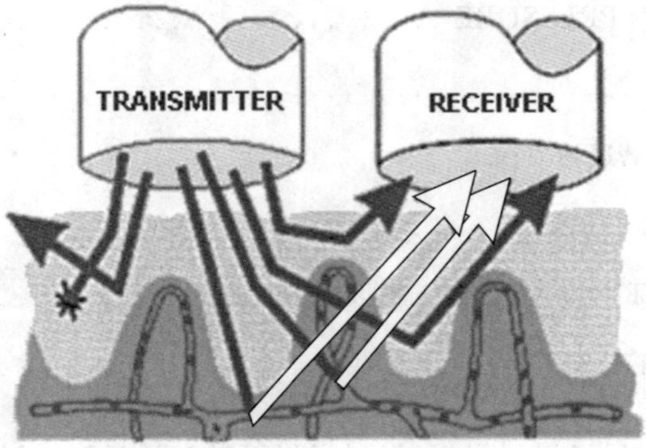

FIGURE 1.

The principle of LDF is that the laser light beam is transported to the tissue via fiber optic lines. Light beams scattered in moving red cells undergo a frequency shift according to the Doppler effect, while beams scattered in static tissue remain unchanged in frequency. A portion of the backscattered light is brought back via another fiber optic line to the instrument where an output signal related to the flow of red blood cells in a specific tissue volume is calculated. The signal from the laser Doppler flowmeter is arbitrary. It cannot give any physiological definition such as the actual number of cells flowing through a given volume of tissue during a given time period. Perfusion values must be compared relative to one another and are not absolute. The best LDF tests are provocation tests that measure and compare the local perfusion before and after a standardized change of the perfusion. This makes the tissue its own reference. Examples of such provocations are:

- Heat test
- Occlusion test
- Posture (leg elevation or lowering)

CLINICAL USE OF LASER DOPPLER FLOWMETRY

Laser Doppler Flowmetry, a non-invasive technique for measurement of tissue perfusion, has become an increasingly familiar technology in hyperbaric medicine and wound management circles. For many years this technology has also been used to evaluate the flow of blood in the capillary beds, particularly in the field of plastic surgery where free flaps are used in reconstructive surgery. The first use of the laser Doppler technique was for retinal blood flow measurements in 1972 demonstrated by Riva et al. Stern first demonstrated the possibility of using LD technique in assessing skin blood flow in 1975.

The technique has recently grown in importance in the diagnosis and treatment of ischemia-related tissue disorders. Valuable information is provided for the following:

- Management of peripheral vascular disease
- Diabetes treatment
- Amputation level determination
- Monitoring therapy
- Plastic surgery (evaluation of flaps)
- Treatment of burns

HEAT PROVOCATION

Skin perfusion is strongly dependent upon skin temperature, and generally the perfusion value in normal tissue will rise during increased heat. With local heat provocation (44 degrees C), vasodilatation is maximized, enabling LDF to assess the tissue reserve capacity and severity of ischemia. The increase of the perfusion measured before and after the local heating is a measure of the tissue reserve capacity. When the tissue reserve capacity is too low, the healing process is compromised.

SKIN PERFUSION PRESSURE

Skin perfusion is another parameter that can be obtained using Laser Doppler Flowmetry. A laser Doppler probe is placed underneath or inside a blood pressure cuff. When the pressure is increased in the cuff, the laser Doppler detects an occlusion. The pressure is slowly released until the perfusion returns. This is the skin perfusion pressure. When the skin perfusion pressure is too low, the healing is compromised. The occlusion may be painful for some ischemic patients.

TOE PRESSURE

Ankle pressure is measured routinely today, but becomes unreliable when the vessels have become hardened and calcified. The pressure taken on the toe is more reliable for these patients. The pressure is measured using a laser Doppler probe and miniature blood pressure cuffs, which inherently can create technical problems in some patients. Laser Doppler instruments used as sensors may avoid most of these difficulties.

COMBINATION WITH tcpO_2

By performing simultaneous measurements of laser Doppler and tcpO_2, more accurate and informative measurements can be obtained. Combining two independent measurements presents additional information for a better diagnosis of problem wounds. This is particularly helpful if the tcpO_2 values are falsely low because of tissue inflammation or edema.

EQUIPMENT

The equipment required to perform a laser Doppler heat provocation study includes at least two channels of laser Doppler with heat-controlled probes, computer components, and appropriate software developed by the manufacturer. All associated equipment and devices must be connected according to the manufacturer's instructions. Most instruments should warm up for at least 20 minutes before taking measurements to ensure maximum accuracy. Care must be taken when using the probes as the fiber optic cables should not be subjected to bends since breakage may occur. The instrument should be placed in a stable location close to the subject being studied. Keep the instrument away from sources of vibration such as ventilation systems or other machines that can cause vibrations since vibrations will cause artifacts. The thermostatic probes have built-in safety elements to help prevent injury to the subject. Probes should be cleaned after each use with a lint-free cloth moistened with alcohol after wiping with an antimicrobial solution. Acetone, alcohol concentration over 70%, or other strong solvents should not be used to clean the probes. Heat sterilization should not be used. Instrument manufacturers usually include a "Trouble Shooting" section in the user's manual. If the instrument fails to work correctly, refer to the user's manual or call the manufacturer.

PATIENT SELECTION AND PREPARATION

Any patient referred to the wound care center is a potential candidate for LDF. Each patient must be assessed as to whether or not the information derived from the study would be useful. Patient selection depends upon trained staff to perform the procedure and physicians who understand and can interpret the results of the data obtained. Blood flow fluctuates in response to metabolic needs, environmental conditions, physical and mental activity, stress, or trauma as well as pharmacologic agents, all of which can affect the study. Therefore, measurements must be made under standard conditions, such as a temperature of 78°F, quiet atmosphere, regulated humidity, and allowing the patient to rest and acclimatize to the room for about 30 minutes prior to beginning the study. This permits the heart to stabilize at its resting rate and allows capillaries to reopen. Successive studies should be done under the same conditions at the same time of day. The patient should be encouraged to avoid hot drinks and tobacco.

PERFORMING THE STUDY

All equipment used for the study is designed and intended for use only according to the manufacturer's instructions. The instrument should be operated only by qualified personnel. Personnel must heed Laser precautions and warning labels must be displayed on the equipment. After the instrument is set up and calibrated, begin preparing the skin for probe placement. The skin must be prepared in much the same way as for transcutaneous oximetry by cleansing with alcohol. However, it is important not to perform tape stripping and shaving as this will create a hyperemic response. Position the probe without pressure where the tip touches the tissue to be studied. If the tissue is occluded by pressure, the readings will be incorrect. Affix the probe with double-sided tape or a fixation ring. Position the fiber optic cable so that it curves gently and is not kinked. Secure the cable in such a way that it does not pull at the tissue or move freely and cause artifacts. Several sites should be monitored simultaneously. Generally, the number of sites measured will determine the number of machines required. After completing the study, remove the probes carefully, taking care not to tear fragile skin. Observe where the probe was placed and report unusual findings on the skin. When using heat provocation, a temperature of 44 degrees C is usually used. Temperatures over 40 degrees C may cause burns in babies and there are time limits to heat provocation in young children and the elderly.

CONCLUSION

LDF estimates the flow of moving particles in the range of laser light penetration. No other technique for monitoring blood flow does this. Information about the microcirculation flow is a critical part of the microcirculatory puzzle. LDF is an easy handling method for real-time monitoring of blood perfusion in almost any tissue, and is an excellent diagnostic tool in lower limb ischemia. LDF appears to be a useful tool for further understanding of microcirculation, early diagnosis of vascular disorders, evaluation of certain therapies, and monitoring patients with particular vascular disorders. LDF also provides a non-invasive method of assessing the dermal effects of systemic pharmacologic therapy, which is data that are extremely important for the wound care clinician. It has also been suggested that quantifiable measurements in dermal flow could be used to assess wound care product performance and wound healing potentials. This technology is currently being used in conjunction with transcutaneous oximetry to assess healing potential in non-healing, chronic wounds. However, the procedure of perfusion evaluation is still under investigation and the results have not been fully validated. LDF is an important tool in the array of technologies used to assess tissue perfusion in patients who are at risk for an ischemic injury.

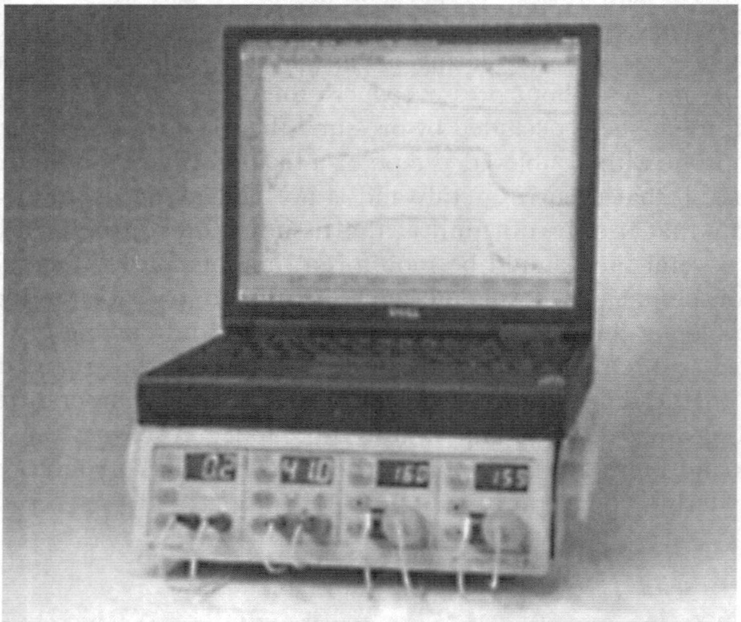

FIGURE 2. PeriFlux System 5000 Main Unit equipped with one LDF Unit, One Temp Unit (for heat provocation), and two $tcpO_2$ Units.

REFERENCES

1. Belcaro G, Hoffman U, Bollinger A, Nicolaides A: Laser Doppler; Med-Orion Publishing Company 1994
2. Krasner D, Kane D: Chronic Wound Care; Health Management Publications, Inc. 1997
3. Nilsson G, et al.: Evaluation of a laser Doppler flowmeter for measurement of tissue blood flow. Vol.BME-27: 597-598, 1980
4. Riva C, Ross B, Benedek GB: Laser Doppler measurements in capillary tubes and retinal arteries. Invest Opthalmol 11:936-944, 1972
5. Sheffield PJ, Dietz D, Posey KI, Ziemba TA, Bakken B: Use of transcutaneous oximetry and laser Doppler with local heat provocation to assess patients with problem wounds. Book of Proceedings, 1st Congress of the Alps-Adria Working Community on Maritime, Undersea and Hyperbaric Medicine, April 2001
6. Stern MD: In vivo evaluation of microcirculation by coherent light scattering. Nature 254:56-58, 1975
7. Tenland T. On Laser Doppler Flowmetry, Methods and Microvascular Applications; Linkoping University Medical Dissertations No. 136, 1982

NOTES

CHAPTER I

PROFESSIONAL ORGANIZATIONS

R.B. GUSTAVSON

UNDERSEA AND HYPERBARIC MEDICAL SOCIETY (UHMS)

www.uhms.org

As stated on the organizational web-site, "The Undersea and Hyperbaric Medical Society (UHMS) is the primary source of information for diving and hyperbaric medicine physiology worldwide."[1] The UHMS is arguably the premier professional organization in the field of hyperbaric medicine for physicians. It has long championed keeping hyperbaric oxygenation in the "mainstream" of medicine.

Originally chartered in 1967 as the Undersea Medical Society, the UMS was formed to provide a professional medical organization for physicians and scientists practicing in the field of undersea and hyperbaric medicine. Although the primary interest of the organization was undersea medicine and hyperbaric medicine was only important as it related to undersea medicine, the UMS saw a need to get involved in clinical hyperbaric medicine. In the early to mid-'70s the indiscriminate use of hyperbaric medicine had reached epidemic proportions, with entrepreneurs treating chronic conditions such as CVA, senility, arthritis, impotence, and other debilitating illnesses hoping for some improvement. This growth in hyperbaric medicine with little concern for the science was of great concern to a number of hyperbaric clinicians. Practitioners and insurers had no guidance to determine when the use of hyperbaric oxygen was appropriate. In 1972, Medicare convened a committee of UMS members with experience in clinical hyperbaric medicine to make recommendations as to the appropriate use. This committee, chaired by George B. Hart, made broad recommendations which did little to change the practice of hyperbaric medicine. In November 1976, the UMS formed an *ad hoc* Committee on Hyperbaric Oxygenation to review the field of clinical hyperbaric medicine and make recommendations on the appropriate use of this modality. Eric Kindwall, M.D. was appointed Chair and he selected 18 members from the scientific and military community to review the field and applicable scientific literature. In May 1977, the committee issued a report that was subsequently approved by the Executive Committee of the UMS. The *ad hoc* Committee had consulted with the Social Security Administration, which administered Medicare, and the Blue Cross/Blue Shield Association to determine their requirements for a "covered" condition and to elicit input on issues they would like to see addressed in the Committee report. The final approved report separated the conditions where hyperbaric oxygenation may or may not be indicated into four categories. The first category included those conditions for which there is no doubt of the benefit of hyperbaric oxygenation. Category Two encompassed disorders where there was a strong physiological basis for using hyperbaric oxygenation, but lacked sufficient data to be included in Category One. The report recommended that third-party payers reimburse these two categories. The third category was classified as investigational and recommended additional studies. Category Four included those with no basis and the benefit of hyperbaric oxygenation was placebo at best.

Also in 1977, the textbook *Hyperbaric Oxygen Therapy* was published under the auspices of the UMS. Authored by numerous international experts in the field, the text was edited by Jefferson C. Davis and Thomas K. Hunt. The former is considered one of founding fathers of clinical hyperbaric medicine and was responsible for setting up the clinical hyperbaric program at the School of Aerospace Medicine at Brooks Air Force Base. Dr. Hunt is a Professor of Surgery and Director of Lab/Clinic Wound Healing Research Lab at University of California-San Francisco. This text represented a significant step in the maturity of clinical hyperbaric medicine as "mainstream" medical practice. UMS and subsequently the UHMS have published professional journals. Beginning in 1974, the UMS published the journal Undersea Biomedical Research with an emphasis on undersea medicine and occasional articles on clinical hyperbaric medicine. In 1980, UMS launched a journal devoted to clinical hyperbaric medicine. Titled *Hyperbaric Oxygen Review*, it was published quarterly and contained abstracts from the literature and one major review article in each issue. Dr. Charles W. Schilling was the moving force behind the publication and the first editor was Dr. Eric P. Kindwall. This was the first journal dedicated to the practice of clinical hyperbaric medicine. In 1986, the UMS Executive Committee decided there was a need for a journal that published original articles in the field and the *Hyperbaric Oxygen Review* was replaced by the *Journal of Hyperbaric Medicine* with Enrico Camporesi as its editor. In January 1993, the *Undersea Biomedical Research* and the *Journal of Hyperbaric Medicine* were combined as the *Undersea and Hyperbaric Medicine* to facilitate listing, archival, and retrieval by the National Library of Medicine.

In 1986, the UMS changed its name to Undersea and Hyperbaric Medical Society to reflect the expanded role of hyperbaric medicine, and its importance and interest in the physiology and clinical application of hyperbaric medicine therapy. The UHMS's stated purpose "is to provide scientific information to protect the health of sport, military, and commercial divers and to improve the scientific basis of hyperbaric oxygen therapy, promote sound treatment protocols and standards of practice, and provide CME accreditation."

Membership includes over 2,000 members in 50 countries. The full membership is available to physicians and scientists involved in diving or hyperbaric research and clinical practice. Associate membership includes nurses, technicians, respiratory therapists, and others who work in the field. UHMS also has many corporate sponsors that support its research and educational agenda.

AMERICAN COLLEGE OF HYPERBARIC MEDICINE (ACHM)

www.hyperbaricmedicine.org

The American College of Hyperbaric Medicine was founded in 1983 by a group of physicians practicing the developing specialty of hyperbaric medicine. Adopting the framework of a medical specialty society, they sought to develop the image of hyperbaric medicine as a distinct medical specialty. Since 1996, the ACHM has represented hyperbaricists before the American Medical Association's Specialty and Service Society. This allows input into the policy-making process in the AMA. It was through this mechanism that the ACHM successfully lobbied the Health Care Financing Administration's efforts to set certification criteria for practicing hyperbaricists. The College is active in public education, regulatory oversight, and support for the ethical use of hyperbaric medicine to assure a scientific basis for its application. AHCM publishes a book on the "best hyperbaric practices" titled *Preferred Practice Protocols for Hyperbaric Medicine,* which is used by practicing hyperbaricists and payors in determining the effective and efficient use of hyperbaric medicine. The College has also published recommendations for the minimum credentialing of hyperbaric physicians.

FOUNDATION FOR THE INTERNATIONAL CONGRESS ON HYPERBARIC MEDICINE (ICHM)

www.ichm.net

The First International Congress on Hyperbaric Medicine was held in Amsterdam, the Netherlands, in 1963 with the founding president, Professor Boerema, presiding. The intent was to provide a forum for researchers in the field to exchange information on their research. Dr. Boerema is remembered in the history of hyperbaric medicine for his research in placing infants with congenital heart disease in a pressurized chamber and "drenching" the tissue with oxygen, allowing the heart to be stopped long enough to be surgically repaired. Dr. Boerema is also recognized for being the first to treat clostridial myonecrosis with adjunctive hyperbaric oxygen. The publication of his studies provided the impetus for an international interest in hyperbaric medicine for treatment of patients for more than just decompression illness and air embolism. The Second Congress was held in Glasgow, Scotland in 1964 with the Third Congress convening in 1965 in Durham, North Carolina. At that time when interest in hyperbaric medicine was lagging, the next scheduled Congress was held in Sapporo, Japan in 1969 and continued every four years until 1987. During the Ninth Congress, in 1987 in Sydney, Australia, the leadership changed the schedule to every three years. Also during the Ninth Congress, the Foundation for the International Congress on Hyperbaric Medicine was chartered, the purpose being to "promote the triennial Congress and improve understanding among the international hyperbaric medicine community."[2]

A permanent office was established in 1990 in the Netherlands to oversee the Congresses.

Membership is drawn from the public at large and includes physicians, scholars, laymen, and philanthropists. However, anyone with an interest in hyperbaric medicine may join. The Foundation reports a core membership of 88 Life Members. Membership in the Foundation for the International Congress on Hyperbaric Medicine insures an invitation to the next triennial meeting of ICHM as well as a subscription to the ICHM newsletter, *Oxygen*. Lifetime Members receive a certificate, suitable for framing, acknowledging their support of the Foundation. Currently, the Foundation offers two types of membership: three-year membership for $50.00 and lifetime membership for $300.00.

The proceedings of all meetings beginning with the 1984 meeting are available and may be purchased on their website. The first seven proceedings are out of print.

NATIONAL BOARD OF DIVING AND HYPERBARIC MEDICAL TECHNOLOGY (NBDHMT)

www.nbdhmt.org

In 1982, The National Association of Diving Medical Technologist (NADMT) was founded as a professional society for Dive Medical Technicians. Numerous attempts were made to include a sixteenth module in the National Association of Emergency Medical Technician's (NAEMT) Emergency Medical Technician certification program. This would recognize the additional training in dive accident management necessary to function as a Dive Medic. The NADMT was concerned about the "independent" nature of DMT's work offshore out of touch with physicians and opted not to include the dive tech module in their program. The NADMT proceeded with their own certification program that became the NBDHMT. The NADMT was renamed the NBDHMT in 1991 to fill the need for a national standard of training and certification for dive medical technicians and hyperbaric technologists. The first certifying exam was administered in San Diego, CA in 1991 concurrently with the UHMS Scientific Meeting. Up through 1996, nurses, respiratory therapists, and hyperbaric technicians with a minimum of 2,000 hours of chamber operation experience could qualify for the exam. In 1996, the minimum qualification increased to include graduation from a UHMS- or NBDHMT-approved course and as of 1999 the 40-hour course has to be approved by the NBDHMT. Certification now requires successful completion of an approved course, the exam, and 480 hours of hyperbaric chamber experience.

REFERENCES

1. www.uhms.org/home.html
2. ICHM Fact Sheet, Foundation for the International Congress on Hyperbaric Medicine, www.ichm.net

CHAPTER II

HYPERBARIC OXYGEN THERAPY ASSOCIATION

S. DeSANTIS

HISTORY

In October 1998, the Federal Register published the initially proposed Outpatient Prospective Payment System (OPPS) Rates by the Health Care Financing Administration (HCFA) for the Medicare Program. Hyperbaric oxygen therapy had a proposed rate of $136 per treatment, potentially a fatal blow to the industry as a whole. As a result of this publication, the Hyperbaric Oxygen Therapy Association (HOTA) was born in November 1998 under the leadership of Jimmy Ledoux, President of Total Wound Treatment Centers, Inc. The original goal of the organization was to focus on the issue of OPPS rates for hyperbaric oxygen therapy. The response needed to be quick as the comment period is open by statute for a brief 60 days.

The original members included manufacturers of hyperbaric equipment, clinical providers of hyperbaric oxygen therapy services, and two hospitals. After the election of the Board of Directors and the development of the bylaws, the organization raised sufficient capital to hire the Lewin Group in Washington, D.C. to assist with the response back to Medicare. The rationale for hiring the Lewin Group was simple. The Lewin Group was the agency hired by HCFA to assist in determining all payment rates for services approved for coverage under OPPS. The process was tedious and intense because of the time constraints in addition to an expense of $80,000. The goal was accomplished and the response was submitted on time. The grueling wait for the adjusted rates hung over the industry like a devastating black cloud.

There were numerous delays on the part of HCFA to publish the final rates in the Federal Register. This was frustrating to hospitals and healthcare providers in general because the Balanced Budget Act required OPPS to be implemented in August 2000. The final rates were eventually published in March 2000, rendering another potentially devastating blow to the industry of hyperbaric oxygen therapy. The new rate was published at $146 with a co-payment of $140, thus leaving Medicare with the responsibility of a $6.00 per treatment payment rate.

Pending the publication of the new rates, the HOTA, Undersea and Hyperbaric Medical Society (UHMS), and the American College of Hyperbaric Medicine (ACHM) were struggling with the Office of Coverage Policy and Clinical Standards at HCFA on coverage, supervision, and credentialing issues. This activity prompted the need to hire a law firm with expertise in healthcare issues and specifically dealing with HCFA. After several interviews and the evaluation of costs and expertise, it was decided to retain the professional services of Hogan and Hartson, L.L.P. based in Washington, D.C. The attorney working with our groups, Darrel Grinstead, J.D., had formerly served as the General Counsel at HCFA immediately prior to his joining Hogan and Hartson. Meetings at HCFA in Baltimore, MD began in 1997 and continue to current date. Some issues were resolved; however, the leadership at the Office of Coverage and Clinical Standards has changed four times since the inception of the efforts begun by UHMS in 1997. The work continues today requiring the perseverance and financial endurance of the industry. Outstanding coverage issues remain and are currently being evaluated by the Agency for Healthcare Research and Quality.

MISSION

The Hyperbaric Oxygen Therapy Association is dedicated to enhancing the understanding, acceptance, and growth of hyperbaric medicine as a proven and cost-effective clinical modality.

GOALS OF THE ASSOCIATION

- To represent all constituents involved in the practice of hyperbaric medicine.
- To work with Congress and the Health Care Financing Administration to establish and clarify coverage and reimbursement policies for hyperbaric oxygen (HBO_2) that are in the best interest of the patients and in the communities we serve.
- To enhance public awareness of hyperbaric oxygen therapy.
- To work proactively on all legislative issues.

CURRENT WORK WITH HCFA

Our current work with HCFA has primarily been shifted over to the Agency for Healthcare Research and Quality. When HOTA and UHMS submitted the formal request in November 2000 for new coverage for the hypoxic wound, the request was accepted by HCFA on December 1, 2000. By statute, HCFA had ninety days to respond. During the first week of March 2001, we were notified that our request for coverage of the hypoxic wound was forwarded to the Agency for Healthcare Research and Quality (AHRQ). The request from HCFA was for a technology assessment to include not just the hypoxic wound but all indications for hyperbaric oxygen therapy. Therefore, the work in this area is just beginning and we are working directly with AHRQ. We have pending issues with HCFA and inadvertent deletion of codes relative to Meleney's ulcer and underlying progressive necrotizing infections. A significant amount of work is also being done with individual fiscal intermediaries in direct relation to physician credentialing requirements and the definition of supervision in some states.

Federally, HCFA pulled its requirements for both of these issues, yet individual fiscal intermediaries claim they have received unspecified directives to implement policy.

DYNAMICS

The dynamics of working with the government require tenacity with a positive attitude. The Balanced Budget Act prohibits judicial involvement; thus, issues without forward movement at HCFA require additional audiences with Congressional leaders. The key committees are the House Ways and Means Committee as it is home to the Health Care Subcommittee, Commerce in the House, and Finance in the Senate. All of these committees render the Congressional oversight of HCFA; therefore, if HCFA is slow to respond or does not respond at all, the oversight committees are prompt in replying to our requests for intervention.

The dynamics of HCFA are seemingly in continual change with turnover of leadership staff. In January 2001, a new Secretary of Health and Human Services was appointed by the Bush Administration, Mr. Tommy Thompson. In May 2001, a new administrator for HCFA was appointed, Mr. Tom Scully. Mr. Scully has previously reigned as the President of the American Hospital Federation, the professional organization representing the for-profit hospitals of America. It is unclear at the writing of this section as to the immediate agenda of the new leadership. As of this writing, it seems as though the first order of business is to rename the Health Care Financing Administration and reorganize the structure into separate product lines. Mr. Scully and Mr. Thompson are vowing to be more responsive to both beneficiaries and to the Congress via several mechanisms that have not been fully disclosed yet.

The course of the next several months will give clarity to the changing dynamics for the next four years.

CODING AND REIMBURSEMENT ISSUES

As stated in the Office of Inspector General (OIG) report of 2000, there is inconsistency from state to state as to the appropriate and covered ICD-9 codes to be utilized by the providers of care, thus causing a fluctuation in reimbursement. The OIG made a recommendation to HCFA that standardization be made possible by the issuance of Federal guidelines, thus facilitating oversight by the intermediaries.

A new code for a hypoxic wound is currently being applied for through an application process made available by the CDC and then considered by HCFA and the AMA. Hearings are held on a semiannual basis for consideration; however, payment cannot be expected for one year after the acceptance and approval of the code. To alter the current process, the venue is an amendment to the Balanced Budget Act possible only through Congress.

There is also variation in some states between Medicare Part A (the hospital) and Part B (physician professional component). This is an issue that by structure should be resolved by the Program Integrity Division of HCFA; however, progress is very slow and Congressional support is being sought to facilitate decision.

COLLABORATIVE EFFORT

The work of the Hyperbaric Oxygen Therapy Association is being performed in a collaborative effort with the Undersea and Hyperbaric Medical Society (UHMS). The role of the physicians is imperative in the publication of Best Practice Guidelines for all of the accepted indications.

While the current request from HCFA to the Agency for Healthcare Quality and Research is very specific to hypoxic wounds, it has also been requested by HCFA to include a technology assessment for all accepted indications as published in the Medicare Coverage Policy (35-10). There are two current technology assessments published, one by the Blue Cross/Blue Shield Association of California, 1999, and one by the Australian Ministry of Health, 2000. While both documents are supportive of the usage of hyperbaric oxygen therapy in the treatment of problem wounds particularly in the diabetic patient, they are not totally in favor of hyperbaric oxygen usage for other indications by virtue of the perception of lack of clinical evidence or double-blinded randomized controlled studies. The Australian document is still a work in process and has not been adopted into policy as of this writing. There have been some intermediary changes in the U.S. based on the California Technology Assessment, but the policies are currently in a comment phase.

It is, therefore, essential that Best Practice Guidelines be published for added continuity of care among the hyperbaric oxygen therapy community. A unified front is necessary to secure respect at the governmental level.

THE FUTURE

Our best efforts will grow forward in conjunction with the UHMS to fortify the awareness of the subspecialty of hyperbaric oxygen therapy by means of educating the fiscal intermediaries via the Medicare Advisory Committees (MCAC), the Congress via the key committees responsible for HCFA oversight, HCFA physicians and analysts, and the Agency for Healthcare Research and Quality.

While the current responsibilities of HCFA are enormous in comparison to our niche in healthcare, it is essential for our work to continue so that our profession remains in the forefront and patients can receive adequate care.

To ensure the strengthening of our position, we need to maintain our lobbying efforts with HCFA, Congress, and the fiscal intermediaries. We are at a critical time in securing our future in healthcare as an excellent adjunct to conventional therapies.

CHAPTER I

HYPERBARIC NURSING EDUCATION

W. McGINN-MERRITT AND M. SKARBAN

INTRODUCTION

"Wisdom begins in wonder." –Socrates

Florence Nightengale wrote in "Notes on Nursing" (1859) that nursing has as its most critical work the caring required to promote the health of the individual. Nursing today is that and so much more. With ongoing changes in the healthcare environment, nurses must develop skills to support technological and assessment competencies required for our profession to survive. The paradox in the future practice for hyperbaric nurses, as well as all healthcare professionals, will be to continue to keep up with this explosion in technology while creating new approaches to care and maintaining or decreasing costs. In order to keep up with these changes, specialize in practice, and remain competent, education is the key. Never has this been more important than now for those who have chosen hyperbaric nursing as their specialty. Education is the single most important element in our profession's future.

The education process is defined as a systematic, sequential, planned course of action consisting of two major interdependent operations: teaching and learning. This has always been compared to the nursing process, and rightly so. The steps of each process run parallel to one another: assessment, planning, implementation and evaluation. As nurses we are adept at the nursing process, and we have long been teachers and learners, formally and informally. This carries with it a huge responsibility. There must be a solid foundation to build on. Only through education and experience can the expert level be reached. Experience does not refer to the passage of time or longevity. Rather, it is the refinement of preconceived notions and theory through encounters with many practical situations that add to that experience. One must recognize that only through this experience can one become an expert. And only through experience can one become competent.

Nursing competence is defined as the ongoing ability to render safe and direct nursing care, and the ongoing ability to make sound judgements upon which that nursing care is based. Competent behavior rests on the use of the scientific method from which the nursing process emanates. Through time, commitment, teaching, and education, we can all move from novice to expert in hyperbaric nursing.

This chapter focuses on entry-level competencies and standards for hyperbaric nursing. Other roles have been included as a knowledge base. This was not an attempt to be exclusionary, but rather a means of concentrating on hyperbaric nursing practice.

Our motivation for writing this chapter was based on our personal belief that hyperbaric nursing has a great destiny, and that this destiny can only be achieved through personal and professional commitment to education of ourselves and our colleagues.

REGULATORY AGENCIES

Why are We Required to have Mandates from Regulatory Agencies?

The hyperbaric medicine environment consists of unique characteristics that are recognized as vastly different from many other medical practices. Some consider it an alternative medicine out of control and without guidelines. Actually, any respected hyperbaric medicine program has to meet several regulatory bodies' standards in order to operate and collect monetary reimbursements. It is imperative that new hyperbaric departmental managers have a clear understanding and become cognizant of not only the medical and legal regulatory agencies' requirements but also the physical and environmental agencies governing over fire, chemical, and pressurized vehicle regulations.

As a nurse involved in the overall care of the patient, you may not understand why you need all of these regulatory bodies or how they impact the care you give. To get a full understanding of the importance of the safety regulations, I would refer you to more in-depth information in the chapter Regulatory and Safety in this book. This information is intended to assist the nursing director in understanding the importance and differences in these agencies.

Joint Commission on Accreditation of Healthcare Organizations (JCAHO)

The most sought-after accreditation of any medical facility in the United States is from the Joint Commission on Accreditation of Healthcare Organizations, more commonly known by its abbreviation JCAHO. The JCAHO mission is to continuously improve the safety and quality of care provided to the public through the provisions of healthcare accreditation and related services that support performance improvement in healthcare organizations. The Joint Commission evaluates and accredits nearly 20,000 healthcare organizations and programs in the United States. An independent, not-for-profit organization, the Joint Commission is the nation's predominant standards-setting and accrediting body in healthcare. Accreditation by the JCAHO is recognized nationwide as a symbol of quality that indicates an organization meets certain performance standards. The standard focus is not simply on what the organization has but on what it actually does to affect the quality of patient care. In other words, if an organization does the right things and does them well, there is a strong likelihood that its patients will experience positive outcomes.

Without accreditation, a medical program may risk the loss of certain federal subsidized funds including Medicare and Medicaid benefits. Healthcare organizations seek the Joint Commission to meet certain Medicare certification requirements; subsequently, JCAHO assists these organizations in improving their quality of care which, in turn, often improves community confidence that provides staff education opportunities, expedites third party payments, often fulfills state licensure requirements, and may favorably influence liability insurance premiums.

Acknowledging the JCAHO requirements, which minimally includes mission or vision statement, purpose, scope of care, qualifications of the hyperbaric team members, general operational policies, and performance standards, should assist you in setting up the standards you design for your department. State and federal regulations differ from the independent scope of care as given by the state licensing boards. Although many states may have different scopes of practices, you will find that in all 50 states there is a consistency to maintain licensed, competent staff in a medical care environment that follows guidance from multiple regulatory disciplines.

Undersea and Hyperbaric Medical Society (UHMS)

During that last few decades, there has been an incredible growth in hyperbaric programs across the United States and internationally. With that growth comes improper, overzealous abusers who use hyperbaric facilities for their own monetary gains, ignoring proper medical research for stability. Historically, these practitioners exaggerated claims and fees, causing questionable payments to those facilities using proper, rational diagnosis. This led to the establishment of the Undersea and Hyperbaric Medical Society (UHMS) in 1972, followed by an increased committee focus on hyperbaric oxygenation in 1976. Today, the UHMS boasts a strong body of professionals dedicated to advocating the proper uses of hyperbaric oxygen therapy through responsible research.

The more we grow, the more we recognize the need for standardizing recommendations for training, responsibility, staffing, credentialing, safety, and quality assurance qualifications in any program. The intent is to improve patient care, optimize outcomes, maintain safety, and create positive effects in our patients' lives. As in any medical specialty practice, it is the responsibility of the provider and the institution that support their practice to ensure competency, quality of care, and safety within the program. The UHMS sets basic guidelines for any hyperbaric team. It is up to the facility, Medical Director, Nursing Management, and Safety Officer to abide by the recommendations and maintain the highest level of ethical and moral standards of practice.

Baromedical Nurses Association (BNA)

Since its infancy, nursing has produced strong leaders to guide and direct safe patient care through the evolution to what is now considered modern medicine. In 1985, hyperbaric practicing nurses discovered a need for comradery between such experts, and wanted to share common knowledge among them while yearning to learn more from their peers. Subsequently, the Baromedical Nurses Association (BNA) was born. Common practices and experiences across the nation were documented, initiating the sharing of stories and helping each other's network, benchmarking outstanding programs and procedures that continue to evolve and escalate beyond today's expectations. The organizational mission is a simple one: to provide nurses with a professional organization to define, develop, maintain, and promote the status and standards of hyperbaric nursing. They have refined a nationally recognized certification exam, better known as the Certified Hyperbaric Registered Nurse, and its complement of the advanced nurse and nurse clinician. It is not recommended that certification be an entry-level pathway, but rather the result of multiple hours of practiced skill and knowledge.

Food and Drug Administration (FDA)

The description of hyperbaric oxygen therapy includes the use of the drug called oxygen. According to the Food and Drug Administration (FDA), oxygen application and devices used to administer oxygen are under FDA jurisdiction. As a result, the hyperbaric chambers are considered prescriptive devices by the FDA in which a physician must be involved in the procurement and administration of the prescribed oxygen treatment.

National Fire Protection Association (NFPA)

As with any drug, there are risks associated with using 100% oxygen within an enclosed, pressurized vehicle. Clearly, we know that oxygen by itself cannot produce a flame, but with the proper fuel, oxygen will intensify the burning capacity incredibly. In 1967, two tragic events led the hyperbaric, as well as the diving and hypobaric communities, to demand development and mandatory regulation toward enforcing fire safety guidelines. In response, the National Fire Protection Association (NFPA) published a tentative safety standard that was revised in 1984 as Chapter 19, "Hyperbaric Facilities" in the *Health Care Facility Manual* (NFPA 99).

American Society of Mechanical Engineers/Pressure Vessels for Human Occupancy (ASME/PVHO)

During the same time frame, the American Society of Mechanical Engineers (ASME) took on the challenge of designing and maintaining proper functions within the hyperbaric chambers. In 1970, they teamed up with hyperbaric chamber experts to develop a new committee called ASME/PVHO (Pressure Vessels for Human Occupancy). They specifically looked at creating safe engineering standards. Immediately after the development of these standards, accidents within the hyperbaric environment drastically reduced, fulfilling their goal.

Center for Disease Control (CDC)

Infection control is a hallmark of interest in any inspector's guide, although it may not be the "white glove" test that many of us are used to. All medical facilities must show a highly effective and workable standard infection control program that includes specific methods for cleaning equipment and how to handle various infectious medical cases. The Center for Disease Control provides guidelines for any infection control item.

Occupational Safety and Health Administration (OSHA)

Another organization that regulates what we can and cannot do is the Occupational Safety and Health Administration (OSHA). This agency of the United States Department of Labor develops and enforces job safety and health regulations. With the NFPA, OSHA regulations deal with fire prevention, protective garments, railings, and other safety issues. Among various other safety issues, OSHA regulates exposure to noise. OSHA's noise requirements in and around the hyperbaric chamber must conform to standards of the Hearing Conservation Amendment. They do not have any direct program or regulation that deals specifically with hyperbaric facilities; however, if you are attached with a medical facility, it is in your best interest to get to know which department is responsible for noise exposure inspections and ensure your work area is up to code for the facility requirements.

HYPERBARIC NURSE TRAINING GUIDELINES

Training guidelines, as defined by the Operations Committee of the Undersea and Hyperbaric Medical Society, are the recommended standard that hyperbaric nurses practice under. The guidelines are designed to help improve medical care and are not intended to be inclusive, to rewrite authoritative texts, or to usurp accepted organizations or certifying bodies. These recommendations were designed to help improve medical care, optimize outcomes, maintain safety, and positively affect the lives of our patients. The following recommendations are entry-level qualifications to practice hyperbaric medicine.

Clinical Hyperbaric Registered Nurse (entry-level)

- Must hold a current nursing license in the state in which the nurse is practicing (certain government agencies may be exempt).
- Must have documentation of successful completion of at least a 40-credit-hour National Board of Diving and Hyperbaric Medicine Technology (NBDHMT) approved Hyperbaric Medicine Introductory Course.
- Must hold current BLS.
- Should have an interest in learning, practicing, and maintaining competency in the field of hyperbaric nursing.

- Should be a clinical hyperbaric registered nurse (CHRN), basic level (when eligible).
- Should obtain a minimum of 20 continuing education units (CEUs) per 2-year time period, with 10 CEUs in the field of hyperbaric medicine/nursing.
- Should hold (ACLS).

Nursing Manager/Director

- Must first meet entry-level training standards as described above.
- Must hold CHRN, basic level: advanced level strongly recommended.
- Should have at least 12 months of recent practical experience in clinical hyperbaric medicine, after meeting the entry-level qualifications and training requirements as delineated in this document for entry level hyperbaric nurse.
- Should have a Bachelor of Science Degree.
- Should have a working understanding of the codes and regulations that govern the operation of a hyperbaric medicine facility.
- Should participate in professional organizations.
- Should maintain a minimum of 30 CEUs per 2-year period with 15 CEUs in the field of hyperbaric medicine/nursing.
- Should be an active participant in education and leadership activities.

Clinical Nurse Specialist

- Must meet all the training standards of the above.
- Must hold a Master's Degree in Nursing.
- Must have 24 months of recent practical experience in clinical hyperbaric medicine with at least 12 months in an advanced or administrative role.
- Must hold CHRN, hyperbaric nurse clinician level (when eligible).
- Should be an active participant in education, research, and leadership activities.

Job Descriptions

Hyperbaric Registered Nurse. Is accountable to the hyperbaric nursing director/manager and is responsible for:

- Assisting in the coordination of hyperbaric staff and patients.
- Assisting in day-to-day operation of the hyperbaric facility.
- Maintaining competencies, continuing education, and certifications as appropriate to the position.
- Performing nursing assessments; developing, implementing, and evaluating nursing plans of care and instructing patient and significant others in appropriate discharge instruction.

- Keeping complete and accurate patient records as they pertain to assessment, treatments, and documentation of care.
- Participating in quality assurance programs.
- Participating in the safety program.
- Participating in active research protocols.

Note: The above statements reflect the general duties and responsibilities considered necessary to describe the principal functions of the job as identified, and shall not be considered as a detailed description of all of the work requirements that may be inherent in these positions.

Hyperbaric Nurse Manager/Director. Is ultimately responsible for the quality of hyperbaric nursing services provided, budgetary oversight, and 24-hour accountability for the hyperbaric unit. Is accountable to the Medical Director and Administration. In addition to the responsibilities listed under hyperbaric nurse, the nurse manger/director:

- Oversees the quality of nursing services rendered in the hyperbaric department and ensures that it meets current standards of practice.
- Ensures safe and adequate staffing for patient volume and acuity.
- Assists the Medical Director with the development of policies, procedures, and protocols for hyperbaric services.
- Assists the Medical Director in the development of a quality assurance program.
- Works in conjunction with the Medical Director and senior staff in the development of orientation and inservice programs for all levels of hyperbaric personnel.
- Works in conjunction with the Medical Director and Safety Director to ensure ongoing and effective safety program.
- Ensures appropriate marketing of the hyperbaric unit.

HYPERBARIC PHYSICIAN TRAINING GUIDELINES

Clinical Hyperbaric Medicine Physician Qualifications and Training (entry-level)

- Must be an M.D. or D.O. graduate holding a valid diploma from an Accredited Medical School.
- Must be Board Certified or Board Eligible in a recognized medical or surgical specialty.
- Must have successfully completed at least a 40-credit-hour, UHMS-approved Hyperbaric Medicine Introductory Course. (Fellowship-trained hyperbaric medicine physician meets this requirement, if holding a certificate of training from an organized, academically based clinical program with a continuous training period of more than 11 months.)

Practice Guidelines (entry-level)

- Must first meet the Qualifications and Training as stated above.
- Must maintain an unrestricted license to practice medicine in the state where the physician delivers hyperbaric medicine therapy. (Certain government agencies may be exempt.)
- Must be specifically privileged to practice hyperbaric medicine in the sponsoring medical institution(s) under the process delineated by the institution's privileging or credentials committee.
- Should be allowed to work unsupervised by his/her medical director only after a period of preceptorship where the physician has demonstrated a consistent competence in standard clinical hyperbaric medicine treatments, procedures, and safety.

Physician Medical Director

- Must first meet the entry-level qualifications, training, and practice guidelines as delineated in this document for Clinical Hyperbaric Medicine Physician.
- Must have a minimum of 12 months of recent credentialed experience in clinical hyperbaric medicine after meeting the entry level qualifications, training, and practice guidelines. (Physician sub-specialty training and certification in undersea and hyperbaric medicine are ongoing, aimed at developing core knowledge and practice into a nationally recognized sub-specialty. It is expected that a future revision of these recommendations will reflect sub-specialty training and certification as a desired level of competence.)
- Should be a physician in good standing in hyperbaric medicine, and support UHMS clinical indications and protocols through a high standard of practice.
- Should have demonstrated leadership, management, teaching, and administrative abilities.

- Should have a working understanding of the codes and regulations that govern the operation of a hyperbaric medicine facility.
- Should support the pursuit of scholarly activities and debate in the field of hyperbaric medicine.

Continuing Medical Education Requirements (Physician CME)

- Should successfully complete and document at least 12 credit hours of Physician Category I CME hours in hyperbaric-medicine-related topics for every 24 months of hyperbaric practice, not including the initial training year.

Job Descriptions

Hyperbaric Physician. Is accountable to the Hyperbaric Medical Director and is responsible for:

Supervision

- Assists in the day-to-day supervision and coordination of the hyperbaric staff.
- Assists in the proper day-to-day operations of the hyperbaric facility.

Clinical

- Consults, examines, selects, and manages patients who could benefit from HBO_2 therapy.
- Keeps complete and accurate records pertaining to the indications, rationale, and progress of the patient treatments.
- Is immediately available to manage patient emergencies which may occur before, during, or after treatments while the patient is in the hyperbaric medicine department.
- Maintains communication with referring medical providers.
- Conducts appropriate patient discharge, follow up, and onward referrals.
- Supports and participates in scheduled hyperbaric medicine/call coverage.

Education

- Assist in the continuing education of all levels of the hyperbaric staff.
- Other duties and responsibilities as deemed appropriate for safe and proper clinical operations.

Medical Director. Is ultimately responsible for the quality of hyperbaric services provided and is accountable to the medical staff and hospital administration for the activities of the hyperbaric center. In addition to the duties listed under hyperbaric physician, the Medical Director is responsible for:

Supervision

- Supervision of the senior clinical and technical staff.
- Assists the senior staff in evaluation and selection of new clinical personnel.

Administration

- Development of policies directing the use and availability of hyperbaric services for therapy and research.
- Supports the establishment of ongoing and effective safety programs.
- Supports compliance with current quality assurance standards.
- Supports the establishment of a program for clinical peer review.
- Ensures that sufficient administrative support is available.
- Designates a qualified physician staff member to act in his/her absence.

Clinical

- Oversees the quality of medical services rendered in the hyperbaric department and ensures it meets current standards of practice.
- Develops and oversees adherence of patient care protocols for hyperbaric oxygen treatments.

Education

- Together with senior clinical and technical staff, assists in the development of an ongoing program for orientation and in-service training for all levels of hyperbaric personnel.
- Supports opportunities for staff members to attain their required continuing medical education.

Research (optional)

- Ensures that clinical research within the facility follows the direction of the Helinski Accords as well as any standing policies of the sponsoring institution.
- Oversees all medical research protocols that may be undertaken in the department.

Note: The above statements reflect the general duties and responsibilities considered to be principle functions of the job as identified, and shall not be considered as a detailed description of all of the work requirements that may be inherent in these positions.

ALLIED HEALTHCARE PROVIDER TRAINING GUIDELINES (ENTRY-LEVEL)

- Must have successfully completed at least a 40-credit-hour, NBDHMT-approved Hyperbaric Medicine Introductory Course.
- Vocational/Practical Nurses and Respiratory Therapy Technicians must be licensed, if required, in their specialty in the state in which they perform their duties.
- Must hold BLS certification.
- Should have a working knowledge of decompression procedures.
- Should be certified by the (NBDHMT) within two years of completing a Hyperbaric Medicine Introductory Course.
- Should participate in professional organizations such as the Associates of the UHMS and the BNA.
- Should attend courses specifically related to the operational hyperbaric safety issues.
- Hyperbaric chamber technicians should have training and/or experience in hyperbaric chamber maintenance, to include a mechanical background where appropriate.

Note: In an emergency, medical personnel may be used as additional tenders for multiplace and monoplace hyperbaric facilities to deliver specialized or specific medical care not routinely in the training of regular hyperbaric staff. Such personnel must be screened by the responsible hyperbaric physician/director and properly oriented to the hyperbaric environment, including safety and emergency procedures, and should function under the supervision of fully trained and responsible hyperbaric staff.

Job Description

General:

- Performs duties under direct supervision of the Technical and Safety Directors or Nurse/Program Manager as is appropriate for the facility.
- Is responsible for the safe and effective operation of the hyperbaric chamber(s) and related support systems.
- Is responsible for day-to-day maintenance of hyperbaric chamber(s) and related support systems.

Knowledge:

- Refer to technical training recommendations for Allied Healthcare Providers.

Job Responsibilities:

- Patient preparation for treatment.
- Reinforce education as it relates to hyperbaric therapy.
- Keep complete and accurate patient records as they pertain to treatment documentation.

- Perform duties and procedures as directed by supervisor/ medical director.
- Perform hyperbaric chamber operations and system maintenance as required.
- Participate in safety program.
- Maintain competencies, continuing education and certification as appropriate.

Safety Director

- Must meet training requirements as designated above.
- Must successfully complete a UHMS- or NBDHMT-approved hyperbaric safety course.
- Must be certified by the NBDHMT within one year of assuming responsibilities of Safety Director.
- Should have at least 12 months experience in clinical hyperbaric chamber operations.

For Responsibilities, see chapter on Safety.

Technical Director

- Must meet the training requirements as designated under Safety Director and Allied Healthcare Provider.
- Must have documented experience of at least five years in hyperbaric facility operations.
- Must be certified by the NBDHMT.

Job Description:

General:

- Responsible for the safe and effective operation, control, and maintenance of the hyperbaric chamber system and supporting components.
- Work closely with the Safety Director to ensure compliance with all department policies and regulatory requirements.
- Ensure that all technical personnel meet standards set by various licensing and regulatory agencies.

Knowledge/Experience:

- Refer to Training recommendations for Allied Healthcare Personnel, Technical Director.

Responsibilities:

- Serves as the hyperbaric facility senior technical representative and ensures that technical personnel comply with published preventative maintenance schedules.

- May serve as the hyperbaric facility Safety Director as required.
- Develops and reviews department policy and procedure and revises operational manuals annually.
- Develops and maintains monthly reports of hyperbaric chamber system maintenance activities and submits same to the Safety and Medical Directors.
- Supervises all hyperbaric technologists to ensure the safe and effective operation of all hyperbaric chambers and related equipment.
- Coordinates and approves all upgrades, modifications, and repairs to the hyperbaric chamber system, including interaction with hospital maintenance personnel and outside contractors, as appropriate.
- Operates all hyperbaric chamber systems and related components.
- Maintains operating and maintenance logs and other required documentation in accordance with hyperbaric facility policy and regulatory requirements.
- Serves as the hyperbaric facility senior technical trainer for full- and part-time personnel. Conducts and participates in in-services related to various technical aspects of the operation of hyperbaric chamber systems and related components.

PROGRAM MANAGER TRAINING GUIDELINES

- Must have documentation of successful completion of at least a 40-credit-hour, NBDHMT-approved Hyperbaric Introductory Course.
- Must have documented experience of at least one year in hyperbaric facility operations.
- Must be certified by the NBDHMT.
- Must hold BLS certification.
- Should have working knowledge of all applicable hyperbaric safety codes.
- Should attend courses specifically related to operational hyperbaric safety issues.
- Should have a working knowledge of decompression procedures.
- Should participate in professional organizations such as Associates of the UHMS and BNA.

JOB DESCRIPTION:

Is responsible for the quality of hyperbaric services provided, budgetary oversight, and 24-hour accountability for the hyperbaric unit. Is accountable to the Medical Director and Administration.

General:

- Oversees the quality of services rendered in the hyperbaric department and ensures that it meets current standards of practice.
- Ensures safe and adequate staffing for patient volume and acuity.
- Assists the Medical Director with the development of policies, procedures, and protocols for hyperbaric services.
- Assists the Medical Director in the development of a quality assurance program.
- Ensures appropriate marketing of the hyperbaric unit.

NURSE STAFFING GUIDELINES

The following staffing guidelines as delineated by the Operations Committee of the Undersea and Hyperbaric Medical Society correlate with the previously described personnel. Staffing levels should be determined by analysis of procedure and volume data, productivity indicators, and acuity. It is the responsibility of the Medical Director, Nursing Director, and/or Program Manger to ensure the safe and proper operations of the unit.

1. A minimum of one CHRN or CHT should be on duty in the clinical area at all times when a patient is receiving treatment.
2. A registered nurse is responsible for ensuring provision of the following nursing duties:
   - Timely RN assessment is required every 24 hours while the patient is receiving treatment.
   - RN supervision of non-physician wound care and treatments.
   - RN attendance of critically ill or emergency patient.
   - RN case management.
3. Staff Mix of licensed and unlicensed personnel.
   - RN-licensed activities:
     - Physical, psychological, and social assessment which requires professional nursing judgement, intervention, referral, or follow-up.
     - Formulation of the plan of nursing care and evaluation of the patient's responses to the care rendered.
     - Specified tasks involved in implementation of the plan of care, which requires professional nursing judgement or intervention.
     - Responsibility and accountability for patient health teaching and health counseling which promotes patient education and involves the patient's significant others in accomplishing healthcare goals.
     - Administration of IVP medications and vasoactive infusions.
   - LVN-licensed activities:
     - Includes all of the unlicensed activities below.
     - Under the RN's direction, supervision of unlicensed personnel may be delegated to the LVN as appropriate.
     - Administration of oral and intramuscular medications, start and manage simple intravenous infusions.
     - Perform sterile treatments under the direction of the RN or physician.
   - Unlicensed activities:
     - Non-invasive and non-sterile treatments.
     - Collection, reporting, and documentation of data.
     - Hyperbaric chamber operation.

- Transportation of the client within the facility.
- Reinforcement of health teaching and planning provided by the RN.

1. Staff Mix determinations should provide for safe care and allow for the following factors:
   - Type and number of hyperbaric chambers to be used (complexity).
   - Anticipated patient treatment load.
   - Types of patient treatments anticipated (routine or emergent).
     - Number of patient treatments to be conducted daily.
   - Location of facility: hospital-based, clinic, or non-affiliated.
   - Experience level of available nursing and technical staff.
   - Degree of ancillary technical support (hospital maintenance staff, etc.).

PHYSICIAN STAFFING GUIDELINES

1. A minimum of two trained and credentialed hyperbaric physicians should be on staff for any full-time Clinical Hyperbaric Medicine Program. One must qualify and be responsible for the duties of the Medical Director.
2. Physician staffing should ensure coverage of the following clinical safety provisions:
   - Twenty-four-hour hyperbaric medicine consultation.
   - Timely and appropriate patient evaluation and treatment.
   - Physician supervision of patient evaluation and treatment.
   - Compliance and maintenance, through personal initiative or appropriate delegation of patient staff, department, and hospital training / safety requirements.
   - Proper administration of the hyperbaric medicine department within recognized local and national standards. (Joint Commission on Accreditation of Healthcare Organizations (JCAHO), UHMS, etc.).
   - Adequate physician rest and recovery time.

Note: Should patient volume or physician responsibilities begin to regularly compromise any one of the above clinical safety provisions, additional qualified physician staffing is required to a level where the provisions are consistently met.

TECHNICAL STAFFING GUIDELINES

The technical staff requirements for a clinical hyperbaric medicine facility will vary depending on the type of chambers used (Class A multiplace or Class B monoplace) and the number of chambers in operation. Also to be considered is the location of the facility (hospital based, clinic, or non-affiliated) as related to the availability of other technical support.

1. A minimum of one CHT or CHRN should be on duty in the clinical area at all times when a patient is receiving treatment.
2. A minimum of one hyperbaric technician should be on duty in the hyperbaric medicine facility when non-treatment chamber operations are ongoing.
3. In accordance with the requirement of NFPA 99, *Health Care Facility Manual*, there must be a designated Safety Director, regardless of the type or number of hyperbaric chambers used. Although not preferred, this position may be combined with that of the Technical Director if the size of the hyperbaric facility does not warrant two distinct positions.
4. In accordance with the requirements of NFPA 99, *Health Care Facility Manual*, Chapter 19, Hyperbaric Facilities, the Safety Director is to work with the hyperbaric Medical Director and the governing body of the parent institution to establish the baseline number and type of technical support required based on the needs of the individual facility. Among other factors to be considered:
    - Type and number of hyperbaric chamber(s) to be used (complexity).
    - Anticipated patient load.
    - Types of patient treatments anticipated (routine or emergent).
    - Location of facility: hospital-based, clinic, or non-affiliated.
    - Experience level of available technical staff.
    - Degree of ancillary technical support (hospital maintenance staff, etc.).

CERTIFICATION IN HYPERBARIC MEDICINE

"Competence promotes confidence, wisdom fosters power"
– author unknown

To be recognized in a specialty skill, physicians train, study, and gain expertise prior to becoming "boarded" in that specific medical entity. Like physicians, nurses and technicians gain proficiency and recognition in their given specialty by applying for and successfully completing certification in that specialty. The following is a discussion regarding what is required for each certification program as recognized internationally and guided under the auspices of the UHMS and affiliated liaisons. It is noted that any of the following certifications are not an entry-level pathway to hyperbaric medicine.

Certified Hyperbaric Technologist (CHT)

Prior to 1981, the diving community had medical technicians working with commercial divers and used during offshore oil and gas exploration. These technicians recognized a need for forming a strong alliance, creating the National Association of Diving Medical Technicians (NADMT). The association created a diving medical technician certification which was quickly embraced and recognized as a needed profession by the government and marine scientific community for recreational-based personnel supporting isolated recompression chambers. Throughout the 1980s, clinical hyperbaric oxygen research exploded. It was no longer just a military- or government-isolated position. Growth expanded in the medical community, and the most frequent use of recompression chambers – decompression sickness – became less than three percent of typical diagnosis. A new birth of a specialized technician grew from the NADMT, largely due to the efforts of the NADMT president, Dick Clarke, in 1991. He recognized the need for a new organization to include diving medicine and hyperbaric medicine. On March 1, 1991, the National Board of Diving and Hyperbaric Medicine Technology (NBDHMT) was born with the addition of the nationally recognized certified hyperbaric technologist (CHT).

Candidates Applying for the CHT Requirements:

- Must be at least 18 years of age with a high school diploma or equivalent
- Open to several disciplines to include therapists, technologist, chamber technicians, physician assistants, diving medical technicians, corpsmen, physiologists, emergency medical technicians, paramedics, life support technicians, researchers, and physicians
- Registered and licensed nurses may also take the CHT although there is a separate process discussed later in this section
- Must have recently worked or currently work in the hyperbaric medicine environment

- Must complete a NBDHMT-approved hyperbaric medicine introductory course (note: must check with NBDMT directly to specify course acceptance)
- Must complete 480 hours of clinical internship of undersea, hyperbaric, or aviation technology/medicine
- Must complete Transcutaneous Oxygen Monitoring (TCOM) Module with validation
- Provide a letter of recommendation from your present employer, administrator, or medical director
- Naval personnel must complete 1000 clinical hours in addition to required, approved training course received in the U.S. Navy due to less emphasis on clinical applications outside diving

Hyperbaric Nursing Certification Origin

In the early years of the Baromedical Nurses Association (BNA) in 1985, the mission included providing nurses with a professional organization to define, develop, maintain, and promote status and standards of baromedical nursing. To signify competence and continued education in our field, the hyperbaric nursing certification examination was developed. It was accepted from the National Board of Diving and Hyperbaric Medical Technology and is now a nationally recognized certifying examination. Recognizing different levels of nursing qualifications prompted the board to design progression in the levels of hyperbaric nursing certifications. Each will be discussed in detail below.

Certified Hyperbaric Registered Nurse

- Registered nurse degree granted from an accredited school of nursing
- Current license in the state of hyperbaric nursing practice
- Minimum of two years clinical experience in acute care setting, in-hospital setting, or one year critical care experience
- Certification of Basic Life Support
- Completion of an NBDHMT-approved primary hyperbaric medicine course
- Minimum of one year hyperbaric experience and a minimum of 200 hyperbaric hours
- Completion of accepted Transcutaneous Oxygen Monitoring (TCOM) Module
- Letter of recommendation from your employer, including validation of hyperbaric experience
- No history of conviction of any of the following within the last five years:

- Felony
- Unethical or unprofessional conduct
- Sexual abuse, molestation, or harassment of a present or former patient or other person
- Use of any drug or intoxicant to a degree which impairs objective professional performance
- Prescribing, selling, or administering any substance except as permitted by law
- Unauthorized disclosure of confidential patient information
- Gross or repeated negligence, or incompetence to perform professional work

Advanced Certified Hyperbaric Registered Nurse

- You may request application for advanced certification when seeking certification or recertification
- In addition to the basic Standards of Certification, you must meet the following:
- Minimum of three years experience in the field of hyperbaric oxygen therapy, working 20 hours or more per week
- Written documentation of two of the following:
    - That you contribute to the administrative activities of the hyperbaric unit/department
    - That you have taught Baromedical Nurses Association Certification Board (BNACB) approved entry-level hyperbaric oxygen therapy courses and/or classes or lectures on hyperbaric therapy
    - That you have primary responsibility for planning/coordinating nursing care for patients undergoing hyperbaric therapy

Hyperbaric Registered Nurse Clinician

- Master's Degree from an accredited academic program in nursing or health-related area
- Minimum of five years experience in the field of hyperbaric oxygen therapy, currently working 20 hours or more per week
- Written documentation of three of the following:
    - Responsible for administrative and nursing care activities of the hyperbaric unit/department
    - Speaker at regional/national hyperbaric conferences and workshops
    - Contributes to hyperbaric materials for regional/national distribution, i.e., journal articles, manuals, videos, etc.
    - Active participation in the BNA, UHMS, UHMS Chapters, and/or UHMS Associates as an officer or committee member
    - Principal investigator or co-investigator in a published hyperbaric or related research study

All certifications are valid for two years and expire on December 31, two years from the year of initial certification. As with any national certification, the BNACB and the National Board of Diving and Hyperbaric Medical Technology (NBDHMT) do not warrant job performance of applicants or registrants. The board may revoke or take action against your application if specific violations occur once certified.

Undersea and Hyperbaric Medicine certification for physicians is possible as a subspecialty board recognized and sponsored by the American Board of Preventive Medicine and the American Board of Emergency Medicine.

ADDITIONAL CORE COMPETENCY REQUIREMENTS

Every medical facility mandates required, minimal educational activities. The educational coordinator must be creative when mirroring the initial/ annual base requirements with the facility requirements. It is best to keep individual education files that include, but are not limited to, the following:

- Job title
- Job description
- Scope of care
- Basic Life Support (BLS) and Advanced Cardiac Life Support (ACLS) certification with expiration date
- Specialty certifications
- General orientation with completion date
- Department-specific orientation with completion date
- Initial skills assessment
- Skill checklist/competency
- Inclusion of Safety Programs to include:
    - Electrical safety
    - Ergometrics/back safety
    - Security
    - Emergency preparedness
    - Infection control
    - Blood-borne pathogens
    - Radiation safety
    - Hazardous materials/waste
    - Fire safety
    - Patient safety
    - Holiday safety
- Annual tuberculin screening with preventive health personnel
- Age-specific competency
- Performance improvement involvement
- Pain management
- Other class/in-service attendance

Your unit-specific policies and procedures should describe unit-based nursing orientation and preceptor programs. It should be based on your individual medical facility's philosophy of personnel education as related to patient care. The accountabilities of the orientee, preceptor, supervisor, clinical coordinator, and others in the educational process should be clearly defined, as well as the description of the evaluation process and the annual requirements.

It is wise to send out an educational needs assessment at least annually to field the overall needs of your staff. You might be surprised at the individual needs that will surface. Give a multitude of examples in every facet of care to include medical treatments, safety items, quality indicators/ programs, and emergency after-hour responsibilities. High risk/low volume activities should be emphasized as well.

To keep the staff active in the orientation process, it is recommended to follow a self-assessment guide closely to assist with thorough training. Reinforcement and evaluation of staff members emphasize your commitment to completing quality orientation while meeting the individual needs of your personnel. A good manager will always follow up deficits in a timely manner.

Transcutaneous Oxygen Monitoring (TCOM) Competency

To complete the certification programs listed above, you must include a course on Transcutaneous Oxygen Monitoring (TCOM). TCOMs are used to support clinical evaluations of hypoxic or poorly healing wounds. As part of the wound care evaluation, the tissues are tested in room air at normobaric conditions, then with 100% oxygen per re-breather oxygen mask, and lastly, if the effects are not clear, a pressure test under hyperbaric conditions will be completed. As discussed in more detail in an earlier chapter, TCOMs are a primary key to evaluating whether hyperbaric oxygen would benefit hypoxic wound-healing. It is the responsibility of the facility to determine competency of persons performing TCOMs. Interpretation of the test should be left up to the medical provider who ordered it. A sample of a TCOM competency as given for completion prior to the precertification process by the National Board of Diving and Hyperbaric Medical Technology (NBDHMT) is as follows:

SAMPLE TCOM COMPETENCY SKILLS LIST

Technical Knowledge of Transcutaneous Oxygen Monitor and Electrodes

Name____________________ **Instructor**________________

Demonstrate knowledge of the following
Principles of transcutaneous oximetry
Applications for $TCPO_2$
Operating functions for the monitor
Settings
Adjustments
Calibration procedure
Procedure for maintaining membrane and electrode
Troubleshooting procedures for alarms and error codes
Anatomy of common $TCPO_2$ sites
How to select $TCPO_2$ site
How to prepare $TCPO_2$ site
How to perform a comprehensive $TCPO_2$ study
Why reference information is obtained

Anticipated normal $TCPO_2$ values			
How to calculate a regional perfusion index (RPI)			
Range of $TCPO_2$ values that would likely result in stating HBO_2 treatment			
Three common testing errors and their effect on $TCPO_2$ values			
How to obtain the subjects consent for $TCPO_2$ procedure			
Demonstrate procedure for inspection of the equipment			
Monitor			
Site temperature setting			
PO_2/PCO_2 setting (if applicable)			
O_2 alarm limits			
CO_2 alarm limits (if applicable)			
Electrode			
Cable is intact			
Membrane change			
Timing of changes			
Technique			
Ancillary equipment			
O_2 source (HP cylinder, Well O_2)			
O_2 delivery (mask or hood assembly)			
Calibration gas (if applicable)			
Demonstrate test procedure			
Conduct $TcPO_2$ study (3 Subjects)	**1**	**2**	**3**
Set up oxygen monitor			
Set site temperature			
Set PO_2/PCO_2 (if applicable)			
Re-membrane electrode (1 time)			
Calibrate electrode			
Prepare the subject			
Brief the subject			
Obtain consent			
Position subject for test			
Prepare the site			
Select the site			
Remove hair and loose skin			
Clean the site			
Adhere electrode to skin			
Collect Data			
Baseline $TCPO_2$ air			
Physiological challenge (any 2 of following)			
Elevated limb			
Ambient 100% O_2			
HBO_2 w/100% O_2			
Record data			
Date sheet or computer			
Calculate RPI			
Remove electrode			
Remove adhesive device			
Clean electrode			
Store electrode			
Perform $TCPO_2$ mapping (3 subjects)			
Troubleshoot equipment			
Alarms			
Error Codes			

CHAMBER SPECIFIC OPERATIONS

Hyperbaric chambers are described in the United States by the National Fire Protection Agency *Health Care Facility Manual* (NFPA 99), as Class-A, human, multiple occupancy; Class-B, human, single occupancy; or Class-C, animal, no human occupancy.

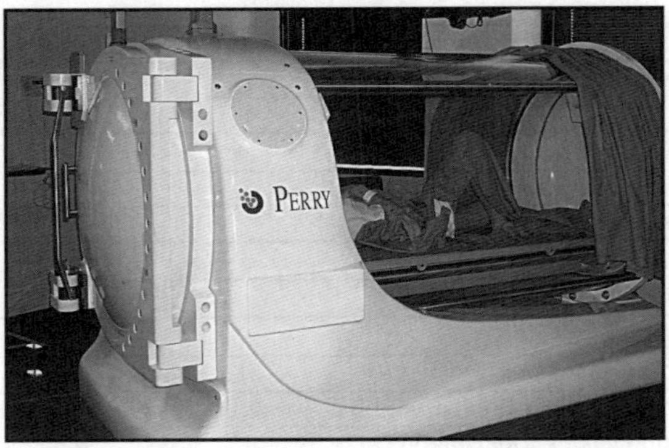

MONOPLACE CHAMBER SPECIFIC OPERATIONS

Monoplace chambers are Class-B human single occupancy chambers. There are currently two basic types of monoplace chamber designs available: the metal and the acrylic cylinder chamber with metal ends. These are single-occupancy vessels with the advantage of operational ease, low maintenance, and low cost of operation. The most prevalent type is the acrylic cylinder chamber, with a significant portion of the chamber body being comprised of a single, acrylic cylinder, held in place by steel tie rods connecting two end caps. To deliver safe, effective, quality, cost-effective care, competency while working in the monoplace hyperbaric environment must be not only established but maintained.

As stated in the introduction, nursing competence is the ongoing ability to render safe nursing care. In addition to core competencies required of all registered nurses, there are additional competencies required of those working in the unique hyperbaric environment. We must be diligent in maintaining these standards, not only upon initial orientation but also in a continual systematic ongoing approach. The following is a sample of a comprehensive skill checklist developed by Dick Clarke, National Baromedical Services Director and Program Director of Hyperbaric Medicine Services at Richland Memorial Hospital. It is specific to the monoplace environment. Successful completion is required during orientation and semiannually for all nurses working in the hyperbaric unit. Additions and modifications to one's individual areas, in accordance with hospital-specific regulations, can be added or modified as deemed appropriate.

Additionally, the competencies can be further broken down into actual equipment-specific operation as indicated by the samples of competencies for the operation of monoplace chambers and duoplace chambers.

FTE & PRN Employee Initial Inservice and Six-Monthly Skills Checklist

Name:______________________________ Date of Hire:________________

Title:______________________________ License Renewal Date:______________

Status: FTE__________ Part time__________ PRN__________ Student__________

SKILLS CHECKLIST TO BE COMPLETED TWICE YEARLY BY JULY 1 AND JANUARY 1

SKILL	**DATE**	**INTIALS OF PRECEPTOR**	**DATE**	**INITIALS OF PRECEPTOR**
1. Chamber Operations (Appropriate Action)				
a. Chamber door opened and closed				
b. Stretcher (rolled out & locked into place)				
c. Ground wire (connected to pt/chamber)				
d. Master valve (turn chamber off/on)				
e. Rate set valve (set per pt comfort)				
f. Pressure set valve (set per prescription)				
g. Gauge (able to convert ATA to psi)				
h. Wall supply valve (identified)				
i. Purge flow rate (set per pt comfort)				
j. Identifies and resolves barotrauma during compression and decompression				
2. Emergency Procedures (explain appropriate action)				
a. Fire- review NFPA guidelines				
b. In-chamber seizure				
c. Emergency decompression of chamber				
-demonstrate appropriate action				
-explain importance of stat c-xray				
-explain prep for "shocking" pt s/p tx				
d. Oxygen toxic episode				
e. Loss of oxygen				
f. Loss of communication				
g. Door safety pin jammed s/p tx				
h. Confinement anxiety				
i. Acute claustrophobia at pressure				
j. Suspected pneumothorax at pressure				

FIGURE 1. Hyperbaric Medicine Competency Skills Checklist

SKILL	**DATE**	**INTIALS OF PRECEPTOR**	**DATE**	**INITIALS OF PRECEPTOR**
3. Equipment Set Up (demonstrates appropriate action)				
a. I.V. Pumps				
~Remove I.V. port "pin" in door				
~Extension set primed in door				
~Abbott infus. pump				
~Ivac 530 infus. pump				
~Ivac infusion pump				
b. NIBP monitor set up				
c. ECG monitor/line set up				
d. Pressure lines (artline/swan) set up				
e. Nebulizer set up				
f. Ventilator set up to chamber/pt				
4. Air Breaks (Identifies purpose for each mask type and demonstrates appropriate set up for each)				
~Free flow mask				
~Face tent				
~Trach collar				
~Demand mask				
5.Charting (documents appropriately for each form)				
a. Nurses notes				
b. Treatment record				
c. Checklist flowsheet				
d. History and physical form				
e. Consent form				
f. Critical care flowsheet				
6. Taking Referrals (demonstrates appropriate action)				
a. Writing new referrals in consult book				
b. Scheduling pts. on daily schedule				
c. Consulting HBO MD for new referrals				
7. Air and Oxygen Cylinders (Awareness)				
a. Location				
b. Opening and closing valve				
c. Interpreting gauges				
d. How to order new cylinders				
e. How to change cylinders				

FIGURE 1. Continued

SKILL	DATE	INTIALS OF PRECEPTOR	DATE	INITIALS OF PRECEPTOR
8. Opening HBO Unit (Actual Experience)				
a. Unforward phones				
b. Wall valve open to all chambers				
c. Open air cylinder				
d. Turn on flwmtrs. for O2 analyzers				
e. Daily inspection checklist completed				
f. Code cart checklist completed				
9. Closing HBO Unit				
a. Forward phones				
b. Chambers cleaned internally				
c. Close air and 02 cylinders				
d. Wall valve closed to all chambers				
e. End-of-day inspection list complete				
f. Lights off and all I.V. pumps plugged in				
g. Patient charges complete				
h. Superbills complete for M.D.				
I. Pt. schedule complete for next day				
j. Doors locked				
10. Maintenance/Infection Control (demonstrates appropriate practice)				
a. Chamber maintenance				
b. Chamber cleaning				
- Mattress, stretcher, EKG cables, ground strap, pillow, and mask cleaned with Tor-HB between every patient				
c. Universal precautions maintained with all patient contact				
d. Neutropenic precautions upheld with all neutropenic patients.				
e. Tor-HB chamber internal surfaces at end of day				
11. Psychometric Test				
a. Test given				
b. Totaled final score				
12. Photographs (demonstrates appropriate practice)				
~ Polaroid camara				
~ Digital camara				
~ Pictures taken of q wound per protocol				

FIGURE 1. Continued

SKILL	DATE	INTIALS OF PRECEPTOR	DATE	INITIALS OF PRECEPTOR
13. Transcutaneous Oxygen Measurement (demonstrates appropriate Skill)				
a. Site preparation				
b. Electrode membrane placement				
c. Trouble shooting				
d. Oxygen challenge				
e. Calculating RPI				
14. Ventilator				
a. Inservice on ventilator				
b. Assembly of ventilator				
c. Ventilator sterilization w/cydex				
d. Operation of ventilator				
15. New Patient Orientation				
a. Risks and benefits explained to patient				
b. HBO procedures explained to patient				
c. Pressure equalization techn's. reviewed				
d. Demonstration usage of masks				
e. Vital signs, lung sounds documented				
f. Tympanic membrane eval documented				
16. Preparation of Patient for HBO Treatment				
a. Explain procedure to patient				
b. Consent signed per pt and M.D.				
c. Dressed in 100% cotton gown only				
d. All contraband items removed				
e. Temperature pretreatment				
f. Ongoing patient assessment				
g. Blood glucose testing/all diabetic pts.				
h. ECG monitor on PRN per patient				
i. Management of drainage tubes				
NG, JP, hemovac, continuous irrigation				
systems, closed drainage systems,				
Colostomy/Ileostomy bags				
j. Saline in ET cuff pre-tx of vent pt				
k. Restraints applied appropriately PRN				
l. Air break system in place				
m. Ground wire attached to pt/chamber				
n. Assuring patient safety/comfort in chamber				
o. Heimlich valve used appropriately PRN				

FIGURE 1. Continued

SKILL		DATE	INTIALS OF PRECEPTOR	DATE	INITIALS OF PRECEPTOR
17. Glucometer					
	a. Certification completed/ renewed PRN				
18. Hospital Manuals and Materials Identified					
	a. HBO policy/procedure manual				
	b. HBO protocol manual				
	c. Hospital policy/procedure manual				
	d. Chamber operation manual				
	e. NBS employee handbook				
	f. Disaster manual				
	g. Infection control manual				
	h. Material data safety sheets				
	i. Patient education materials				
	j. Occurrence reports				
	k. Telephone system				
	l. Fax machine				
	m. Consult book				
19. Wound Care (demonstrates appropriate action)					
	~Wound assessments				
	~Infection control				
	~Sterile technique per patient need				
	~Detection of wound changes				
20. Patient Care Guidelines					
	a. Confidentiality				
	b. Infection control				
	c. Patient scheduling				
	d. Age-specific knowledge				
	e. Patient follow-up				

Supervisor/Date	Supervisor/Date

Comments, assessments of competence, goals, planned methods to obtain goals, and objectives as indicated:

FIGURE 1. Continued

HYPERBARIC MEDICINE

Name:________________________________ **Title:**____________________

Date:________________________________ **Unit:**____________________

Method:____________________ **Actual Clinical Performance:/ Simulated**

Clinical Performance for Sechrist Chamber Operation

Employee Signature: ____

Evaluator Signature: ____

Key: M=Meets **DNM** =Does Not Meet

COMPETENCY: General Operation : **Sechrist Chamber**	M	D N M	A/S
1) Open door fully			
2) Position dolly rails and secure to chamber applying brakes			
3) Release latch and slide bed of stretcher out on to rails, be sure latch clicks into lock position			
4) Position patient on stretcher			
5) Apply antistatic bracelet			
6) Release latch and slide bed of stretcher into chamber until latch re-engages			
7) Release brakes and disconnect dolly rails from chamber			
8) Close door and latch			
9) Turn on gas selection panel to oxygen			
10) Turn on master valve on chamber			
11) Confirm rate set is on 1			
12) Select ATA on set pressure valve			
13) Chamber will automatically go to selected pressure at selected rate (note time is related to rate and ATA, i.e., 15 minutes to get to 2 ATA at rate of 1 PSIG/minute)			
14) After reaching pressure, chamber will automatically maintain set pressure for duration of treatment			
15) When treatment time has elapsed, adjust pressure set to zero. Chamber will decompress at rate set in # 11			
16) When pressure gauge reads less than 2 PSIG turn off master valve			
17) When no red shows on chamber pressure indicator open door slowly to allow for pressure relief			
18) Repeat steps # 2 and # 3			
19) Remove antistatic bracelet			
20) Assist patient from stretcher			

FIGURE 2. Competency-Based Performance Program for Sechrist Chamber Operation

HYPERBARIC MEDICINE

Name:______________________________ **Title:**____________________________
Date:______________________________ **Unit:**____________________________
Method: __________ **Actual Clinical Performance:/ Simulated Clinical Performance**
Employee Signature:____
Evaluator Signature:____

Key : **M**=Meets **DNM** =Does Not Meet

COMPETENCY: General Operation: **ETC Chamber**	**M**	**D N M**	**A/S**
1) Insert key and turn on (1/4 turn clockwise)			
2) After computer self test, sign on			
3) Enter patient profile			
4) Open door fully			
5) Position dolly rails and secure to chamber applying brakes			
6) Release latch and slide bed of stretcher out on to rails, be sure latch clicks into lock position			
7) Release brake, disengage stretcher, lower stretcher to appropriate position (using pneumatic foot pedal) for safely assisting patient onto stretcher			
8) Position patient on stretcher			
9) Apply antistatic bracelet			
10) Raise stretcher (using pneumatic foot pedal) to allow dolly rails to line up to chamber rails, apply brakes			
11) Release latch and slide bed of stretcher into chamber until latch re-engages			
12) Release brakes and disconnect dolly rails from chamber			
14) Assure gas selection panel on oxygen			
15) Press start profile			
16) Chamber will automatically go to preprogramed/preselected profile (note time is related to rate and ATA, i.e., 15 minutes to get to 2 ATA at rate of 1 PSIG/minute)			
17) After reaching pressure, chamber will automatically maintain set pressure for duration of treatment.			
18) When treatment time has elapsed, chamber will automatically start decompression cycle at preprogramed rate.			
19) When profile is complete, alarm will sound and chamber door may be safely opened (this will silence alarm)			
20) Repeat steps # 4, 5, 6, 7			
21) Remove antistatic bracelet			
22) Assist patient from stretcher			

FIGURE 3. Competency-Based Performance Program for ETC Chamber Operation

AGE-SPECIFIC RECOMMENDATIONS

The Joint Commission on Accreditation of Healthcare Organizations (JCAHO) requires that anyone with patient contact be annually evaluated by their supervisor for age-specific competencies. The evaluation requires assessment for competency with measurable, specific criteria.

As healthcare professionals providing nursing care in the hyperbaric environment, we care for people of all ages and all stages of growth and development. People have unique healthcare needs that result from the physical, emotional, intellectual, spiritual, and cultural aspects of their developmental level. To plan and provide individualized care, the hyperbaric nurse must understand the normal behavior pattern for each developmental level. The following is a sample evaluation of age-specific competency that covers seven cycles of human growth and development from infancy to later maturity. Please see the Age-Specific Consideration chapter in this book for further information on the topic.

DUOPLACE CHAMBERS SPECIFIC OPERATIONS

The United States National Fire Protection Agency's (NFPA) publication, the *Health Care Facility Manual* (NFPA 99), describes the duoplace chamber as a Class A multiplace chamber, unlike the monoplace chamber – a Class B single occupancy chamber. Although slightly larger in size than monoplace chambers in some cases, duoplace chambers are designed to treat a patient while accompanied by a medical attendant. One such chamber, named the Reneau (now Proteus), was designed to go to six atmospheres absolute (ATA) and was constructed out of stainless steel. Another manufactured example, the Sigma II type, is acrylic with a 3 ATA capacity. With this model, constant patient attendance is possible during single patient treatments.

These duoplace chamber examples compress with air, and the patient breathes 100% oxygen by either a tight-fitting mask or a specially designed plastic, latex-free, tight-fitting hood with neck ring. Space requirement for the duoplace chamber is only slightly larger than a monoplace chamber yet allows for constant access to the patient in up to 6 ATA pressurization. The disadvantages include a higher cost for personnel per patient treatment, risk of decompression sickness for the inside medical staff, and the inability to treat more than two patients at one time. Training and competency would mirror those of a multiplace system. We will be discussing multipace chambers next.

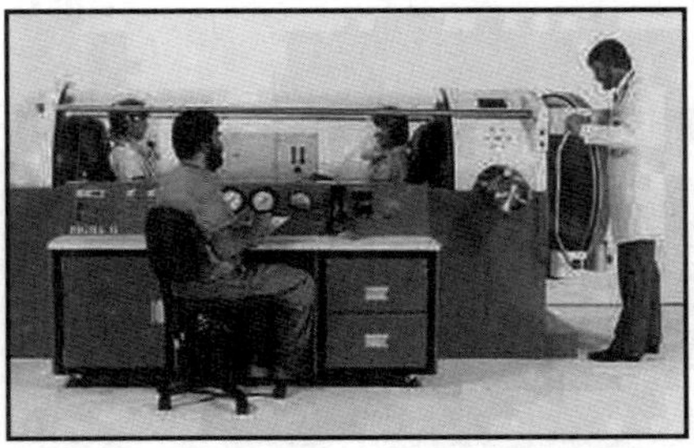

FIGURE 4. Duoplace Chamber

MULTIPLACE CHAMBERS SPECIFIC OPERATIONS

The National Fire Protection Agency (NFPA) describes any multiplace chamber as Class A. These chambers are engineered and custom-made in many unique styles and shapes depending upon the size needed, work pressure maximum, multi-compartments, and number of occupancy. These chambers accommodate 2-18 patients depending on use of gurneys, wheelchairs, or other seating arrangements. There is always a medical attendant available with a minimum of one hyperbaric trained staff member accompanying the patient(s).

Due to the large occupancy space, it is cost effective to compress these multiplace chambers with air while the patient breathes 100% oxygen by a tight-fitting mask, a hood that covers the entire head and is attached to a tight-fitting, latex-free neck ring seal, or an endotracheal tube.

Temperature control is important but not critical in the clinical therapy chambers since constant pressure is maintained through continuous ventilation. This continuous ventilation is required by the fire code to control oxygen levels. Safety standards must be adhered to as delineated in the ASME/PVHO agency requirements.

The advantage of the multiplace chamber, as with the duoplace chamber, is the ability to provide constant patient attendance and assessment. Unlike the duoplace chamber, the multiplace chamber can treat more than three patients per session. Disadvantages of the multiplace chamber include the high capitalization and personnel costs, as well as large space requirements. The inside medical attendant is at risk for decompression sickness. If the patient is at high risk with high acuity, they may need more than one-on-one medical attention during the treatment.

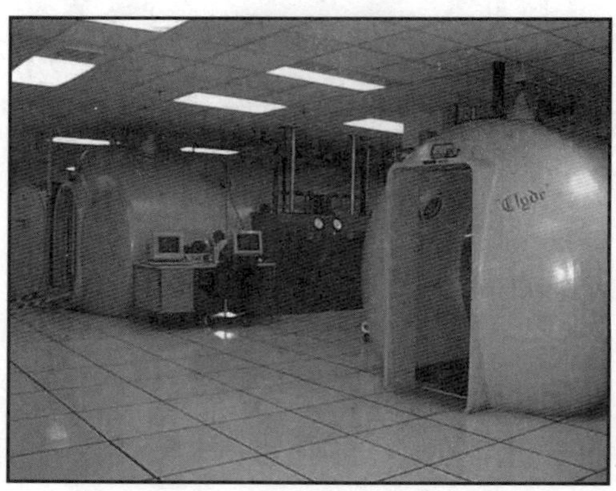

FIGURE 5. Multiplace Chamber

Verifying and maintaining competency in the multiplace hyperbaric environment is required. The following is a suggested example of a skills checklist that you may put into action in your department:

Name: ____

CATEGORY	**AGE-SPECIFIC** (Initial & Date)	**CONTENT GIVEN** (Initial &Date)	**ORIENTATION EXPERIENCE** (Initial & Date)	**DEMONSTRATE COMPETENCY** (Initial & Date)
CHAMBER OPERATORS				
1. Demonstrates activation and use of emergency air systems:				
A. Primary				
B. Secondary				
2. Compressors:				
A. States type, function, and identifies piping components				
B. Demonstrates starting and stopping				
C. Explains loading system, demonstrates use, changes loading 90-125, 125-90				
D. Explains purpose and use of water cooling system				
E. Demonstrates isolation of compressor				
F. Demonstrates isolation of volume tanks				
G. Demonstrates use of electrical resets and emergency power transfer switch				
3. Patient Support Systems				
A. Demonstrates set-up and use of Marquette Tram				
B. Demonstrates calibration and use of Beckman Oxygen Analyzer				
C. Explains and demonstrates application of suction at pressure and on surface				
D. Demonstrates set-up, application, and use of regulators, flow-meters, masks, hoods, ET tubes, ventilator, heated aerosol				
E. Demonstrates use of phone and intercom				
F. Explains reasoning for line isolation monitor and hubble plugs, location of circuit breakers				
G. Demonstrates use of medical locks				

Date: _________ **Primary Preceptor Name:** ____________________**Supervisor:**____________

FIGURE 6. Multiplace Chamber Operator Competencies Outline (sample)

CATEGORY	AGE-SPECIFIC (Initial & Date)	CONTENT GIVEN (Initial & Date)	ORIENTATION EXPERIENCE (Initial & Date)	DEMONSTRATE COMPETENCY (Initial & Date)
CHAMBER OPERATORS				
4. Multiplace Control Panel Operations:				
A. States how panel is organized				
B. Describes how each component functions				
C. Demonstrates pressurization, and holding at pressure by using: **1.** Manual mode **2.** Automatic mode **3.** Computer/profile mode **4.** Hand valves				
D. Explains what a treatment profile is and when they are used				
E. Routine operating procedures **1.** Verbalizes theory and demonstrates use of chamber fans/chillers/heaters **2.** Demonstrates use of chamber lights **3.** Demonstrates proper use of bottom timer and event timers **4.** Demonstrates ability to lock in equipment and personnel belongings **5.** Recognized appropriate profile for each disease category and explains their use **6.** Correctly completes paper work including Record of Dive, USN Record of Dive, log book, treatment record **7.** Figures correct decompression				
5. Demonstrates Theory/Tables:				
A. States gas laws, history of table formulation, and theory is tissue gas loading				

Date: ______________________________

Primary Preceptor Name: ______________________________

Supervisor: ______________________________

FIGURE 6. Continued

REFERENCES

1. Susan B. Bastable. Principle of Teaching and Learning, Nurse as Educator. Jones and Bartlett Publisher, Inc 1997 pp. 4-9.
2. Patricia Benner. Excellence and Power in Clinical Nursing Practice, From Novice to Expert. Addison-Wesley Publishing Company 1984.
3. Eleanor Sullivan. Issues, Opportunities and Challenges, Creating Nurses Futures. Mosby 1999 p. 69.
4. Margretta Styles. Towards a New Endowment. On Nursing, C.V. Mosby 1982.
5. Patrick N. Kimbrell. Operations Committee Report, Undersea and Hyperbaric Medical Society, January 2000.
6. Wilbur T. Workman. Hyperbaric Facility Safety: A Practical Guide, pp. 2-4, Best Publishing Company 1999.
7. Birchenall, J., and Streight, M. (1993) Care of the Older Adult. 3rd Ed. Philadelphia. J.B. Lippincott.
8. Colarrusso, C., and Nemiroff, R. (1996) New Dimensions in Adult Development, New York: Basic Books Inc.
9. Deppoliti, D., Johnson, D., Kohlbrenner, J., Lewis, L., Pond, M., and Samsel, T. (1995) Human Growth and Development Self Learning Packet. Developed at Joseph's Health Center.
10. Erikson, E.H. (1963) Childhood and Society (2nd ed.) New York: Norton.
11. Fowler, J.W. (1981) Stages of Faith: The psychology of human development and the quest for meaning. New York: Harper and Row.
12. Gilligan, C. (1982) In a Different Voice. Cambridge, MA: Harvard University Press.
13. Havighurst, R.J. (1972) Developmental Tasks of Education. New York: David McKay.
14. Kozier, B., Erb, G., Blais, K., and Wilkinson, J. (1995) Fundamentals of Nursing.
15. Whaley, L., and Wong, D. (1995) Nursing Care of Infants and Children (5th ed.) St. Louis: Mosby.
16. Wilson, A.H. (1994) Nursing Care during Hospitalization. In C.L. Betz, M. Hunsberger, and S. Wright, Family Centered Nursing Care of Children (2nd ed.) pp. 717-781. Philadelphia: W.B. Saunders Company.
17. ANSI/ASME PVHO, Safety Standard for Pressure Vessels for Human Occupancy, 1996 edition, American Society of Mechanical Engineers, 345 East 47th Street, New York, NY 10017.
18. Hyperbaric Medicine Practice, Kindwall, E.P. Editor, Second Edition 1999, Best Publishing Company.
19. NFPA 99: Health Care Facilities Handbook, (1999) National Fire Protection Association.
20. Sheffield, P.J., and Desautels, D.A. Hyperbaric and Hypobaric Chamber Fires: A 73-year Analysis. Undersea and Hyperbaric Medicine, 1997; 24(3): 153-164.
21. Bookspan, Jolie (2000) Hyperbaric Medical Review for Board Certification Exams.

INTERNET SITES

1. Baromedical Nurses Association at http://www.hyperbaricnurses.org/hyml/certification.html

2. Nursing World, The American Nurses Credentialing Center at http://www.nursingworld.org/ancc/fags.htm July 6, 2001 16:14 P.M.

3. National Publications Council, Continued Nursing Competence, National Council Fact Sheet at http://www.ncsbn.org/files/publications/positions/cont4.asp July 6, 2001 1600

4. National Baromedical Services, Inc. at http://www.baromedical.com

5. Joint Commission on Accreditation of Healthcare Organizations (JCAHO) at http://www.jcaho.org or http://www.qmsonline.com/jcaho

6. Undersea and Hyperbaric Medical Society at http://www.uhms.org

7. Global Hyperbaric Resource Project at http://www.hyperbaric-forum.com

8. Health Care Financial Administration (HCFA): Medicare, Medicaid, and the State Children's Health Insurance Program at http://www.hcfa.gov

NOTES

CHAPTER I

INTERNATIONAL NURSING COLLEAGUES

W. McGINN-MERRITT

INTRODUCTION

Great discoveries and improvements invariably involve the cooperation of many minds.—Alexander Graham Bell (Inventor)

Hyperbaric nursing is a unique specialty with a substantial body of knowledge that binds us together. We practice in a complex environment that requires a high level of expertise. Although regulations are different for each country, and individuals practice within their own set of values, there remains this body of knowledge that we all share.

In order to be successful we must keep in mind the following: The foundation for success requires the recognition and acceptance of differing societal and personal views. It also includes the capacity to accept differing opinions and still come together in the accomplishment of purposes that can be agreed upon. Nursing is no different from other professions in that the major concern is the quality of practice. It does not matter where we come from, or how we live; we can all agree on these basic principles.

The specialty of hyperbaric nursing was formally recognized with the founding of "The Baromedical Nurses Association" in June 1985. The goals were to provide nurses practicing in the field of hyperbaric medicine a formal organization within which ideas could be exchanged, educational opportunities promoted, and professional networking developed. Today we have members in Europe, Asia, Africa, South and Central America, and the South Pacific.

The 2000-2001 Baromedical Nurses Association Membership reflects the diversity of our organization. With members from all over the world it has become quite clear that despite our personal differences, our passion for the high quality standards for hyperbaric nursing are very much the same.

This chapter hopes to offer the reader an insight into the practice standards of our nursing colleagues. Information on hyperbaric nursing practice was requested from over 50 countries. Included is the information from those who responded, as well as from literature review. The content of original submissions was changed as little as possible.

While hyperbaric nursing remains in its infancy, it is clear with the dedication of so many people working towards a common goal that it will not remain so for very long.

AUSTRALIA, NEW ZEALAND, SOUTHEAST ASIA

The practice of Hyperbaric Medicine in this region mostly utilizes multiplace chambers, with the majority of those being military-based. The Hyperbaric Technicians and Nurses Association Inc. (HTNA) was formed in Australia on August 29, 1992 and incorporated on March 4, 1993. Its purpose is to provide and encourage the exchange of information, standardize practice and protocols within the technical and nursing communities, educate and inform the recreational diving industry, and encourage research in order to advance the scientific basis of the practice. The executive committee has representatives from Tasmania, Victoria, New South Wales, Australian Capitol Territory, Queensland North, Queensland South, Northern Territory, Western Australia, South Australia and Auckland, New Zealand.

As with many areas there is a large, diverse background among regions, and therefore the level of medical care, training, and education varies. In general standards are military-based. Singapore, Australia, and New Zealand are the most advanced in this region for developing standards and training. There is a current industry guideline, The Hyperbaric Oxygen Therapy Facility Industry Guidelines (HOTFIG), which has been accepted by two major bodies. These are HTNA and the Australian-New Zealand Hyperbaric Medicine Group (ANZHMG), the latter being a subcommittee of the South Pacific Underwater Medical Society (SPUMS).

Nurse training has been established utilizing HTNA guidelines for registered nurses. Formal education as a Registered Nurse is a prerequisite to enter a course for hyperbaric nursing. This is required for both the inside and outside attendants. The course is 40 hours with a further period of clinical orientation. The course is similar to the Certified Hyperbaric Technician Course with RN-specific protocols emphasized. The Medical Director of the unit is directly responsible for the staffing mix and levels; however, guidelines are recommended by the Hyperbaric Oxygen Therapy Facility Industry Guidelines. Continuing education is left up to individual facilities to provide. Two regional conferences are conducted by SPUMS (diving medicine) and HTNA. Many also attend the Undersea and Hyperbaric Medical Society (UHMS) and the Eastern European Underwater and Baromedical Society (EUBS) meetings.

BELGIUM

Hyperbaric Medicine is still in an early development phase in Belgium. The reasons are twofold. First, the reimbursement program for hyperbaric treatments and wound care is poorly organized. In life-threatening situations, such as carbon monoxide intoxication and/or soft tissue infections, only the first two sessions are reimbursed. Second, the education in hyperbaric medicine in nursing and medical schools is very poor. As a consequence, installing a hyperbaric medicine unit in a hospital is not an attractive option.

As an answer to this problem, in December 1993 the Advisory Committee for Hyperbaric Oxygen in Belgium (ACHOBEL) was constituted as a professional organization of 12 hospitals with attached hyperbaric centers. The main goals are to increase knowledge of the actual standards of hyperbaric medicine (European Consensus Conference of Lille 1994), and to convince third-party payers and the government of adequate reimbursement toward actual needs. An additional goal of ACHOBEL is to increase education of the medical community, nurses, and technical staff.

Today, several nurses have been trained and certified by ACHOBEL. Others are trained by programs in some university-based hyperbaric units, as in Antwerp which has a multiplace chamber (Hytech, The Netherlands) with a daily sessions activity, a 24h/7d availability, and a trained staff. Wound care education programs exist and are organized by WSC departments.

Compared with other countries, there is no traditional use of hyperbaric technicians to perform hyperbaric sessions. In Belgium, hyperbaric nurses provide a central role during hyperbaric treatments. They perform the chamber pressurization and decompression, accompany and encourage patients, perform TCOM measurements, and do the wound dressings if necessary. Because most chambers are placed in the emergency department or the intensive care unit, the nurses also have tasks in these units and the majority of them have good experience in intensive care patient management.

An organization for hyperbaric nurses in Belgium does not exist at the time of this writing, although intentions are growing, perhaps in a European context. In the near future, HBO settings will become more and more autonomous units in a multidisciplinary setting of wound care. Actually, the need for wound care settings, with HBO treatment facilities, lives in the mind of hospital directors, still in an undiagnosed pregnancy, but the child will be born.

EUROPE

An attempt was made in Europe to establish a European Baromedical Nurses Association, but due to multiple difficulties this has not happened. The physicians and nurses are members of the EUBS and UHMS, and to a degree the BNA, and follow those recommended guidelines.

European Baromedical Nursing requirements: A basic education and a formal nursing degree are required. Special courses for hyperbaric nurses are recommended, but they are not required. The hyperbaric nurse is subject to the regulations of working under pressure as established by the European Union.

The hyperbaric nurse performs the usual nursing functions with variations characteristic of the hyperbaric activity. Specific education in critical care is important. Knowledge of other specializations as appropriate is recommended, but not required, such as traumatology and wound care. Special courses on diving and hyperbaric medicine are essential. Nurses require approximately 120-160 hours of modular training with emphasis on critical care. The nurse may receive the necessary training in the same institution from the Medical Director and/or Medical Staff.

Hyperbaric Nursing Education includes:

1. General principles of decompression theory, diving technique, and pneumatics
2. Hyperbaric technique
3. Safety and preventative measures
4. Operation of monoplace hyperbaric chambers
5. Intensive critical care of patients
6. Other aspects inherent in both diving and hyperbaric medicine

As in all fields of health and medicine, hyperbaric nurses must complete and continue their education by reading specialized texts and attending courses and congresses. Their affiliation to specialized societies is highly recommended and recognized.

GERMANY

The German Society of Diving and Hyperbaric Medicine (GTUM) is an organization of physicians who acknowledge diving and hyperbaric medicine as a specialty. They are waiting for a specialty board in Diving and Hyperbaric Medicine to be installed by the German Physician Association. The GTUM published the second edition of "Quality Standards for Hyperbaric Oxygen Therapy" in August 1996 that contains the recommendations of a Joint Commission of the German Society of Anesthesiology and Critical Care Medicine. It was the first attempt to regulate hyperbaric facility safety in Germany.

Hyperbaric Nurse

Qualifications:

- Registered Nurse
- 2 years of training or experience in Anesthesiology/Critical Care
- 160 hours of training in Diving and Hyperbaric Medicine:
  - Participation in Diving Medicine Course A (40 hours) according to GTUM regulations
  - Participation in Diving Medicine Course C (40 hours) according to GTUM regulations
  - Two weeks practical experience at a hyperbaric facility working according to GTUM standards (80 hours)

Job Definition:

- Independent execution of hyperbaric oxygen therapy by order and under direct supervision of a qualified physician
- Monitoring and care of patients during therapy
- Consultant to patients for the particularities of hyperbaric oxygen therapy
- Initiation of an emergency hyperbaric treatment until a physician is on site

All personnel of a hyperbaric facility are required to participate in CME activities in the field of hyperbaric medicine and related fields. Training in emergency procedures and emergency medicine knowledge, together with practical exercises at the chamber, are required.

The minimum staffing requirements during hyperbaric oxygen therapy according to standards of GTUM are:

- One physician with minimal qualification as "Hyperbaric Oxygen Physician"
- One nurse with minimal qualification as "Hyperbaric Nurse"
- One chamber operator

HONG KONG

The Hong Kong Diving and Hyperbaric Medical Society (HKDHMS) is a nonprofit organization. The society was established with the objectives of encouraging the study and advancement of the science and practice of diving and hyperbaric medicine, as well as maintaining the good practice of diving and hyperbaric medicine by ensuring the highest professional standards of competence and ethical integrity.

A subcommittee of Hyperbaric Nursing exists as a specialty division dedicated to promoting quality care in clinical hyperbaric nursing and strengthening ties with patient families and the community to achieve this purpose. This is accomplished through health education to the public and healthcare professionals; promotion of research activities to support evidence-based nursing practice; and implementation of agreed practice standards of clinical hyperbaric nursing care, as listed below.

1. To define and promote standards of clinical hyperbaric nursing practice.
2. To provide clinical hyperbaric nurses with educational opportunities in the form of continuing education(Basic Training, Advanced Training, and certification examinations).
3. To support and facilitate clinical hyperbaric nursing research.
4. To work collaboratively with other health-related organizations towards the improvement of hyperbaric nursing.
5. To provide rapid information dissemination and effective communication networks to and on the behalf of clinical hyperbaric nurses.

IRAN

Hyperbaric treatment in Iran is under the control of the armed services. Nurses who practice hyperbaric medicine do so under the direction of the armed forces, usually navy physicians. Hyperbaric treatment is used mainly to treat decompression sickness and arterial gas embolism. Military nurses must have four years of training after high school. They must be registered and licensed.

JAPAN

All guidelines for hyperbaric medicine in Japan are determined by the Japanese Society for Hyperbaric Medicine (JSHM).

JSHM's Education for Nurses

PREREQUISITES:

- Japanese national license as a clinical engineer or nurse
- JSHM membership history for more than two continuous years
- Employment as a full-time employee at time of application
- Clinical experience in HBO practice
- History of attendance at two JSHM educational courses

For those entering HBO, the JSHM training system has been operating a training course for many years. Currently, it is open only to hyperbaric engineers and nurses because the curriculum was prepared as part of a postgraduate education for the engineering staff. It consists of lectures by many HBO experts and practical drills in real hyperbaric facilities. The course is a two-year program. In the first year, the fundamental curriculum is taught, and in the second year, the clinical program is covered.

LATIN AMERICA

Hyperbaric chambers have been used in Latin America from the early 1900s, with civilian clinical units starting in the '60s and '70s. Due to a large diversity of countries (39), it has been a challenge to standardize guidelines for training, staffing, construction, and operation of hyperbaric chambers as well as accepted and investigational conditions. The Latin American Chapter of the Undersea and Hyperbaric Medical Society (LACUHMS) is making efforts to accomplish this goal.

The majority of chambers are multiplace because most of the people working in HBO have naval backgrounds and the cost of oxygen is very high, especially in Central and South America. Although there are standards in the area for multiplace chambers (pressure vessels), there are minimal standards for PVHO. The challenge for Latin America is to create minimum standards for safe facilities, adequate staffing, appropriate training, and then to enforce these regulations.

Operating hospital-based Hyperbaric Medicine Units are usually well-staffed with technicians, nurses, or paramedics and one or more trained physicians. The most common hyperbaric medicine units are free standing, and normally have a technician and a physician available during treatment.

The Safety Committee of the LACUHMS, chaired by Ruben Campuzano, is presently working to create minimum safety standards and is expected to have them available at the end of 2001. Also, the LACUHMS is working in conjunction with the National Board of Diving and Hyperbaric Medical Technology (NBDHMT) to create the first CHT courses in Spanish. The curriculum of the course is being prepared by E. Cuauhtémoc Sánchez, M.D., and Renie Guilliod, M.D., The first grandfathered exam is expected to take place in May, and the first course should start in August of 2001.

Although training in Latin America is still "hands on," México is setting the standards for the area. The first Latin American certified nursing course (240 hours) accredited by a University (National Autonomus University of México – UNAM) has recently been approved. The course has 120 hours of theory and 120 hours of practice, 30 of these including a research project on clinical applications of hyperbaric oxygenation. The course was created by Guillermina Silva, R.N., from the Hospital Angeles del Pedregal Hyperbaric Unit.

UNAM has also approved the first subspecialty one-year course (fellowship) for physicians created by E. Cuauhtémoc Sánchez, M.D. This has opened the door to create the first Board on Hyperbaric Medicine accepted by the Academy of Medicine in México.

Cuba is the only country that has had a national hyperbaric program that incorporated training for technicians, nurses, and physicians. This program was created and is managed by Rafael Castellanos, M.D. The objective is to spread this type of course in all countries of Latin America to create a minimum standard of training for all the area, under the guidance of the Latin American Chapter of the UHMS. We are very close to accomplishing this goal, but there is still a lot of work to do.

MALAYSIA

There is only one clinical Hyperbaric Chamber in Malaysia, and that is located in the Lumut Armed Forces Hospital, Royal Malaysian Naval Base, 32100 Lumut, Perak, Malaysia.

It is a two-compartment Galleazzi chamber: Capacity is five seats in first compartment, two seats at the entry lock, and ten seats at the second compartment (walk-in door).

Our DMTs are trained locally. We run a six-week DMT course for our Medical Assistant and/or Staff Nurses. After that, those who are transferred to our unit undergo on-job training (apprenticeship).

The six-week course is run by both myself and another Diving Medical Officer, with our ENT surgeon and another Diving Medical Officer giving some lectures.

We have, on average, twelve patients receiving daily treatments. Another ten patients are being treated under our research program.

SOUTH AFRICA

Southern African Undersea and Hyperbaric Medical Association (SAUHMA)

SAUHMA was developed in 1992 by a group of physicians interested in HBO. This association follows the safety and medical recommendations of the UHMS. Subsequent development of a training program was undertaken by Frans J. Cronje, the Diving and Hyperbaric Medicine staff training course (DHMSTC) for specialty training of physicians, nurses, EMTs, and chamber technicians. In November 1998, the South African Bureau of Standards formed a technical committee to introduce clinical HBO standards. This will facilitate mandating of minimum safety and training standards in the future.

The training and credentialing for hyperbaric nurses has not yet been fully implemented. The South African Nurses Council has been asked to validate hyperbaric nursing as a subspecialty.

To date, three categories have been accepted by SAUHMA for HBO nursing competence:

I. Assistant Hyperbaric Nurse
- Minimum orientation to nursing care in the HBO environment
- Medically fit to dive (multiplace)
- Function under the direct supervision of a hyperbaric nurse
- Orientation course as recommended/provided by respective HBO department

II. Hyperbaric Nurse
- Nurses who have successfully completed a minimum of 50 hours of academic training in clinical hyperbaric medicine through a course recognized by SAUHMA and/or UHMS
- Clinical experience in the HBO environment
- Medically fit to dive (multiplace)
- May provide patient care within the scope of their practice for routine HBO treatments

III. Certified Hyperbaric Nurse

- Successful completion of 50 hours (minimum) academic training in clinical hyperbaric medicine through an approved SAUHMA and/or UHMS course.
- 480 or more hours of clinical hyperbaric medicine experience
- Successful completion of CHRN (Certified Hyperbaric Registered Nurse) exam offered by the Baromedical Nurses Association
- Medically fit to dive (multiplace)
- May provide care to all types of patients during treatment within their scope of practice. (Experience in trauma, intensive care, surgery, is considered)

All categories are dependent on the specific needs of the hyperbaric facility and as determined by the Medical Director.

A register is maintained of all nurses actively involved in hyperbaric medicine based on the above-mentioned categories. This adds to the credibility and recognition of hyperbaric nursing as a subspecialty. It also stimulates interest and creates career opportunities within this field of nursing.

SWEDEN

Introduction

In Sweden there are five hospitals with 24-hour on-call hyperbaric medicine departments that can take care of patients in need of acute care. All units have multiplace chambers equipped for intensive care, but they also treat patients with non-acute indications. The physicians and nurses in charge of the units are educated in hyperbaric medicine according to their professional levels and to the standards of Swedish Hyperbaric Medicine Society and Baromedical Nurses Association of Sweden. Each hyperbaric center is responsible for the education of the staff according to the local, national, and international regulations.

The hyperbaric medicine unit at the Karolinska Hospital, Stockholm Sweden, was established in 1990. Our referral base includes about 4.5 million people and we are fully prepared for the civil defense and fire services in the region.

The unit has one multiplace chamber and two monoplace chambers (Sechrist). In the monoplace chambers we treat patients with non-acute indications as well as spontaneous-breathing patients with acute indications. The monoplace chamber is pressurized with 100% oxygen, allowing the patient to breathe oxygen without a mask or hood. Through-hull penetrators allow ECG, invasive or non-invasive monitoring, and intravenous fluid administration.

Patients receive pure oxygen administered by mask or endotracheal tube in the multiplace chamber, in which we treat patients who need hands-on intensive care. The chamber is compressed with air and is equipped for acute care support, with a Servo 900 C ventilator, a Siemens 930 infrared end-tidal CO_2 analyzer, and a Propaq 106 monitor measuring ECG, pulsoximetry, and invasive/non-invasive blood pressure. Infusion pumps and monitors are battery-powered whereas the ventilator and CO_2 analyzer is driven by low voltage. Electrical safety requires that the 220v power supply is placed on the outside of the chamber. The chamber has a built-in breathing system (BIBS) with individual oxygen, air, or mixed gas supply lines for up to eight patients. In 2000, we had about 1400 treatments in the monoplace chambers and around 100 treatments in the multiplace chamber.

Personnel

The hyperbaric unit has two nurses and one assistant nurse working full-time, taking care of both out-patients and in-patients. The staff are also in charge of acute treatments during daytime.

We have 24-hour on-call with two physicians and one nurse. All together we have approximately 25 physicians and 50 nurses trained for working with hyperbaric medicine. They are all educated in the fields of anesthesiology/intensive care and hyperbaric/diving medicine.

A treatment in the multiplace chamber always requires one physician and one nurse inside with the patient. One doctor runs the chamber from the outside.

Academic Requirements and Degrees

The nurses are Registered Nurses, specialized in critical care (CCRN) or anesthesiology (CRNA), and have at least one year of experience in their special fields.

The nurses who work full-time in HBO also have a two-week course including hyperbaric and diving medicine, physiology, clinical HBO, acute and non-acute indications, and practical examples.

The nurses who are on-call have their permanent employment in the intensive care unit, the department of anesthesiology, or in the pre-hospital setting. These nurses have specific training which includes: one day in basic clinical and practical HBO, subjected to the regulations of work under pressure in accordance to the rules of Swedish diving safety guidelines, and one day of practical training at the hyperbaric unit.

Academic Continued Education

Karolinska Hospital organizes an annual two-week national course in Hyperbaric and Diving Medicine, and every third year the international Karolinska Postgraduate course. We also have continuing lectures in HBO and discussions of case reports.

Associations and Societies

The Baromedical Nurses Association of Sweden was established in 1994. One of our aims is to recommend adequate education for nurses who work with hyperbaric medicine and to develop safety guidelines for nurses and patients undergoing hyperbaric treatments.

Once a year, we arrange a one- or two-day meeting together with the Swedish Hyperbaric Medical Society, where members from the different centers lecture, present case reports, and discuss research and news in the field of hyperbaric medicine.

The Swedish Hyperbaric Medical Society and Baromedical Nurses Association of Sweden work closely together and prepare guiding principles for hyperbaric medicine in Sweden.

All the Swedish HBO units operate in line with the recommendations of the two HBO organizations in Sweden, according to the European Committee for Hyperbaric Medicine (ECHM) and Undersea and Hyperbaric Medicine Society (UHMS) standards.

SUMMARY

It is apparent the only legal requirement to practice hyperbaric nursing that we share worldwide is a valid nursing license, and in most cases a desire to practice in the field. Beyond this, every country has a wide range of standards governing nursing practice in the hyperbaric environment. These standards range from none, other than a nursing license, to advanced credentialing and certification. While most countries have a physician-driven organization supporting hyperbaric medicine, few focus on nursing standards. It is therefore essential that the Baromedical Nurses Association avail itself to assist and support all professional nurses in the delivery of quality hyperbaric nursing care. As technology fuels the globalization of our organization, connecting with colleagues is no longer a major undertaking. We encourage the countries of the world to utilize this valuable resource. Through these developed alliances, we can ensure that information is shared for the benefit of all working in the hyperbaric environment.

It is a proven fact that nurses are the number-one resource in every nation's healthcare system. It is therefore imperative that nurses take the initiative in evaluating the outcomes of their practice. This requires an evaluation of nursing activities, clinical practice, education, research, management, and policy development. It is up to us individually and collectively to create a network of knowledge and support to improve the standards for the entire world.

The Baromedical Nurses Association is a dynamic system of interacting parts and coordinating units that must continue to work together to upgrade the quality of hyperbaric nursing. Each of us has the ability to touch other lives, which in turn touch yet more lives, and so one by one we come together and the future of hyperbaric nursing is shaped.

REFERENCES

1. G. Oriani, A. Maroni, F.Wattel, Personal, Professional and Educational Requirements for the Staff of a Hyperbaric Medical Centre, Handbook on Hyperbaric Medicine 1996.
2. J. Desola, Section 3.4, pp. 869-870.
3. Wilbur T. Workman, Staffing and Training Issues in Europe, Hyperbaric Facility Safety: A Practical Guide 1999 Best Publishing, Peter H.J. Mueller Chapter 5.5, pp. 278-280.
4. Eric P. Kindwall, Harry T. Whelan, Hyperbaric Nursing, Hyperbaric Medicine Practice Second Edition 1999,Valerie Messina, George Weyenberg, Joan Cwiklinski, Dianne Norkool, Best Publishing, Chapter 16, pp. 381-382.
5. Wilbur T. Workman, Hyperbaric Facility Staffing and Training in Japan, Hyperbaric Facility Safety: A Practical Guide 1999 Best Publishing, Hideyo Takahashi Chapter 5.7, pp. 309-311.
6. Wilbur T. Workman, Training and Credentialing Standards for Hyperbaric Medicine in South Africa, Hyperbaric Facility Safety: A Practical Guide 1999 Best Publishing, Frances J. Cronje Chapter 5.3, pp. 246-248.
7. Hong Kong Diving and Hyperbaric Medical Society, March 26, 2001 http://www.hkhyperbaric.com/HKDHMS.htm
8. The Hyperbaric Technicians and Nurses Association, Inc. 1995 http://www.users.bigpond.com/HTNA/Committee.htm (February 2001)
9. The International Council of Nurses, April 26, 2001 http://www.icn.ch/ (April 2001)

INDEX

D

E

F

U

V

W-Z